Y0-CAJ-235

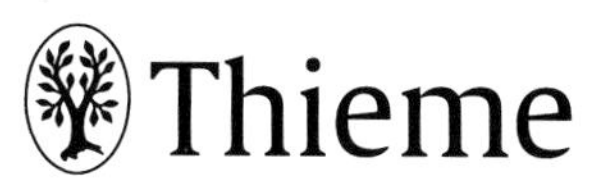
Thieme

Dx-Direct!

Direct Diagnosis in Radiology

Spinal Imaging

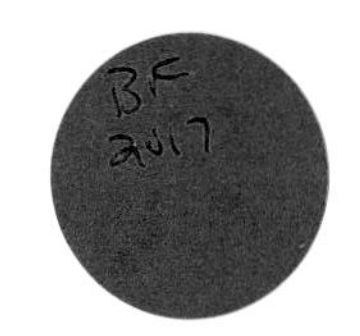

Professor Herwig Imhof, MD
Department of Radiology
Division of Osteoradiology
Medical University Vienna
Vienna General Hospital (AKH)
Vienna, Austria

With contributions by

Benjamin Halpern, Andreas M. Herneth, Klaus M. Friedrich,
Michael Matzner, Christina Mueller-Mang, Iris-Melanie Noebauer-Huhmann,
Daniela Prayer, Oliver Sommer, Florian Wolf

327 Illustrations

Thieme
Stuttgart · New York

Library of Congress
Cataloging-in-Publication Data

Wirbelsäule. English.
Spinal imaging / [edited by] Herwig Imhof ; with contributions by Benjamin Halpern ... [et al. ; translator: John Grossman ; illustrator, Emil Wolfgang Hanns].
p. ; cm.
Includes bibliographical references and index.
ISBN 978-3-13-144071-6 (TPS : alk. paper) – ISBN 978-1-58890-560-4 (TPN : alk. paper)
1. Spine–Imaging. 2. Spinal cord–Imaging. 3. Spine–Diseases–Diagnosis. 4. Spinal cord–Diseases–Diagnosis . I. Imhof, H. (Herwig) II. Halpern, Benjamin. III. Title.
[DNLM: 1. Spinal Diseases–diagnosis–Handbooks. 2. Diagnostic Imaging–methods–Handbooks. 3. Spinal Cord Diseases–diagnosis–Handbooks.
WE 39 W798s 2007a]
RD768.W5513 2007
617.4'8207548–dc22 2007023541

This book is an authorized and revised translation of the German edition published and copyrighted 2006 by Georg Thieme Verlag, Stuttgart, Germany. Title of the German edition: Pareto-Reihe Radiologie: Wirbelsäule.

Translator: John Grossman,
Schrepkow, Germany

Illustrator: Emil Wolfgang Hanns,
Schriesheim, Germany

Rüdigerstrasse 14, 70469 Stuttgart, Germany
http://www.thieme.de
Thieme New York, 333 Seventh Avenue,
New York, NY 10001, USA
http://www.thieme.com

Cover design: Thieme Publishing Group
Typesetting by Ziegler + Müller,
Kirchentellinsfurt, Germany
Printed by APPL, aprinta Druck,
Wemding, Germany

ISBN 978-3-13-144071-6
(TPS, Rest of World)
ISBN 978-1-58890-560-4
(TPN, The Americas) 1 2 3 4 5 6

Important note: Medicine is an ever-changing science undergoing continual development. Research and clinical experience are continually expanding our knowledge, in particular our knowledge of proper treatment and drug therapy. Insofar as this book mentions any dosage or application, readers may rest assured that the authors, editors, and publishers have made every effort to ensure that such references are in accordance with **the state of knowledge at the time of production of the book.**
Nevertheless, this does not involve, imply, or express any guarantee or responsibility on the part of the publishers in respect to any dosage instructions and forms of applications stated in the book. **Every user is requested to examine carefully** the manufacturers' leaflets accompanying each drug and to check, if necessary in consultation with a physician or specialist, whether the dosage schedules mentioned therein or the contraindications stated by the manufacturers differ from the statements made in the present book. Such examination is particularly important with drugs that are either rarely used or have been newly released on the market. Every dosage schedule or every form of application used is entirely at the user's own risk and responsibility. The authors and publishers request every user to report to the publishers any discrepancies or inaccuracies noticed. If errors in this work are found after publication, errata will be posted at www.thieme.com on the product description page.

Benjamin Halpern, MD
Department of Radiology
Division of Osteoradiology
Medical University Vienna
Vienna General Hospital (AKH)
Vienna, Austria

Andreas M. Herneth, MD
Professor
Department of Radiology
Division of Osteoradiology
Medical University Vienna
Vienna General Hospital (AKH)
Vienna, Austria

Klaus Friedrich, MD
Department of Radiology
Division of Osteoradiology
Medical University Vienna
Vienna General Hospital (AKH)
Vienna, Austria

Michael Matzner, MD
Department of Orthopedics
Medical University Vienna
Vienna General Hospital (AKH)
Vienna, Austria

Christina Mueller-Mang, MD
Department of Radiology
Division of Neuroradiology
Medical University Vienna
Vienna General Hospital (AKH)
Vienna, Austria

Iris-Melanie Noebauer-Huhmann, MD
Department of Radiology
Division of Osteoradiology
Medical University Vienna
Vienna General Hospital (AKH)
Vienna, Austria

Daniela Prayer, MD
Professor
Department of Radiology
Division of Neuroradiology
Medical University Vienna
Vienna General Hospital (AKH)
Vienna, Austria

Oliver Sommer, MD
Central Department of Radiology
Lainz Hospital
Vienna, Austria

Florian Wolf, MD
Department of Radiology
Division of Osteoradiology
Medical University Vienna
Vienna General Hospital (AKH)
Vienna, Austria

1 Congenital Malformations

Christina Mueller-Mang, Daniela Prayer, Klaus M. Friedrich, Michael Matzner

Arnold–Chiari Malformation 1
Lumbarization and Sacralization .. 4
Diastematomyelia 6
Tethering 9
Sacrococcygeal Teratoma 13
Meningocele, Myelomeningocele . 16
Vertebral Malformations 21
Klippel–Feil Syndrome 26
Kyphosis 29
Scheuermann Disease 33
Scoliosis 36
Malrotation 40

2 Trauma

Christina Mueller-Mang, Daniela Prayer, Klaus M. Friedrich, Florian Wolf, Michael Matzner, Herwig Imhof

Spinal Injury—Magerl Classification 43
Vertebral Fractures—Causes 45
Dens Fracture 48
Flexion Fracture of the Cervical Spine 51
Burst Fracture of the Spine 54
Chance Fracture (Seat Belt Fracture) 58
Jefferson Fracture 60
Hangman's Fracture 63
Spinal Cord Trauma 66
Syringohydromyelia 69
Anterior Subluxation 73
Insufficiency Fracture of the Sacrum 76
Stress Phenomena in the Spine 79
Stress Fractures in Ankylosing Spondylitis 83

3 Degenerative Disorders

Iris-Melanie Noebauer-Huhmann, Benjamin Halpern, Michael Matzner, Herwig Imhof

Disk Degeneration 87
Degenerative Disk Disease—Modic I 90
Degenerative Disk Disease—Modic II 93
Spondylosis Deformans—Modic III 96
Disk Herniation 100
Bulge, Protrusion, Extrusion, Sequestration 103
Disk Calcification and Vacuum Phenomenon 108
Facet Joint Degeneration 111
Uncovertebral Osteoarthritis 116
Synovial Cyst 118
Hypertrophy of the Ligamenta Flava 120
Baastrup Disease 121
Spondylolisthesis and Pseudospondylolisthesis 123
Degenerative Spinal Stenosis 126
Diffuse Idiopathic Skeletal Hyperostosis 131

4 *Inflammatory Disorders*

Christina Mueller-Mang, Daniela Prayer, Andreas M. Herneth, Oliver Sommer, Michael Matzner, Herwig Imhof

Rheumatoid Arthritis 133
Rheumatoid Arthritis–Chronic Trauma 138
Psoriatic Spondyloarthropathy ... 141
Reiter Syndrome 144
Ankylosing Spondylitis 147
Ankylosing Spondylitis–Ligament Calcification and Bamboo Spine 152
Ankylosing Spondylitis–Fractures 154
Acute Bacterial Spondylitis 158
Tuberculous Spondylitis 166
Epidural Abscess 172
Granulomatous Inflammations of the Spinal Cord 175
Arachnoiditis 178
Acute Transverse Myelitis 182
Spinal Multiple Sclerosis 186

5 *Tumors*

Andreas M. Herneth, Christina Mueller-Mang, Daniela Prayer, Michael Matzner, Herwig Imhof

Hemangioma 190
Osteoid Osteoma 195
Osteoblastoma 198
Osteochondroma 201
Aneurysmal Bone Cyst 204
Giant Cell Tumor 208
Langerhans Cell Histiocytosis 212
Malignant Tumors 215
Bone Metastases 216
Multiple Myeloma 222
Chordoma 226
Ewing Sarcoma 229
Lymphoma 232
Nerve Sheath Tumors 237
Leptomeningeal and Intramedullary Metastases 240
Meningioma 244
Ependymoma 248
Astrocytoma 252
Hemangioblastoma 256

6 *Vascular Disorders*

Christina Mueller-Mang, Daniela Prayer

Epidural Hematoma 259
Arteriovenous Malformation 262
Arterial Spinal Cord Infarction .. 266

7 *Postoperative Disorders*

Andreas M. Herneth, Michael Matzner, Herwig Imhof

Failed Back Surgery Syndrome .. 270
CSF Fistula 272
Peridural Fibrosis 275
Rapidly Progressive Osteoarthritis (After Intersegmental Fusion) 277
Complications of Spinal Instrumentation 280

8 *Metabolic Disorders*

Andreas M. Herneth, Herwig Imhof

Senile and Postmenopausal Osteoporosis 287
Paget Disease 291
Spinal Epidural Lipomatosis 293

Index 295

ACE Angiotensin converting enzyme
ADEM Acute disseminated encephalomyelitis
AFP Alpha-fetoprotein
A-P Anterior-posterior
AVF Arteriovenous fistula
c-ANCA Cytoplasmic antineutrophil cytoplasmic antibody
CSF Cerebrospinal fluid
CT Computed tomography, computed tomogram
DD Differential diagnosis
DEXA Dual-energy x-ray absorption
DISH Diffuse idiopathic skeletal hyperostosis
DSA Digital subtraction angiography
DWI Diffusion-weighted imaging
FDG-PET Fluoro-18-deoxyglucose positron emission tomography
HIV Human immunodeficiency virus
MRI Magnetic resonance imaging
NSAID Nonsteroidal anti-inflammatory drug
P-A Posterior-anterior
PCR Polymerase chain reaction
PD Proton density
PET Positron emission tomography
PNET Primary neuroectodermal tumor
Q-CT Quantitative CT
SPECT Single photon emission computed tomography
STIR Short tau inversion recovery
TNF-α Tumor necrosis factor α
TSE Turbo spin echo

Definition

- **Epidemiology**
Rare malformation of the posterior cranial fossa and craniocervical junction (underdevelopment of the endochondral occiput) • Autosomal inheritance pattern.
- **Etiology, pathophysiology, pathogenesis**
Chiari I: Displacement of the cerebellar tonsils caudal to the foramen magnum (McGregor line) • Associated with cervical syringomyelia (syringohydromyelia) and atlantooccipital fusion (25–50% of cases) • May occur in combination with scoliosis and kyphosis (42% of cases).
Chiari II: Small posterior cranial fossa • Portions of the cerebellum, fourth ventricle, and medulla oblongata are caudally displaced • Hypoplastic pons associated with spinal dysraphism (most often lumbar myelomeningocele).
Chiari III: Very rare • Type II malformation combined with an occipital or high cervical encephalocele.
Chiari IV: Very rare • Aplasia or severe hypoplasia of the cerebellum • Small brainstem • Enlarged CSF spaces in the posterior cranial fossa.
Caution: In published literature, the term "Arnold–Chiari" is used for both Chiari I and Chiari II malformations.

Imaging Signs

- **Modality of choice**
  - MRI: Sagittal • Axial • CSF flow measurement (Chiari I).
  - Prenatal ultrasound or fetal MRI.
- **MRI findings**
Chiari I: Descent of the cerebellar tonsils (> 5 mm caudal to the foramen magnum) • Malformation of the bony skull base is common (shortened clivus) • The fourth ventricle appears normal or elongated • The posterior cranial fossa is not too small • There are no associated cerebral malformations • Secondary hydrocephalus may result from blockage of CSF drainage in the foramen magnum • Syringomyelia is present in 50–75% of cases • Abnormal CSF pulsation (CSF flow measurement).
Chiari II: Early diagnosis on fetal MRI (associated malformations) • Closed or open dysraphism (more often lumbar than cervical) • Portions of the cerebellum and medulla oblongata are displaced into the spinal canal • Hypoplasia of the posterior cranial fossa with parietooccipital microgyria • Callosal dysgenesis • Hypoplastic, flattened pons • Enlargement of the prepontine cisterns • Beaklike extension of the quadrigeminal plate • Hydrocephalus • Syringomyelia (hydromyelia) extending past C1.
- **Prenatal and postnatal ultrasound findings**
Chiari II: Caudal displacement of the cerebellum • Hydrocephalus.

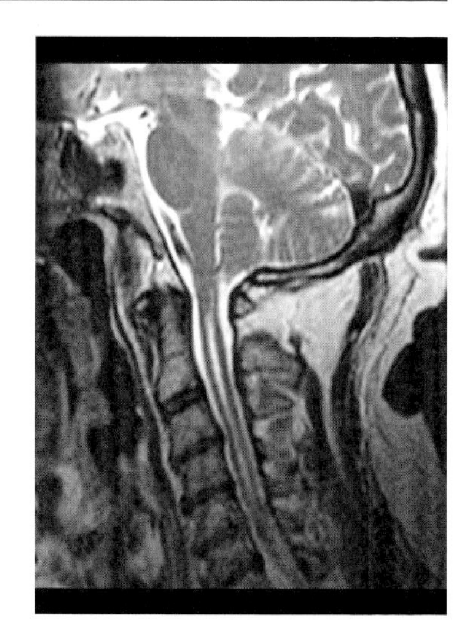

Fig. 1.1 A 57-year-old man with a history of pain in both upper extremities for many years, now accompanied by sensory deficits on the left side. MR image of the craniocervical junction (sagittal, T2). The image shows elongation and cervical descent of the cerebellar tonsils accompanied by cervical hydromyelia (Arnold–Chiari I).

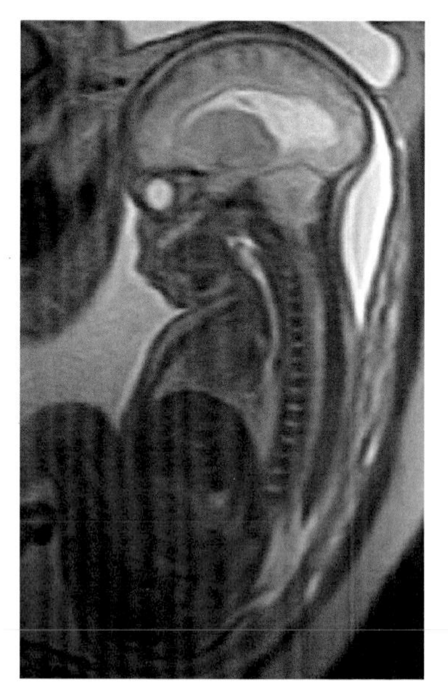

Fig. 1.2 Fetal MR image (sagittal, T2, single-shot fast-spin echo). A small posterior cranial fossa with caudal displacement of the cerebellum, enlarged ventricles, and lumbar myelomeningocele (Chiari II).

Clinical Aspects

- **Typical presentation**
  Chiari I: Up to 50% of all cases are asymptomatic • Herniation > 12 mm is almost invariably symptomatic • Pain on movement of the head and neck • Gait ataxia • Caudal cranial nerve symptoms • Sleep apnea.
  Chiari II: Myelomeningocele • Paralysis of the lower extremities • Sphincter dysfunction • Obstructive hydrocephalus • Brainstem compression.
- **Therapeutic options**
  Chiari I: Patients with symptoms require suboccipital craniotomy or dorsal resection of C1 to decompress the spinal cord • Conservative treatment is indicated in the absence of syrinx.
  Chiari II: Hydrocephalus is treated by shunting • Surgical closure of the myelomeningocele (sometimes this may be done prenatally, in which case there will be near normal development of the posterior cranial fossa).

Differential Diagnosis

Acquired hydromyelia from another cause	
Descent of the cerebellar tonsils	– Basilar invagination (osteogenesis imperfecta, Paget disease, acromegaly, Klippel–Feil syndrome) – Chronic petrosal vein shunt, elevated intracranial pressure

Selected References

Gammal TE, Mark EK, Brooks BS. MR imaging of Chiari II malformation. Am J Röntgenol 1988; 150: 163–70
Osborn AG. Diagnostic Neuroradiology. Philadelphia: Mosby 1994; 15–24, 66

Definition (Transitional Lumbosacral Vertebra)

Sacralization: The border between the sacrum and lumbar spine is shifted one segment cranially.
Lumbarization: The first sacral vertebra develops as a lumbar vertebra.
Cranial shifts are more common than lumbarization. Sacralization can also occur unilaterally. A full-spine radiograph is required to clearly identify the malformation as lumbarization or sacralization. Wherever this is not feasible or not indicated, the term "transitional lumbosacral vertebra" is preferred.

Imaging Signs

- **Modality of choice**
  - Conventional radiographs or CT.
  - MRI (when neurologic symptoms are present).

Clinical Aspects

- **Typical presentation**
  Asymmetric transitional lumbosacral vertebrae, in particular, are often accompanied by spinal symptoms.
- **Therapeutic options**
  Physical therapy.

Selected References

Brossmann J, Czerny C, Freyschmidt J. Grenzen des Normalen und Anfänge des Pathologischen in der Radiologie des kindlichen und erwachsenen Skeletts, 14th ed. Stuttgart: Thieme 2001

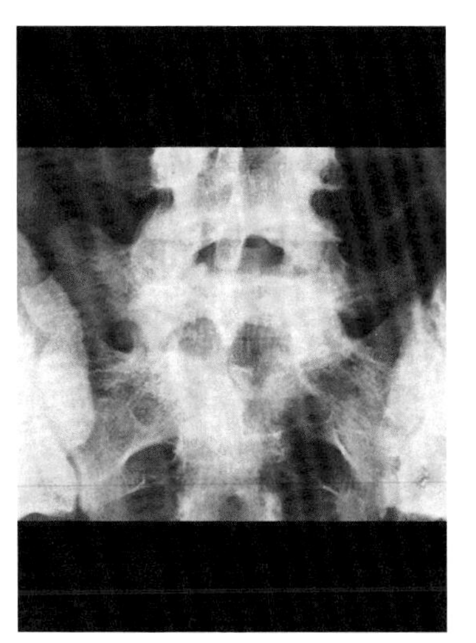

Fig. 1.3 Conventional radiograph of the lumbosacral junction (A-P, detail). Asymmetrical transitional lumbosacral vertebra.

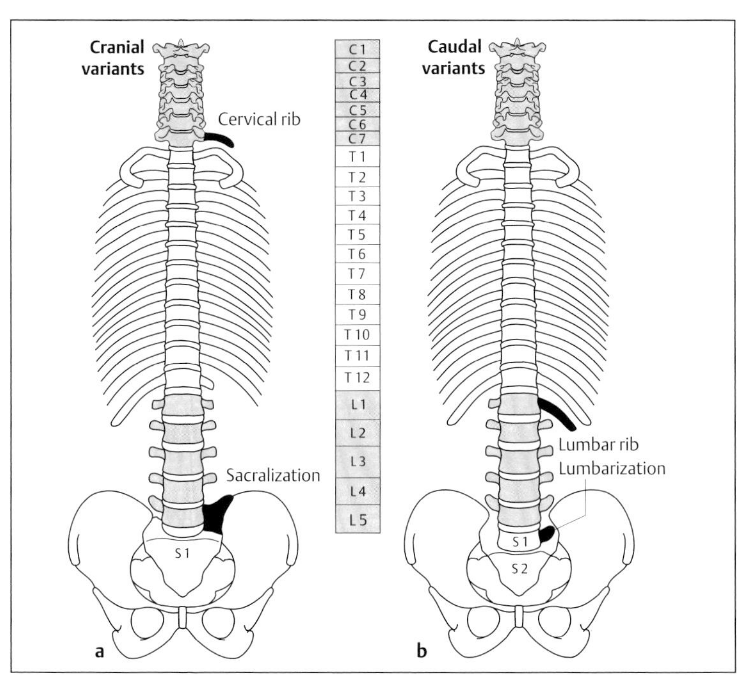

Fig. 1.4 a, b Schematic diagram: Sacralization (**a**); lumbarization (**b**).

Definition

▸ **Epidemiology**
Rare closed spinal dysraphism • Most common in the lumbar and thoracic spine • More common in men than in women (4:1).

▸ **Etiology, pathophysiology, pathogenesis**
Characterized by development of a sagittal cleft in the spinal cord.
Type I (diastematomyelia with a septum): The spinal cord is split by a bony or cartilaginous septum or "spur" extending between the vertebral body and arch • Each hemicord has its own dural tube and separate subarachnoid space • The hemicords may be asymmetrical.
Type II (diastematomyelia without a septum): The two hemicords are contained in a single dural tube, occasionally separated by a fine cartilaginous septum.
Cutaneous stigmata: Hypertrichosis, hemangioma, lipoma, dermal sinus • Associated with bony malformations (85% of cases): Fused vertebrae, hemivertebrae, "butterfly" vertebrae, scoliosis (up to 60% of cases) • Associated hydromyelia (30–40% of cases), especially with type I • Associated myelomeningocele.

Imaging Signs

▸ **Modality of choice**
MRI:
- Sagittal: T1, T2 (skin surface also visualized).
- Coronal: With severe scoliosis.
- Transverse: T2-TSE with 3-mm slice thickness in the region of the bony defects, slice thickness of 5–10 mm over the rest of the spinal cord (associated hydromyelia); T1 with 3-mm slice thickness over the bony defects.
- Contrast administration is indicated when intraspinal soft tissue components are present (cartilaginous structures can develop into fibromatous tumors) or for postoperative imaging (to exclude inflammation): Sagittal and transverse T1-weighted sequences with fat suppression.
- Cerebral MRI to identify associated anomalies.

▸ **MRI findings**
The two hemicords are visualized with their common or separate dural tubes and/or a bony spur • Associated hydromyelia or adherent lipomas are seen • Vertebral dysplasia is visualized • The precise craniocaudal extent of the malformation is seen • Prenatal examination is also possible.

▸ **CT findings**
Three-dimensional visualization of the bony anomalies • CT myelography can demonstrate the cleft spinal cord when MRI is contraindicated • Useful for visualizing associated bony malformations and reconstruction in all planes.

▸ **Ultrasound findings**
Prenatal diagnosis and postnatal examination through the bony aperture.

▸ **Conventional radiography findings**
A bony spur and vertebral dysplasia may be seen.

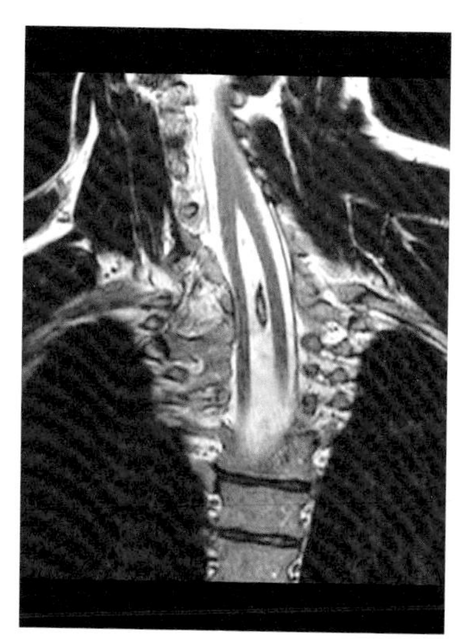

Fig. 1.5 A 25-year-old patient with a history of scoliosis since childhood presented with increasing sensory deficits and weakness in the right hand, and beltlike bands of pain. MR image of the cervicothoracic region (coronary, T2). Two narrow hemicords are separated by a bony septum (type I diastematomyelia with septum).

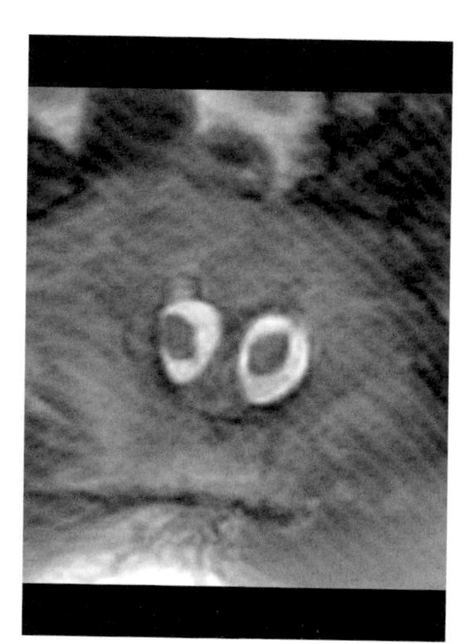

Fig. 1.6 MR image of T1 (axial, GRE). Hemicords are visualized. Adhesions to the bony septum are seen on the right.

Clinical Aspects

- **Typical presentation**
  Often only becomes symptomatic in adults • Scoliosis • Discrete atrophy or weakness in one or both lower extremities • Progressive paraparesis • Bladder and bowel dysfunction.
- **Therapeutic options**
  Surgical intervention immediately after the diagnosis to avoid irreversible damage to the nerve tissue • Resection of a bony spur or fibrous septum • Correction of a tethered cord.

Differential Diagnosis

Hydromyelia	– May present a similar picture where axial and coronal slices are not obtained

Selected References

Pang D et al. Split cord malformation. Part I: A unified theory of embryogenesis for double spinal cord malformations. Part II: Clinical syndrome. Neurosurgery 1992; 31: 214–217, 481–500

Songio-Cohen P et al. Prenatal diagnosis of diastematomyelia. Childs Nerv Syst 2003; 19: 555–566

Tortori-Donati P et al. Magnetic Resonance Imaging of Spinal Dysraphism. Topics Mag Res Im 2001; 12: 375–409

Definition

- **Epidemiology**
  Almost always congenital • Most commonly occurs in preadolescence (7–12 years) • *Predilection:* lumbosacral region.
- **Etiology, pathophysiology, pathogenesis**
  "Tethered cord" is not a morphologic symptom but a clinical syndrome consisting of:
  - Pain and/or sensory deficits in the lower extremity.
  - Spastic gait.
  - Muscle atrophy.
  - Occasionally bladder and bowel dysfunction.
  - Occasionally club foot.
- **Etiology**
  Adherence of the spinal cord to the dura prevents the cord from ascending normally and results in increasing traction • Intradural lipoma or lipomyelomeningocele • Split cord malformation (diastematomyelia) • Dermal sinus • Fibrotic lipomatosis ("fatty filum") • Myelomeningocele • Arachnoiditis • Posttraumatic condition.

Imaging Signs

- **Modality of choice**
  MRI:
  - Sagittal: T1, T2 (skin surface also visualized).
  - Coronal: With severe scoliosis.
  - Transverse: T2-TSE with 3-mm slice thickness in the region of the bony defects • Slice thickness of 5–10 mm over the rest of the spinal cord (associated hydromyelia, diastematomyelia; T1 with 3-mm slice thickness over the bony defects).
  - Contrast administration is indicated where intraspinal soft tissue components are present (cartilaginous structures can develop into fibromatous tumors) or where there is postoperative inflammation: Sagittal and transverse T1-weighted sequences with fat suppression.
  - Cerebral MRI to exclude associated malformations.
  - CSF flow study.
  - Fetal MRI: To assess the prognosis.

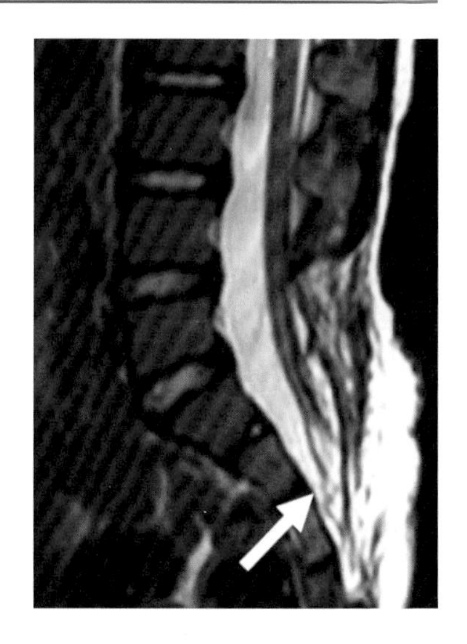

Fig. 1.7 A 4-year-old boy with spastic gait and bladder dysfunction. MR image of the lumbar spine (sagittal, T2). There is no typical conus medullaris, the spinal cord is elongated and fixed within a lipoma at the level of S2.

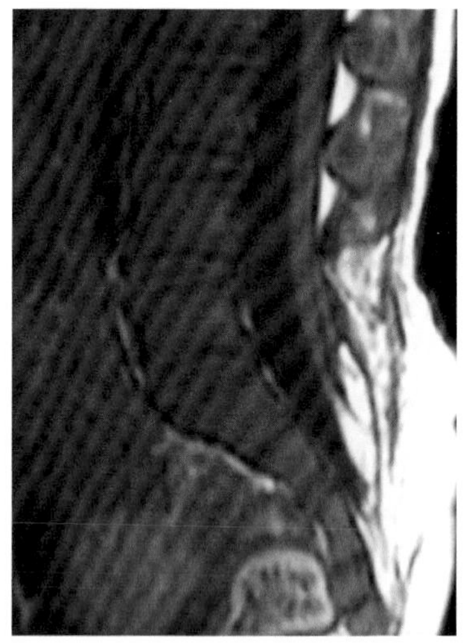

Fig. 1.8 MR image of the lumbar spine (sagittal, T1). Lipoma fused with the short, thick fibers of the cauda equina ("thickened fatty filum").

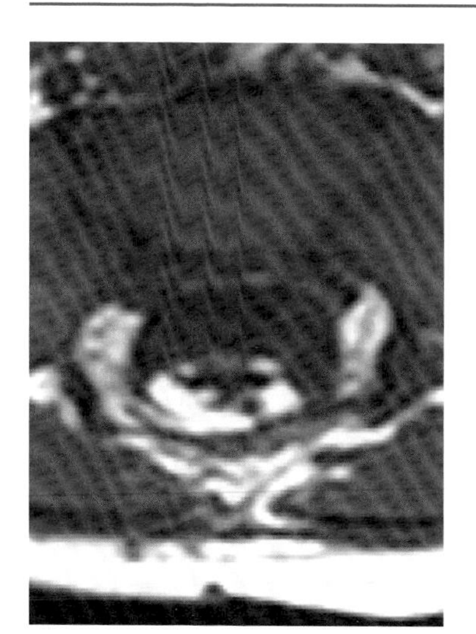

Fig. 1.9 MRI of S1 (axial, T1). Neural structures are fixed within the lipoma.

- **MRI findings**

  Descent of the conus medullaris (normal position at 8–10 weeks after birth is approximately L1–L2) • *Changes in the shape of the conus medullaris:* Elongated and thinned without the physiologic bulb-shaped expansion of the spinal cord at the level of the conus medullaris • *Filum terminale:* Thickened and shortened • Underlying pathology is visualized.
- **CT findings**

  Three-dimensional reconstruction to visualize associated bony malformations • Urodynamic study • Evaluation of compromised bladder function • *CT myelography:* Evaluation of descent of the conus medullaris when MRI is contraindicated.
- **Ultrasound findings**

  Fetal examination to assess prognosis • In the presence of instability in a newborn (when MRI is not feasible) • Prenatal detection of dysraphism • Direct visualization of tethering (through a bone aperture after a laminectomy).
- **Radiographic findings**

  Visualization of associated bony anomalies: Spina bifida, fused vertebrae, rib malformations • Evaluation of scoliosis.

Clinical Aspects

- **Typical presentation**
  Increasing muscle weakness • Heightened muscle tone, spasticity • Unsteady gait • Rapidly progressive scoliosis • Increasing bladder and bowel dysfunction • Back and leg pain • Leg deformity.
- **Therapeutic options**
  Surgical intervention is indicated only in worsening neurologic symptoms or pain resistant to therapy • *Primary goal:* Prevention of further neurologic deficits; postoperative improvement of neurologic function is a secondary aim that is often not achieved • Mobilization of the fixed spinal cord • Resection of scar tissue • Laminectomy where indicated • *Surgical complication rate:* 1–2% (infection, bleeding, worsening of neurologic symptoms) • Tethering recurs in 10–20% of all cases, especially where the initial surgery is performed at an early age (growth of spinal column).

Differential Diagnosis

Drop metastases	– History (underlying malignancy) – Difference in patient age
Associated malformations with tethering	

Selected References

Cornette L et al. Closed spinal dysraphism: a review on diagnosis and treatment in infancy. Eur J Paediatr Neurol 1998; 2: 179–185

Gupta SK et al. Tethered cord syndrome in adults. Surg Neurol 1999; 52: 362–370

Kim MJ et al. Tethered spinal cord with double spinal lipomas. J Korean Med Sci 2006; 21: 1133–1135

Sarwark JF et al. Tethered cord syndrome in low motor level children with myelomeningocele. Pediatr Neurosurg 1996; 25: 2

Yamada S, Won DJ. What is the true tethered cord syndrome? Childs Nerv Syst 2007; 23: 371–375

Definition

- **Epidemiology**
  Most common congenital neoplasm, usually diagnosed before birth • Benign in 80–85% of cases • *Mortality:* 15–35% • *Localization:* Lesions are usually intradural and extramedullary, rarely intramedullary (2% of cases) • More common in females than males (3:1); malignant subtype is more common in males.
- **Etiology, pathophysiology, pathogenesis**
  Mixed tumor with tissue components from all three germ layers • Arises from pluripotent cells of the node of Hensen • The tissue components exhibit varying degrees of maturation.
  Staging classification:
  - Type I: Spreads beyond the fetus.
  - Type II: External and presacral spread.
  - Type III: Small external component, primarily intrapelvic and intraabdominal tumor spread.
  - Type IV: Completely presacral tumor.

  Currarino triad:
  - Sacral anomaly.
  - Anal atresia or stenosis.
  - Presacral tumor (benign teratoma in 40% of all cases, anterior meningocele in 47%).

Imaging Signs

- **Modality of choice**
  MRI:
  - Sagittal: T1, T2, STIR.
  - Coronal: T2.
  - Axial: T2.

  Abdominal study (CT or MRI): Evaluation of ventral spread (into the abdominal cavity).
- **General**
  Inhomogeneous solid-cystic mass in the region of the sacrum and distal lumbar spine, occasionally extending into the intrapelvic and intraabdominal regions • Secondary hydronephrosis due to compression • Polyhydramnios.
- **MRI findings**
  Cysts: Homogeneously hyperintense (T1 and T2) with high protein content, or hypointense (T1) and hyperintense (T2) with serous content, occasionally septate • *Solid nodules:* Enhance with contrast • *Fatty components:* Fat suppression with a STIR sequence • *Calcified deposits:* Markedly hypointense on T1 and T2.
- **Ultrasound findings**
  Hyperechoic (solid) areas with inclusions of or peripheral anechoic (cystic) components • *Calcifications:* Hyperechoic foci with acoustic shadows.

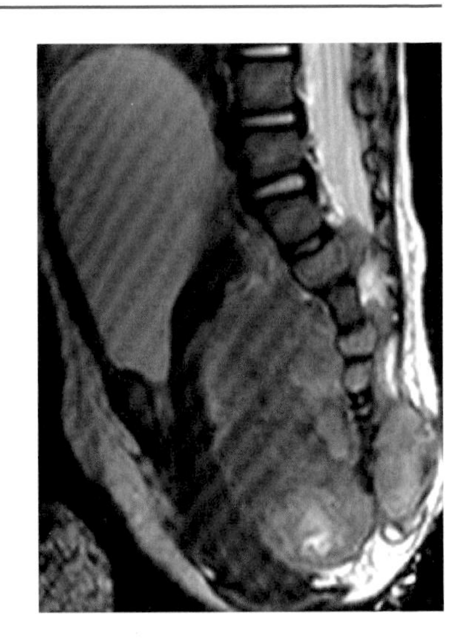

Fig. 1.10 Newborn with a known a sacrococcygeal mass detected by prenatal ultrasound. Pelvic MR image (sagittal, T2). Mass with a larger component anterior to the spine than posterior to the spine, exhibiting inhomogeneous signal; the caudal spine is completely present.

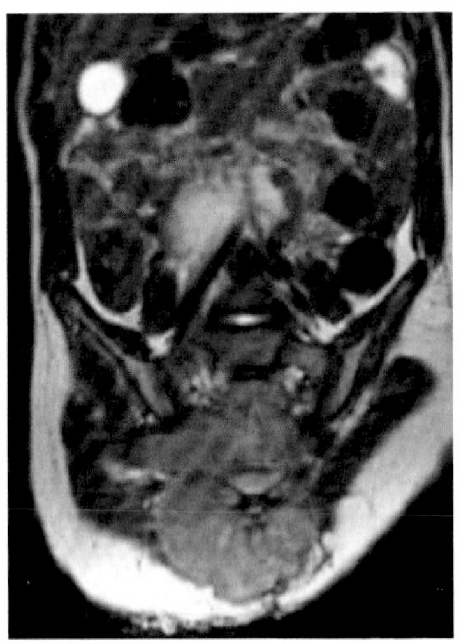

Fig. 1.11 MR image of the sacrum (coronal, T2). Tumor spread is visible in the sacrum.

Clinical Aspects

- **Typical presentation**
  Hydrops fetalis: Results from intrauterine complications such as polyhydramnios and tumor hemorrhage. Fatal prognosis where hydrops occurs prior to the 30th week of pregnancy (93% mortality) • Postpartum morbidity resulting from associated congenital anomalies (10% of cases), compression of adjacent organs (such as the urogenital tract), recurrent tumor, intraoperative and postoperative complications.
- **Therapeutic options**
  In cases of hydrops, birth should be induced as soon as the lungs are sufficiently mature • Radical resection of the tumor including the coccyx is indicated prior to birth or within the first week of life • *Fetal interventions:* Tumor resection, cyst aspiration, reduction of the amnion.

Differential Diagnosis

External tumors: myelomeningocele	– Spina bifida located higher and further dorsal
Intrapelvic tumors	– Ovarian, mesenteric cysts – Bowel dilation or duplication – Cystic neuroblastoma
Solid tumors	– Chordoma – Neurogenic tumors – Lipoma – Hemangioma – Malignant melanoma

Selected References

Avni FE et al. MR imaging of fetal sacrococcygeal teratoma: diagnosis and assessment. AJR Am J Roentgenol 2002; 178: 179–183
Feldman M et al. Neonatal sacrococcygeal teratoma: multiimaging modality assessment. J Pediatr Surg 1990; 26: 675–678
Hedrick HL et al. Sacrococcygeal teratoma: prenatal assessment, fetal intervention, and outcome. J Pediatr Surg 2004; 39: 430–438

Definition

Spinal dysraphism: Developmental anomaly with incomplete closure of the neural tube • A third of dysraphic anomalies are open and two-thirds are closed.
Meningocele: Accounts for 2.4% of all closed dysraphic anomalies • Herniation of a CSF-filled sac lined with dura and arachnoid through a posterior spina bifida • Completely covered by skin • Incomplete dysraphism with incomplete closure of the vertebral arch (spina bifida) is common. Often there is associated superficial skin pathology (indentation, hypertrichosis, etc.) • Spina bifida is usually clinically insignificant • Lesion usually does not contain any nerve structures (rarely nerve roots of the filum terminale will pass through a large meningocele) • Not an indication for immediate surgery.
Meningomyelocele: Most common type of open spinal dysraphism (98.8% of cases) • Herniation of the incompletely developed spinal cord and meninges through a bony defect in the posterior vertebral structures with projection of these neural structure above the surface of the skin (neural placode) • Often combined with an abnormally small posterior cranial fossa, caudal herniation of cerebellar tissue, and hydrocephalus (= Chiari II malformation) • Imaging studies are useful primarily for postoperative follow-up and visualizing associated malformations; hydrocephalus in the setting of a Chiari II malformation may develop only after closure of the meningomyelocele • *Neurosurgical emergency:* Surgical closure is indicated within 48 hours to avoid infection of the exposed spinal cord and an increase in neurologic dysfunction • Lumbar and lumbosacral regions are most often affected • More common in women than in men.

Imaging Signs

▸ **Modality of choice**

MRI:
- Sagittal: T1, T2 (skin surface also visualized).
- Coronal: With severe scoliosis.
- Transverse: T2-TSE with 3-mm slice thickness in the region of the bony defects. Slice thickness of 5–10 mm over the rest of the spinal cord (associated hydromyelia, diastematomyelia); T1 with 3-mm slice thickness over the bony defects.
- Contrast administration is indicated when an intraspinal soft tissue component is present (cartilaginous structures can develop into fibromatous tumors) or when there is postoperative inflammation: Sagittal and transverse T1-weighted sequences with fat suppression.
- Cerebral MRI to exclude associated malformations.
- CSF flow study where tethering is suspected.
- Fetal MRI: To assess the prognosis.

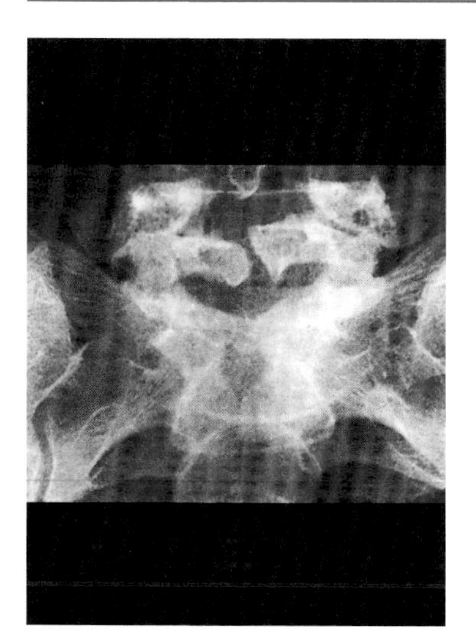

Fig. 1.12 Conventional radiograph of the lumbosacral junction (A-P, detail). Spina bifida at L5.

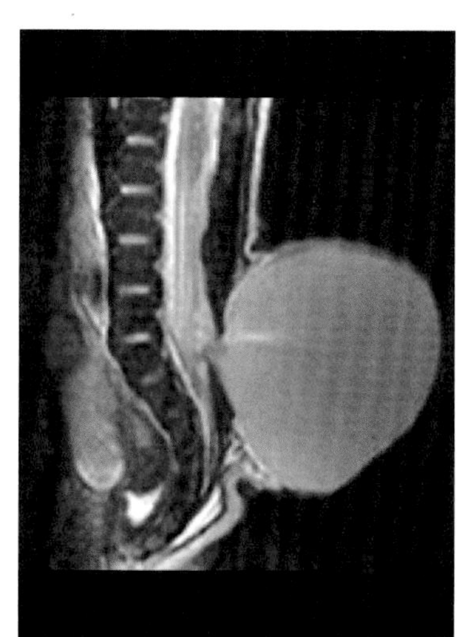

Fig. 1.13 Findings at birth included a sacral mass. Motor function in the child's legs was normal. MR image of the lumbosacral region (sagittal, T2). Myelocele sac containing CSF but otherwise empty. Intraspinal descent of the conus medullaris with short straight cauda equina fibers that are fixed to the caudal end of the dural sac.

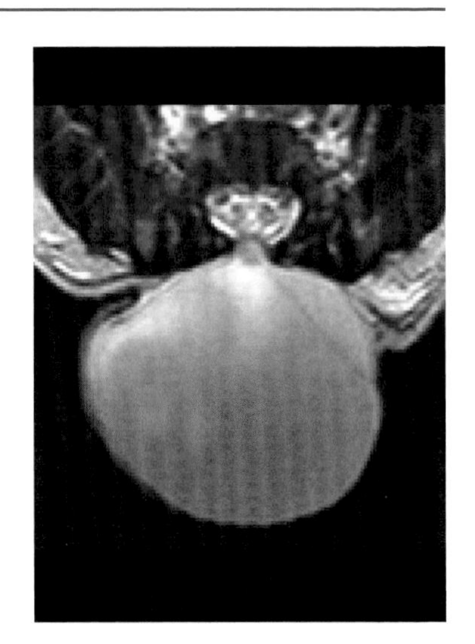

Fig. 1.14 MR image of L5 (axial, T2). Bony defect is occluded by a connective tissue structure (operative report) through which a CSF-filled sac has herniated. Septa are present but there are no neural structures. These structures lie entirely within the spine. The anterior CSF spaces are not enlarged. The myelocele sac is covered by a thin layer of skin along its margins.

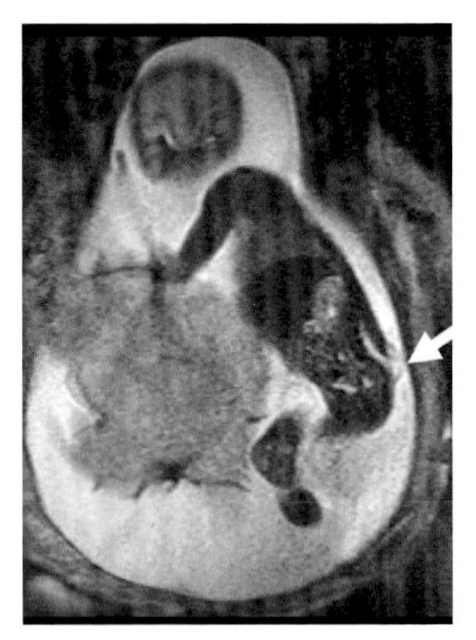

Fig. 1.15 Ultrasound examination in the 20 th week of pregnancy detected spina bifida. MR image of the fetus and pelvis (coronal, T2). Sacral myelocele sac with neural structures coursing along its apex. The axial T2-weighted sequence shows the broad-based bony defect and neural structures within the myelocele (arrow).

▶ **MRI findings**

Clinical indication • Preoperative evaluation • Anatomic characterization of the constituent components of the malformation and their relation to the nerve roots • Identification of morphology and entity • Identification of coexisting diastematomyelia (such as hemimyelomeningocele) • Postoperative visualization of complications • *Hydrocephalus:* 48–72 hours postoperatively • *Recurrent tethering:* Strands of scar tissue fix the spinal cord to the dura • *Arachnoid cysts:* Sequela of postoperative adhesions • Slightly hyperintense to CSF (elevated protein content) • Fine wall • No flow artifacts in contrast with CSF • *Dermoid and epidermoid cysts:* Occur as a result of intraoperative inclusion of epidermal cells, as a primary lesion, or in association with a dermal sinus • Slightly hyperintense to CSF on T1- and T2-weighted images • Superinfection enhances with contrast • *Caution:* Rupture leads to toxic meningitis • *Syringomyelia (syringohydromyelia):* Primarily responsible for worsening postoperative neurologic symptoms, leads to rapidly progressive clinical scoliosis.

▶ **CT findings**

Three-dimensional reconstruction to visualize associated bony malformation.

▶ **Conventional radiographs**

Visualization of bony defect (spina bifida) • Evaluation of scoliosis.

▶ **Ultrasound findings**

Prenatal detection of dysraphism • Fetal ultrasound to assess the prognosis • To evaluate the conus medullaris and filum terminale in newborns with instability (where MRI is not feasible) • Amniocentesis • Elevated AFP.

Clinical Aspects

▶ **Typical presentation**

Meningocele: Usually clinically asymptomatic (no primary spinal cord lesion) • *Caution:* Pressure sores can ulcerate to form open lesions • Tethered cord syndrome with progressive neurologic symptoms.

Meningomyelocele: Reddish raised exposed nerve tissue in the middle of the back • Sensorimotor deficits in the lower extremity • Bladder and bowel dysfunction • Rarely psychomotoric retardation • Severity of the different symptoms varies.

▶ **Therapeutic options**

Meningocele: Immediate closure of the meningocele where ulcerating pressure sores are present • Elimination of a tethered cord syndrome.

Meningomyelocele: Neurosurgical emergency • Mobilization of the placode • Closure of the soft tissue defect • Fetal surgical procedures are being tested.

Differential Diagnosis

Open spinal dysraphism	– Myeloschisis (= myelocele): Very rare. Because the subarachnoid space does not extend to the level of the defect, the neural placode lies at skin level or slightly recessed. – Hemicord with myelocele or myelomeningocele: Malformation affects only one hemicord
Closed spinal dysraphism	– Lipomyeloschisis: Subcutaneous intraspinal lipoma adhering to the neural placode – Lipomyelocele: Subcutaneous extraspinal lipoma adhering to the neural placode – Lipomyelomeningocele: Subcutaneous lipoma, usually adhering asymmetrically to the neural placode. Myelocele on the contralateral side – Terminal myelocystocele: Central canal expanded to form a terminal cyst (syringocele) – Cervical myelocystocele: Dorsal wall of the central canal is displaced and communicates with a meningocele – Cervical myelomeningocele: Fibrous neurovascular cord is displaced into a meningocele through a posterior wall defect

Selected References

Rossi A et al. Imaging in spine and spinal cord malformations. Eur J Radiol 2004; 50: 177–200

Schijman E. Split cord malformation: report of 22 cases and review of literature. Childs Nerv Syst 2003; 19: 106–108

Tortori-Donati P et al. Magnetic Resonance Imaging of Spinal Dysraphism. Topics Mag Res Im 2001; 12: 375–409

Definition

Partial or complete malformation of the vertebrae • Abnormal vertebral segmentation and fusion.
Total aplasia: Absence of both ossification centers. Very rare.
Lateral hemivertebra: Failure of ossification of one of the two ossification centers. A distinction is made between the primordium of a hemivertebra exhibiting a vertebral arch of normal length (hemisoma) and the primordium of a hemivertebra with half an arch (hemispondylus). This is often associated with scoliosis and deformities of the bony thorax.
Butterfly vertebra (partial ventral or dorsal cleavage): Failure of fusion of the individual ossification centers.
Persistent notochord: The remnant divides the vertebral body into two halves; the clefts of the ventral and dorsal halves extend to the notochord canal.
Total sagittal cleavage: This very rare deformity is incompatible with life.
Congenitally fused vertebrae: Partial or total fusion of adjacent vertebrae due to failure of segmentation; partial fusion anomaly type A: Fusion in the anterior third of the vertebral body; type B: Fusion in the posterior third of the vertebral body with or without fusion of the vertebral arches and facet joints.

Imaging Signs

- **Modality of choice**
  - MRI: Multiplanar T1-weighted and T2-weighted sequences • Coronal slices are particularly important in severe scoliosis.
  - CT: Three-dimensional reconstructions can be obtained for preoperative planning.
- **General**

  Radiographic signs of butterfly vertebra: Viewed in the coronal plane, the two halves of the vertebra taper toward the unfused center to produce a shape resembling a butterfly.
  Radiographic signs of lateral hemivertebra: Viewed in the coronal plane, one half of the vertebra tapers toward the center while the other half is absent, producing a nearly triangular or wedge shape.
  Radiographic signs of fused vertebrae: The A-P diameter of the fused vertebrae is diminished, often in combination with narrowing in the area of the disk interspace, which is either absent or underdeveloped. Fused vertebrae are about as high as two normal vertebrae including the interspace. In 50% of cases, the facets joints are also fused. The spinous processes can be malformed or fused as well.
  Localization: C2–C3 > C5–C6 > T12–L1 > L4–L5.

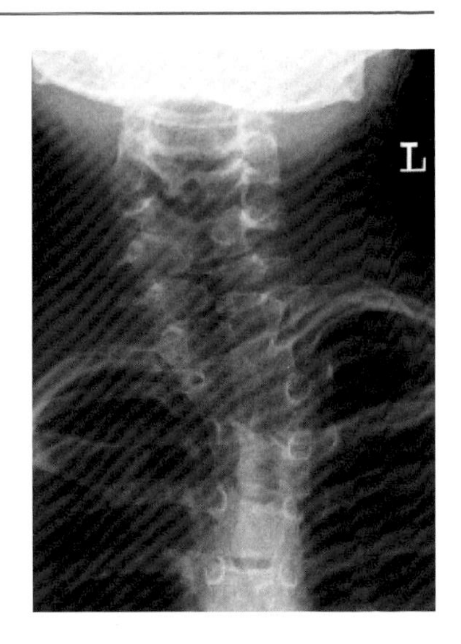

Fig. 1.16 Conventional A-P radiograph of the cervicothoracic junction of an 11-year-old boy. Left hemivertebra at T3, asymmetrical cervical vertebrae from T2 to the occiput, and complex segmentation and fusion anomalies.

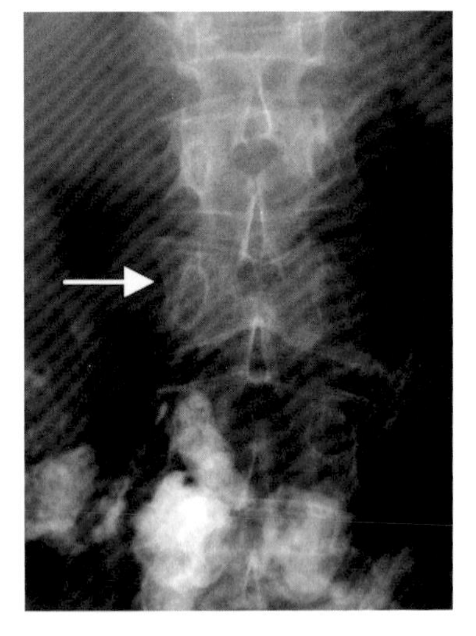

Fig. 1.17 Conventional radiograph of the lumbar spine (A-P, detail) of a 20-year-old patient. Incidental finding of a butterfly vertebra (arrow); additional findings include residual contrast agent projected on the adjacent caudal vertebra, which is also visualized.

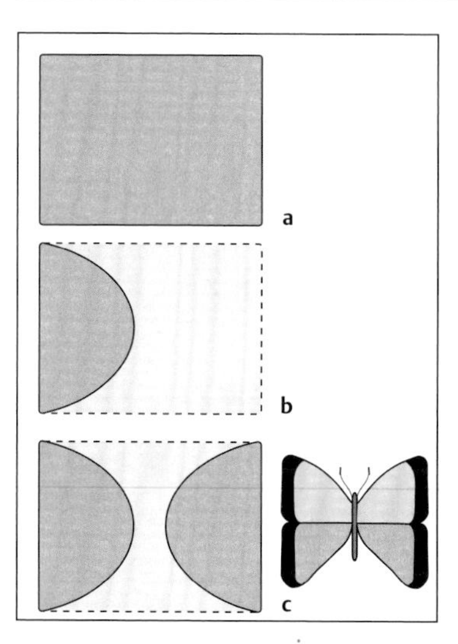

Fig. 1.18 a–c Schematic diagram of vertebral malformations (coronal view). Normal vertebra (**a**); lateral hemivertebra (**b**); butterfly vertebra (**c**).

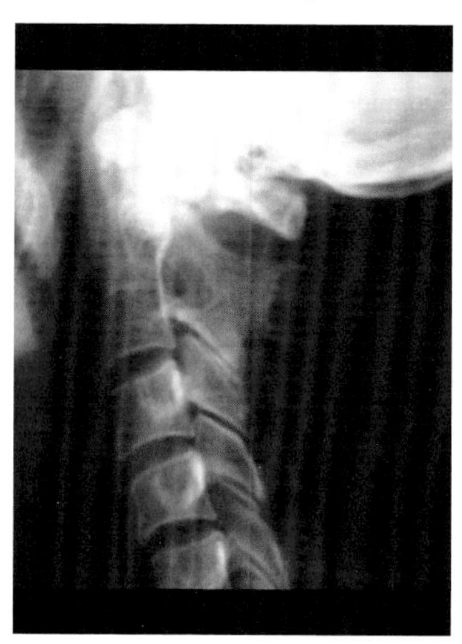

Fig. 1.19 A 25-year-old woman with limited mobility in the cervical spine and congenital vertebral fusion at C2–C3. Conventional lateral radiograph of the cervical spine.

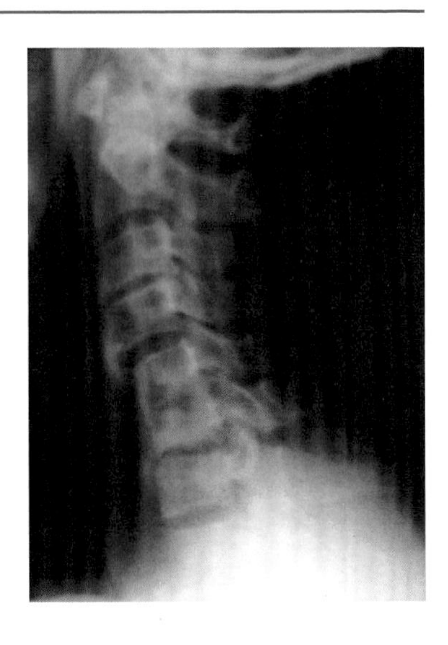

Fig. 1.20 A 39-year-old man with vertebral fusion at C5–C6 in status post spondylitis. Conventional lateral radiograph of the cervical spine.

- **Radiographic findings**
  Primary imaging study to identify and determine the level of vertebral malformations • May be used to evaluate associated scoliosis where indicated • Typical butterfly, wedge, and fusion deformities are well visualized • Examiner can determine whether the abnormal vertebrae are supernumerary or have replaced normal vertebrae.
- **CT findings**
  Axial slices are obtained to evaluate dysraphism of the posterior structures and vertebral fusion anomalies • Coronal and sagittal reconstructions are useful for evaluating cleft vertebrae and hemivertebrae, and for preoperative planning.
- **MRI findings**
  Detection and evaluation of lipomas, diastematomyelia, or spinal cord compression • Evaluation of the spinal cord and exiting nerve roots.

Clinical Aspects

- **Typical presentation**
  Usually asymptomatic • Often detected on radiographs obtained to evaluate scoliosis • Fused vertebrae may be associated with early osteochondrosis, especially in the caudally adjacent segments • Spinal stenosis is rarely encountered.
- **Therapeutic options**
  Conservative treatment • Surgery (resection and/or fusion) is indicated only for severe cases.

Differential Diagnosis

Cleft vertebrae and hemivertebrae	– Fracture: Usually there is a history of trauma. Two pedicles each per vertebra. Presence of an irregular fracture line lacking a cortical boundary. Associated soft tissue edema often present.
Congenitally fused vertebrae	– Isolated anomaly – Klippel–Feil syndrome – Basal cell nevus syndrome (Gorlin syndrome) – Fibrodysplasia ossificans progressiva
Acquired vertebral fusion anomalies (no vertebral "waist" height of affected vertebra often reduced, especially anteriorly)	– Spinal fusion – Posttraumatic – Ankylosing spondylitis – Post bacterial spondylitis – Severe osteochondrosis – Juvenile rheumatoid arthritis – Alcoholic fetopathy

Selected References

Brossmann J, Czerny Ch, Freyschmidt J. Grenzen des Normalen und Anfänge des Pathologischen in der Radiologie des kindlichen und erwachsenen Skeletts. Stuttgart: Thieme 2001

Tortori-Donati P, Fondelli MP, Rossi A, Raybaud CA, Cama A, Capra V. Segmental spinal dysgenesis: neuroradiologic findings with clinical and embryologic correlation. Am J Neuroradiol 1999; 20: 445–456

Definition

▸ **Epidemiology**

Sporadic occurrence • 1 in 42 000 births • Familial genetic component • Females are affected slightly more often than males • *Age range:* Usually 10–30 years.

▸ **Etiology, pathophysiology, pathogenesis**

Congenital malformation of the cervical spine with failed segmentation of two or more vertebrae • *Predilection:* C2–C3 > C5–C6 > craniocervical and thoracolumbar junctions.

Imaging Signs

▸ **Modality of choice**

Conventional radiographs:

- Stress radiographs in maximum flexion and extension are important for evaluating instability.

MRI:

- To exclude spinal cord or nerve root compression.

Abdominal ultrasound or CT:

- To determine whether abdominal organs are affected.

▸ **General**

Vertebral fusion involving one or more segments with a narrow, rudimentary disk interspace. Often the facet joints and spinous processes are also fused • The vertebral body exhibits a shallowly concave "waist" at the level of the fused disk interspace.

▸ **Radiographic findings**

Visualization of typical cervical vertebral stenosis • *Findings on stress radiographs:* Lack of mobility in the affected segment, often with compensatory hypermobility in adjacent segments • Degenerative changes are often present in the adjacent segments • There may be a bony connection with the shoulder (extending from the scapula to the spinous process, vertebral arch, or transverse process of one or more lower cervical vertebrae).

▸ **CT findings**

Evaluation of the width of the spinal canal (stenosis due to degenerative changes in the adjacent segments or widening of the spinal canal in the presence of syringomyelia).

▸ **MRI findings**

Evaluation for possible disk protrusion, spinal or nerve root compression, and presence of Chiari I syndrome.

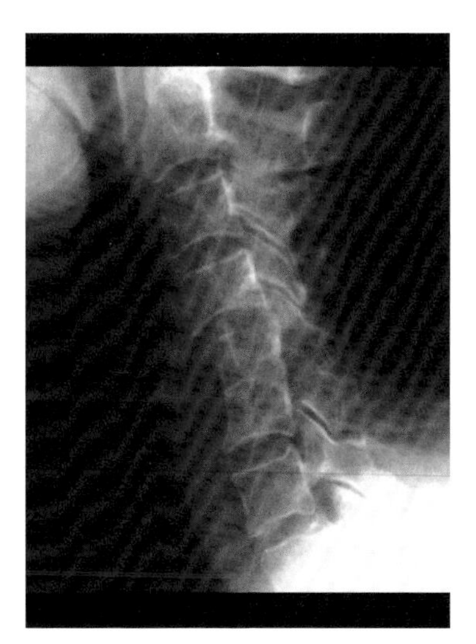

Fig. 1.21 A 22-year-old woman with limited mobility in the cervical spine and chronic pain radiating from the cervical spine. Clinical findings included short neck. Conventional lateral radiograph of the cervical spine (detail). Synostosis at C5–C6 with rudimentary anterior disk interspace, narrowing of the fused C5–C6 vertebrae ("waist"), early degenerative changes in the adjacent segments (especially C4–C5).

Clinical Aspects

- **Typical presentation**
  Triad:
  - Short neck.
  - Low posterior hairline.
  - Limited mobility in the cervical spine.

  Some patients are asymptomatic whereas others show neurologic symptoms as infants and children • After age 30, symptoms arise due to degenerative changes and instability in the adjacent spinal segments • Often associated with other anomalies (Sprengel deformity or elevated scapula, cervical ribs, pterygium colli, spina bifida, cleft palate, etc.).
- **Therapeutic options**
  Initial conservative therapy • Surgery (spinal fusion) is indicated for severe pain despite conservative therapy and with increasing instability.

Differential Diagnosis

Juvenile rheumatoid arthritis	– Inflammatory manifestations are usually present at other sites also – History
Post diskitis	– History – No "waist" – Irregular endplates
Ankylosing spondylitis	– Typical, usually continuous, syndesmophytes – Symmetric involvement in the sacroiliac joints
Surgical spinal fusion	– History – No "waist"

Selected References

Baba H, Maezawa Y, Furusawa N, Chen Q, Imura S, Tomita K. The cervical spine in the Klippel-Feil syndrome. A report of 57 cases. Int Orthop 1995; 19: 204–208

Guille JT, Miller A, Bowen JR, Forlin E, Caro PA. The natural history of Klippel-Feil syndrome: clinical, roentgenographic, and magnetic resonance imaging findings at adulthood. J Pediatr Orthop 1995; 15: 617–626

Reiser M, Peters PE. Radiologische Differenzialdiagnose der Skeletterkrankungen. Stuttgart: Thieme 1995

Definition

Posteriorly convex curvature of the spine • The normal thoracic kyphosis develops naturally by 6 years of age as the child begins to walk upright • When the curvature exceeds the range of normal kyphosis (25–45°) it is considered abnormal kyphosis.

- *Arcuate kyphosis (long arc):* In Scheuermann disease, ankylosing spondylitis, senile kyphosis, and postural deficiency.
- *Angular kyphosis (short arc):* In spondylitis, compression fractures, pathologic fractures, tumors, and congenital wedge vertebrae.

Imaging Signs

- **Modality of choice**
  Conventional radiographs.
- **Radiographic findings**
  A lateral view with the patient standing helps determine the extent of deformity • Lateral view in hyperextension is taken to evaluate flexibility • Measurement is similar to the Cobb method used for scoliosis; the distance measured extends from the superior endplate of the third thoracic vertebra to the inferior endplate of the twelfth thoracic vertebra.
- **CT and MRI findings**
  These can be very useful for identifying the cause of kyphosis.

Clinical Aspects

- **Typical presentation**
  Asymptomatic • Functional impairments • Obstructed vision • Pain due to increased degenerative changes • Neurologic deficits.
- **Therapeutic options**
  Conservative treatment (corset, physical therapy, pain therapy) • Surgical management (correction, spinal fusion).

Differential Diagnosis

Postural kyphosis	
Scheuermann disease	– Note Schmorl nodes, Edgren–Vaino sign, Knutsson sign.
Congenital kyphosis	– Note vertebral malformations such as posterior hemivertebrae
Neuromuscular kyphosis	– Palsies, etc.
Myelomeningocele	
Posttraumatic kyphosis	– History
Iatrogenic kyphosis	– Post laminectomy, excision of vertebra – Post radiation therapy

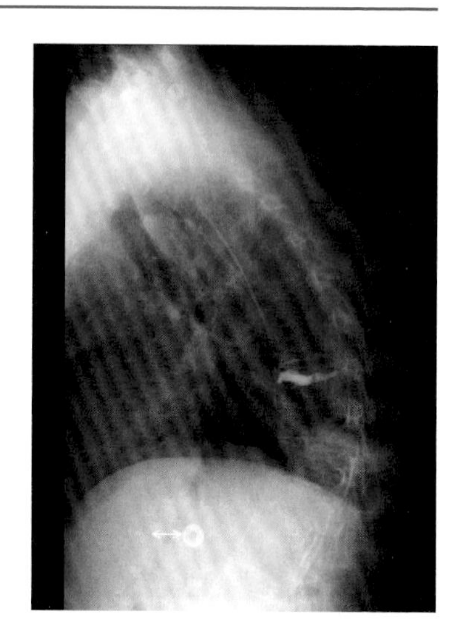

Fig. 1.22 A 74-year-old man with known ankylosing spondylitis and increasing gibbus, post vertebroplasty. Conventional lateral radiograph of the thoracic spine of T9. Calcification of the longitudinal ligaments, slightly barrel-shaped vertebral bodies and abnormally increased thoracic kyphosis.

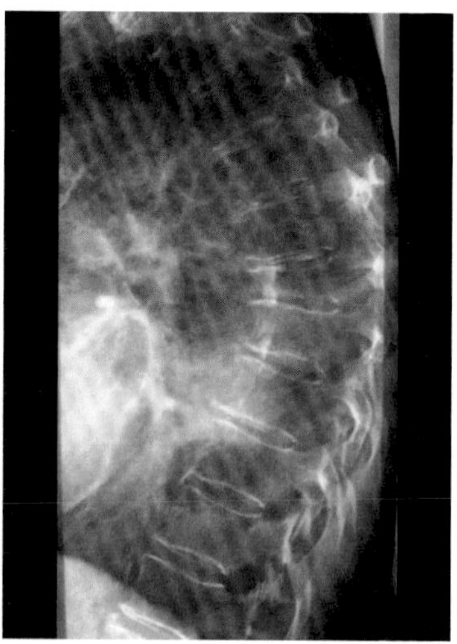

Fig. 1.23 A 74-year-old woman with gibbus and known osteoporosis. Conventional lateral radiograph of the thoracic spine. Vertebral height in the mid-thoracic spine is reduced especially anteriorly, leading to abnormally increased thoracic kyphosis, "osteoporotic kyphosis."

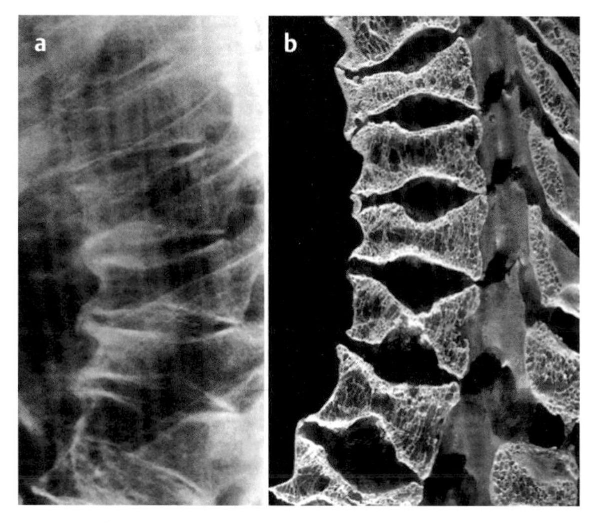

Fig. 1.24 a, b An 83-year-old woman with gibbus. Conventional lateral radiograph of the thoracic spine (detail). Diffusely osteopenic rarefied bone structure with multiple vertebrae significantly reduced in height and showing marked degenerative changes, leading to abnormally increased thoracic kyphosis (**a**). Section of specimen showing corresponding changes (flattened and fishlike vertebrae) (**b**).

Kyphosis due to metabolic disease	– Osteoporosis – Osteogenesis imperfecta – Collapse of individual vertebrae
Kyphosis in skeletal dysplasia	– See vertebral malformations
Kyphosis in ankylosing spondylitis	– Involvement of sacroiliac joints, calcification of paravertebral ligaments
Collagen disorders	– Patient history
Kyphosis due to tumor	– Often secondary blastoma
Kyphosis with inflammatory disorders	– Spondylitis
Idiopathic kyphosis	
Senile kyphosis	– Significant narrowing of the disk interspaces with sclerosis along the adjacent endplates and later ankylosis; multiple vertebrae significantly reduced in height, typically with a flattened shape

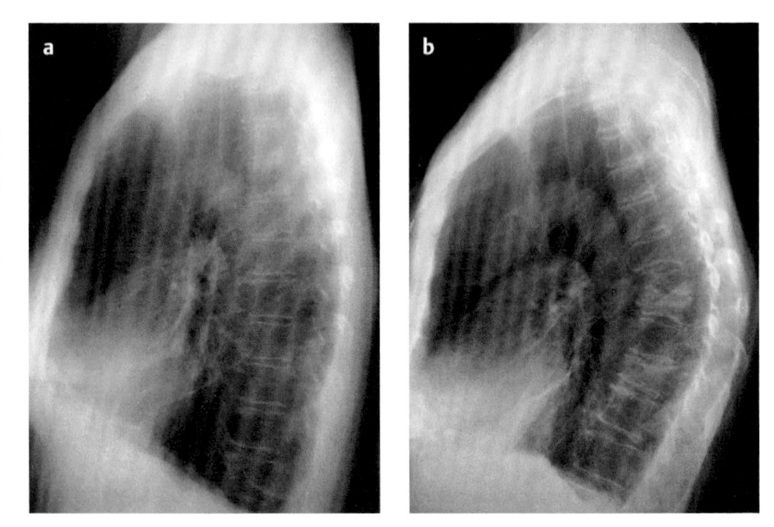

Fig. 1.25 a, b A 60-year-old woman with known osteoporosis presented for follow-up radiograph (after 1 year) with bronchial asthma. Conventional lateral chest radiograph. Abnormal kyphosis of the thoracic spine with osteoporotic vertebral collapse in the mid-thoracic spine, "osteoporotic kyphosis."

Selected References

Jäger M, Wirth CJ. Praxis der Orthopädie. Stuttgart: Thieme 1986

Kormano M, Burgener FA. Radiologische Differentialdiagnostik in Orthopädie und Rheumatologie. Stuttgart: Thieme 1995

Definition

- **Epidemiology**
  Most common spinal disorder in adolescents (10% of the population); usually occurs at 10–18 years • Increased familial incidence.
- **Etiology, pathophysiology, pathogenesis**
  Structural and growth disturbance of the vertebral endplates and disk margins leads to abnormal kyphosis in adolescence • Caused by chronic repetitive trauma to immature bone.

Imaging Signs

- **Modality of choice**
  Conventional radiographs (supplemented by MRI when disk protrusion is suspected).
- **General**
  Reduction in disk height (more pronounced anteriorly) • Three or more thoracic vertebrae with barrel-like convex anterior margins (Knutsson sign) and/or a wedge shape • *Later:* Schmorl nodes (= chondroid disk defects in the region of the vertebral endplates) • Edgren–Vaino sign (exostoses on the endplate of the adjacent vertebra, opposite the cartilaginous nodules) • Separation of marginal ridges from the vertebral body and increased thoracic kyphosis (> 40°) • Sequelae characterized by degeneration and fusion of the anterior portions of the vertebrae can occur • 15% of patients also have scoliosis • *Location:* Usually in the thoracic spine and thoracolumbar junction, < 5% in the lumbar spine, very rarely in the cervical spine.
- **Radiographic findings**
  Detects the signs described above • Used to measure the kyphosis.
- **CT findings**
  Better visualization of the changes in the vertebral endplates.
- **MRI findings**
  Visualization of the frequently associated degenerative changes in the affected disks (disk narrowing, T2 signal loss, possible protrusion) • Schmorl nodes are hypointense on T1-weighted images, hypointense or hyperintense on T2-weighted images • Bone marrow edema may be present around the lesion.
- **Nuclear medicine**
  Bone scan may be normal or there may be increased focal uptake.

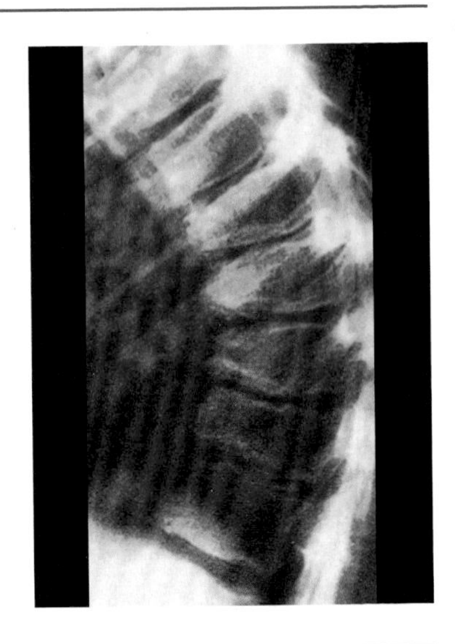

Fig. 1.26 Conventional lateral radiograph of the thoracic spine (detail) of a 20-year-old man with gibbus and back pain. Abnormal kyphosis of the thoracic spine with anteriorly reduced vertebral height. The anterior margins of the vertebrae are irregular: Scheuermann disease.

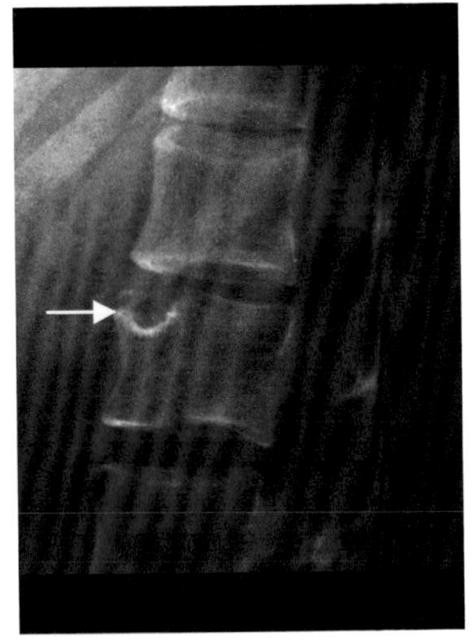

Fig. 1.27 Conventional lateral radiograph of the thoracic spine (detail) of an 18-year-old man with recurring back symptoms. Depression with sclerotic margins in the anterior portion of the superior endplate of vertebra L2 (arrow; Schmorl nodules); there is a corresponding circumscribed bony projection in the inferior endplate of vertebra L1: Scheuermann disease.

Clinical Aspects

- **Typical presentation**
  Typical clinical presentation (thoracic kyphosis) • Increasing pain in the thoracic spine with exercise • Neurologic symptoms (kyphosis, disk protrusion) are rare.
- **Therapeutic options**
  Conservative treatment and regular follow-up until 25 years of age (for kyphosis < 50° in an immature skeleton) • Corset (for kyphosis < 70° in an immature skeleton) • Surgery (spinal fusion; for kyphosis > 75° in an immature skeleton or > 60° in a mature skeleton, with severe uncontrollable pain or neurologic deficit).

Differential Diagnosis

Postural kyphosis	– Normal vertebral endplates, returns to normal when spine is extended
Congenital kyphosis	– Additional vertebral abnormalities are present
Compression fracture	– Fracture line, bone marrow edema
Tuberculous kyphosis	– Extensive destruction of the vertebral endplates, soft tissue and bone marrow edema, and occasionally fused vertebrae
Kyphosis in osteogenesis imperfecta tarda	– Vertebra plana, severe osteopenia
Ankylosing spondylitis	– Pathology in the sacroiliac joints
Cartilaginous nodules on the vertebral endplates	– In the anterior half of the vertebra in Scheuermann disease – In the posterior half of the vertebra in impaired regression of the notochord

Selected References

Ali RM, Green DW, Patel TC. Scheuermann's Kyphosis. Curr Opin Pediatr 1999; 11: 70–75

Tribus CB. Scheuermann's Kyphosis in adolescents and adults: diagnosis and management. J Am Acad Orthop Surg 1998; 6: 36–43

Wenger DR, Frick SL. Scheuermann kyphosis. Spine 1999; 4: 2630–2639

Definition

- **Epidemiology**

  Occurs in 2–4% of the population • Females are affected about five times as often as males • Most often diagnosed in childhood or adolescence.

- **Etiology, pathophysiology, pathogenesis**

  Scoliosis is defined as an abnormal lateral curvature of the spine.

  Classification according to plane of curvature:

  - Right or left scoliosis (lateral deviation in the coronal plane).
  - Rotoscoliosis (rotation in the axial plane).
  - Kyphoscoliosis and lordoscoliosis (kyphotic and lordotic components in the sagittal plane).

  Classification by shape:

  - S-shaped scoliosis (double deviation with curve and reverse curve).
  - C-shaped scoliosis (single curve without reverse curve).

  End vertebrae: The most proximal and distal vertebrae of a curve • The vertebra at which the curve changes direction to become the reverse curve • The vertebra with the greatest tilt toward the concavity and usually the one least rotated.

  Neutral vertebra: The vertebra in a curve which exhibits no rotation (its alignment often matches that of the end vertebra).

  Apical vertebra: The vertebra in a curve which is furthest from normal position and exhibits the greatest rotation.

  Structural curve: Remains present in lateral bending views • Morphologic vertebral changes are seen (wedge vertebra, rotation).

  Nonstructural (functional) curve: Usually only slight, not progressive, and disappears completely with ipsilateral bending.

  Primary curve: Largest structural curve.

  Secondary curve: Lesser curve.

  Compensatory curve: Curve located above or below the main curve.

Imaging Signs

- **Modality of choice**

  Conventional radiographs.

  CT studies with coronal, sagittal, and possibly three-dimensional reconstructions may prove helpful in preoperative planning.

  Supplementary MRI studies may be obtained when bone and spinal cord pathology is suspected (coronal and sagittal T1-weighted and T2-weighted slices, and also axial T2-weighted slices at the level of the suspected pathology).

- **Radiographic findings**

  A-P view with the patient standing (from occiput to sacrum) to measure the severity of scoliosis • Lateral view with the patient standing to evaluate additional abnormal curves in the sagittal plane (required during initial examination as well as preoperatively and postoperatively) • Preoperative lateral bending views differentiate between structural and nonstructural curves • Cobb method of scoliosis measurement. The Cobb angle is determined as follows: Draw a line in the

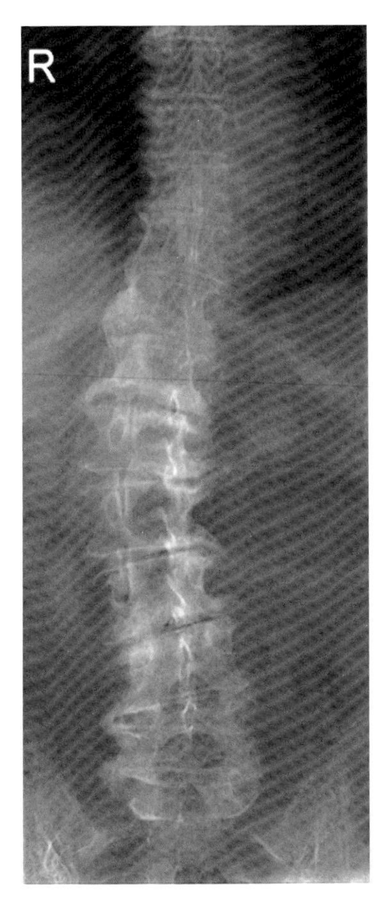

Fig. 1.28 A 61-year-old man with chronic lower back pain. Conventional A-P radiograph of the lumbar and lower thoracic spine: Severe multisegmental degenerative changes (narrowed disk interspaces, subchondral sclerosis, osteophytes) with right convex scoliosis.

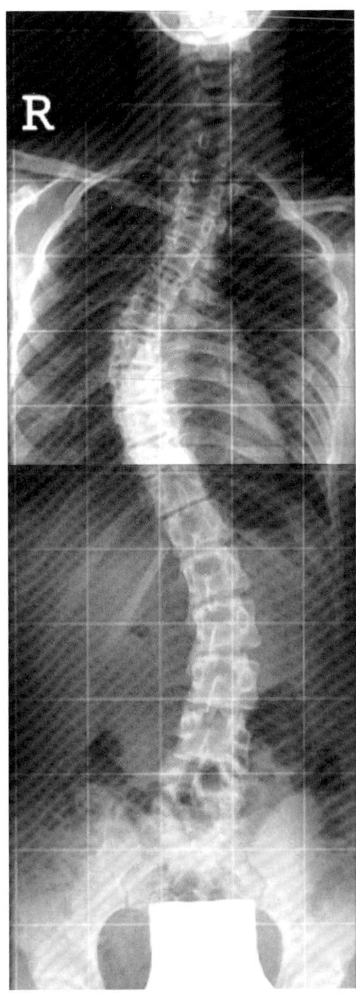

Fig. 1.29 A 16-year-old girl with S-shaped scoliosis. Conventional A-P radiograph obtained with patient standing (overlaid with grid).

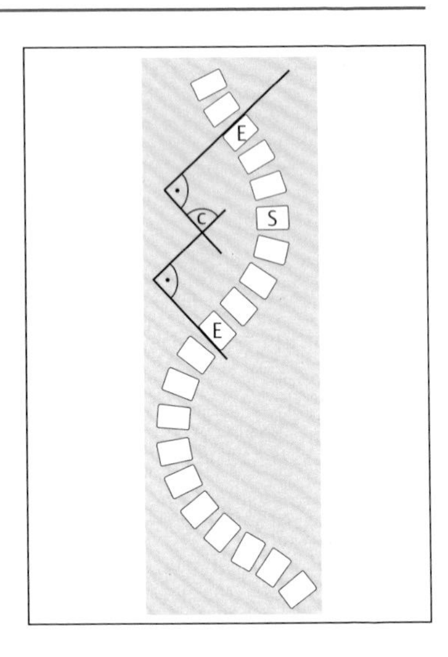

Fig. 1.30 Schematic diagram of coronal view of S-shaped scoliosis showing left and right scoliosis, the Cobb angle (c), end vertebrae (E), apical vertebra (S).

plane of the proximal endplate of the cranial end vertebra and perpendicular to its longitudinal axis, and another similar line in the plane of the distal endplate of the caudal end vertebra, and then measure the angle where these two lines intersect • Follow-up studies are usually indicated at intervals of about 4–6 months (be alert to the radiation dose).

- **CT findings**
  Demonstrates complex congenital bony anomalies • Can exclude tumors, infectious pathology, and postoperative complications.
- **MRI findings**
  To detect bone and spinal cord anomalies and exclude tumors and infectious pathology • Useful especially for atypical idiopathic scoliosis (left convex thoracic curve) and congenital scoliosis.

Clinical Aspects

- **Typical presentation**
  Idiopathic scoliosis is usually asymptomatic • Painful scoliosis usually involves an abnormality • Degenerative disk changes are common • The rare cases of severe scoliosis may involve instability, neurologic symptoms, and breathing problems.

▸ **Therapeutic options**
- For slightly abnormal curvature (< 25°): Physical therapy.
- For moderately abnormal curvature (25–50° in the thoracic spine or 25–40° in the lumbar spine): Corset and physical therapy.
- For severely abnormal curvature (> 50° in the thoracic spine or > 40° in the lumbar spine): Surgical management.

Differential Diagnosis

Idiopathic	– Most common form, classic S curve, progresses with growth
Neuropathic	– Paralytic scoliosis in polio, meningomyelocele, and secondary to trauma or tumor, etc.
Myopathic	– In muscular dystrophy
Congenital	– With vertebral malformations
Metabolic	– Rickets, osteoporosis
With tumor	– Painful curvature with short radius: MRI indicated
Degenerative	– In adults, degenerative changes in the disks and facet joints
Compensatory	– With leg length difference; see pelvis
Post spondylitis	– Painful curvature, usually with short radius
Congenital syndromes without vertebral malformations	– Neurofibromatosis, Ehlers–Danlos syndrome, Marfan syndrome, osteogenesis imperfecta
Scheuermann disease	– Usually slight scoliosis

Selected References

Cassar-Pullicino VN, Eisenstein SM. Imaging in Scoliosis: What, Why and How? Clinical Radiology 2002; 57: 543–562

Greenspan A. Skelettradiologie. München: Urban & Fischer 2002

Hedequist D, Emans J. Congenital scoliosis: a review and update. J Pediatr Orthop 2007; 27: 106–116

Definition

Usually malrotation involves several spinal segments with simultaneous lateral curvature to the contralateral side • Rarely there is rotation of a single vertebra, commonly associated with morphologic anomalies (especially asymmetry of the facet joints) • DD should consider diskogenic, arthrogenous, and reflexive causes.

Imaging Signs

- **Modality of choice**
  Conventional radiographs.
  MRI may be carried out to evaluate whether the rotation also involves spinal stenosis, or if there is nerve root compression or a diskogenic cause.
- **Radiographic findings**
  An A-P view is obtained to evaluate whether the rotation is multisegmental or involves only a single vertebra, and to determine the extent of vertebral rotation • Vertebral rotation can be measured by determining the position of the pedicles or spinous process relative to the imaginary midline of the vertebra or relative to the lateral contours of the vertebra • These methods of measurement are usually not suitable for determining whether rotation has increased.
  Signs of rotation: The rotated vertebra is tilted toward the contralateral side • The spinous process shifts toward the contralateral side • The contralateral pedicle may be projected outside the lateral margin of the vertebra whereas the ipsilateral pedicle is projected within the vertebra • The facet joint on the contralateral side is narrowed, and widened on the ipsilateral side • The facet joint spaces are projected on the vertebra to the side opposite the direction of rotation.
- **CT findings**
  The degree of rotation with respect to the adjacent vertebrae can be measured.
- **MRI findings**
  The width of the spinal canal, disk, and nerve roots can be measured.

Clinical Aspects

- **Typical presentation**
  May be asymptomatic or involve localized or radiating pain.
- **Therapeutic options**
  Depending on the cause and severity of symptoms, treatment is conservative or surgical (for example with severe scoliosis).

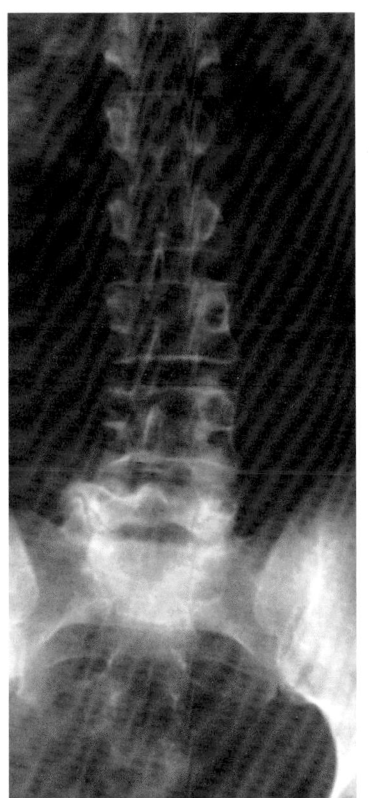

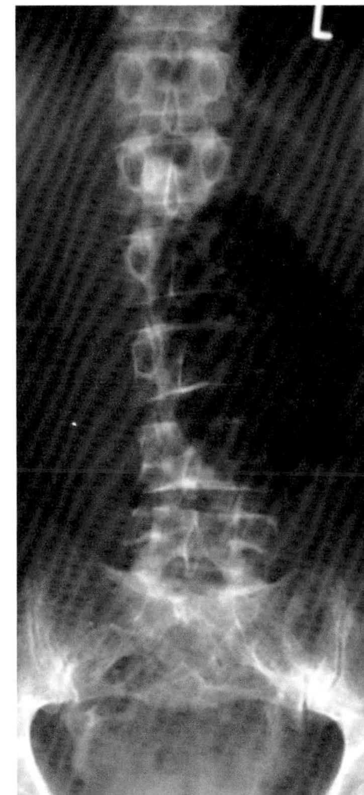

Fig. 1.31 A 39-year-old man with low back pain. Conventional A-P radiograph of the lumbar spine. Partial sacralization of the L5 vertebra with right pseudarthrosis. The spinous process of vertebra L4 (and to a lesser extent that of L3) is shifted slightly to the right. Findings suggest slight leftward rotation of vertebrae L3 and L4 due to partial fusion of a transitional vertebra.

Fig. 1.32 A 45-year-old man with low back pain. Conventional A-P radiograph of the lumbar spine. Slight left convex curve in the lumbar spine. The spinous processes of vertebrae L3, L4, and L5 are shifted slightly to the right. Findings suggest slight leftward rotation of vertebrae L3, L4, and L5 combined with slight left convex scoliosis.

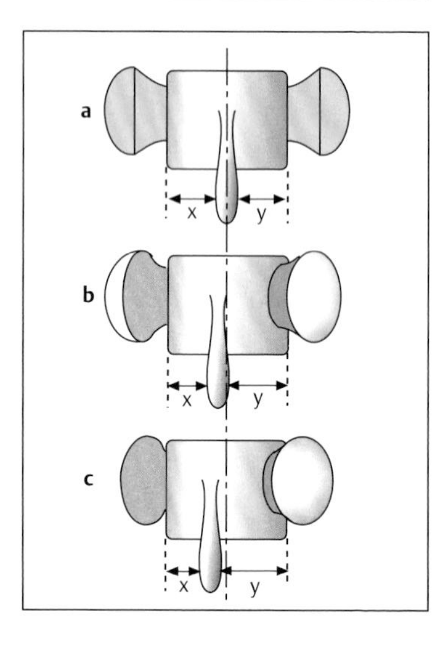

Fig. 1.33 a–c Schematic diagram of coronal view of vertebral rotation.
To evaluate rotation, note the distance between the spinous process and the lateral outer contour of the vertebral body. Where distance X equals distance Y, there is no rotation (**a**). Where distance X is not equal to distance Y, rotation is present (**b, c**).

Differential Diagnosis

Trauma	
Rotation with scoliosis	
Rotation with specific morphologic anomalies	– Facet joint asymmetry
Rotation with blockage due to diskogenic, arthrogenous, or reflexive causes	

Selected References

Gutmann G, Biedermann H. Funktionelle Pathologie und Klinik der Wirbelsäule. Stuttgart: Gustav Fischer 1992
Nash CL Jr, Moe JH. A study of vertebral rotation. J Bone Joint Surg Am 1969; 51: 223–229

General

The severity of the injury increases from type A to type C, as it does within the subdivisions of each specific type of fracture • Type A and type B injuries are often occur together • Today, the Magerl classification is preferred to the Denis three-column classification • The Magerl classification structure provides a more precise indication of the degree of instability/stability of the fracture than previous classifications • Only compression fractures without involvement of the posterior margin are definitively classified as stable • Involvement of the posterior margin is often poorly visualized on conventional plain films • Generous criteria should be applied when determining whether CT is indicated.

Type A

- **Mechanism**
  Compression.
- **Radiologic characteristics**
  Reduced height of vertebra • Fissured vertebra • Increased interpedicular distance • Intraspinal fragments.

Type B

- **Mechanism**
  Distraction.
- **Radiologic characteristics**
  Distance between spinous processes increased • Subluxation or dislocation of the facet joints • Abnormally high posterior vertebral margin • Transverse fractures • Fragments avulsed from the posterior corners of the vertebral body.

Type C

- **Mechanism**
  Rotation.
- **Radiologic characteristics**
  Vertebrae laterally displaced • Asymmetry of the pedicles • Spinous processes displaced • Fractures of the transverse processes • Unilateral subluxation, dislocation, and/or fracture of posterior parts of the vertebra • Unilateral rib fracture or dislocation.

Selected References

Magerl F, Aebi M, Gertzbein SD, Harms J, Nazarian S. A comprehensive classification of thoracic and lumbar injuries. Eur Spine J 1994; 3: 184–201

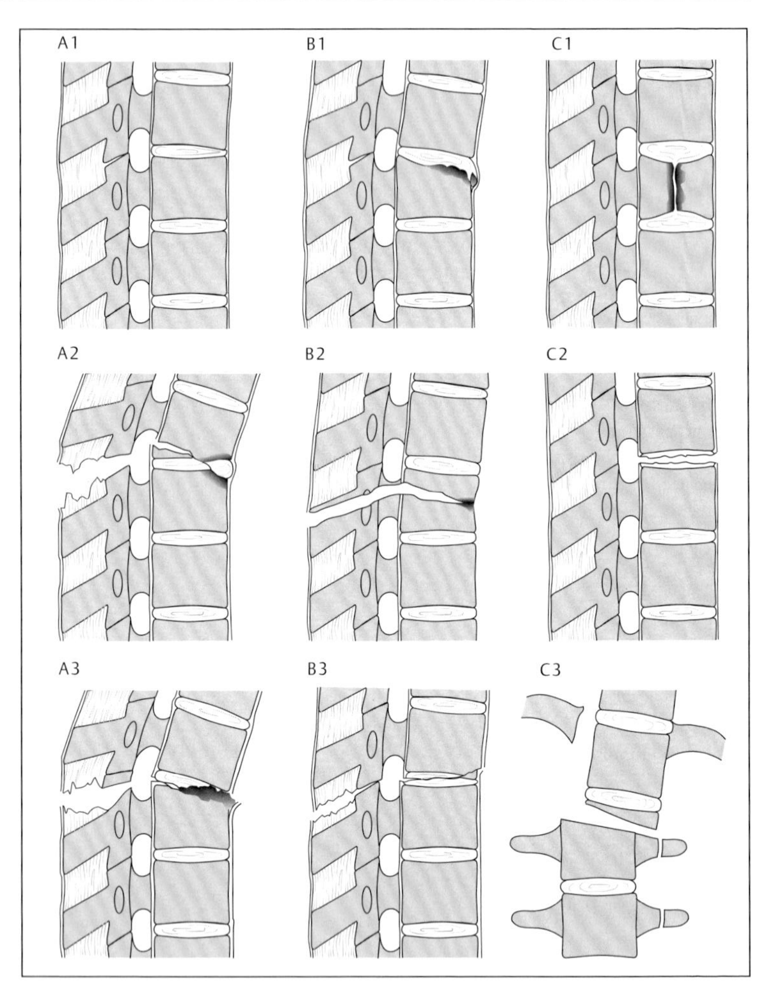

Fig. 2.1 to 2.3

Type A: A1—Impaction fractures, stable. A2—Cleavage fractures, usually stable. A3—Burst fractures, stability varies.

Type B: B1—Posterior ligament tear with disk involvement and associated type A injury. B2—Posterior bony ligament avulsion with fracture of the vertebral body or intervertebral disk or associated type A injury. B3—Torn intervertebral disk with subluxation or fracture of the articular processes, with spondylolysis or posterior dislocation. All type B injuries are unstable.

Type C: C1—Type A injury with rotation. C2—Type B injury with rotation. C3—Rotational shear fractures. All fractures in group C are highly unstable.

Definition

- **Epidemiology**
  The annual incidence of vertebral fractures in women over 70 years of age is 21%; after 80 years it is 50% • Women are affected twice as often as men.
- **Etiology, pathophysiology, pathogenesis**
  Symptoms range from circumscribed upper back pain to distal neurologic deficits.
  Traumatic: High-energy trauma produces a fracture in previously healthy bone.
  Osteoporotic: Slight trauma or everyday activity produces a fracture in weak, osteoporotic bone. Typical sites include the middle and lower thoracic or upper lumbar spine • Fishlike or wedge-shaped vertebrae • Vertebral collapse also occurs elsewhere in the spine • Intravertebral gas phenomenon • Findings include radiodense bands in the endplates (callus formation) • Osteopenic bone structure.
  Malignant: Even normal exercise or slight trauma causes a fracture of the vertebra, whose stability is compromised by a primary or secondary malignant process, such as metastasis or multiple myeloma.
  Pathologic fracture: Fracture from normally inadequate loading.
  Insufficiency fracture: Fracture with abnormal bone structure.

Imaging Signs—Osteoporotic Fracture

- **Modality of choice**
  Conventional A-P and lateral radiographs.
  MRI (DWI where indicated).
- **Radiographic findings**
  Typical sites include the middle and lower thoracic or upper lumbar spine • Fishlike or wedge-shaped vertebrae • Vertebral collapse also occurs elsewhere in the spine • Intravertebral gas phenomenon • Findings include radiodense bands in the endplates (callus formation) • Osteopenic bone structure.
- **MRI findings**
  Diffuse bone marrow edema in an acute fracture • Occasionally there is a halolike paravertebral soft tissue edema • Fluid sign • Gas phenomenon in the vertebral body or in the regions of the facet joints • Edematous changes recede and are increasingly converted to fatty marrow • Elevated diffusion coefficient.

Imaging Signs—Malignant Fracture

- **Modality of choice**
  Conventional A-P and lateral radiographs.
  MRI (DWI where indicated).
- **Radiographic findings**
  Inhomogeneous vertebral density is a sign of metastatic involvement • Vertebral arches are also affected • Atypical localization. (solitary fractures above T7 in particular are suspicious) • Often there is a unilateral reduction in height on the A-P film.

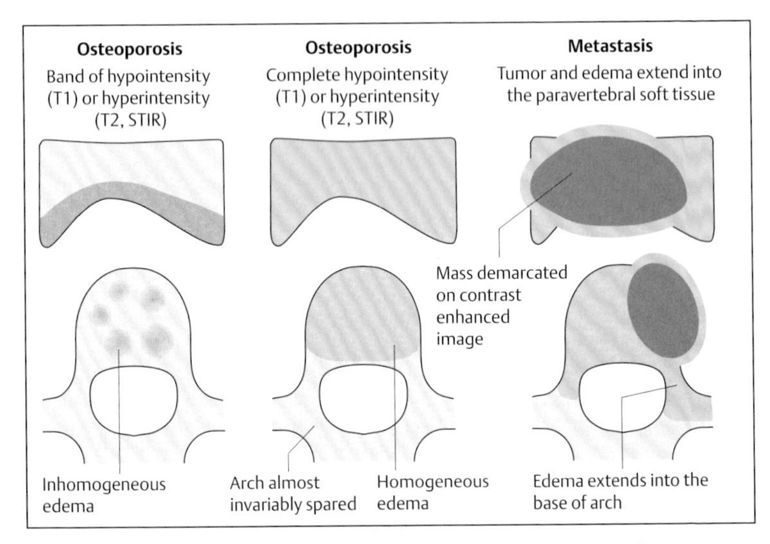

Fig. 2.4 Distinguishing osteoporotic vertebral fractures from metastatic fractures on MRI.

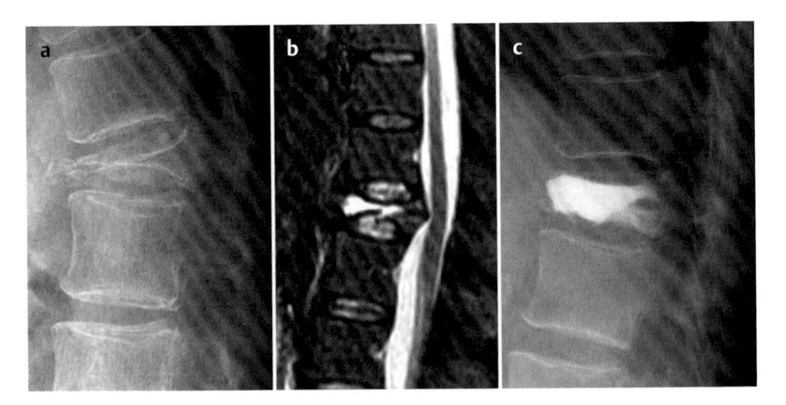

Fig. 2.5 a–c Conventional radiographs (**a**). Osteoporotic compression fracture with vertebral wedge deformity. MR image (sagittal, STIR) (**b**). Acute vertebral collapse with significant edema. Follow-up radiograph after kyphectomy (**c**).

▸ **CT findings**

Focal or epidural soft tissue mass.

▸ **MRI findings**

Solid enhancing mass extending past the margins of the vertebra • Compression of the vertebra pushes the tumor into the paravertebral soft tissue, creating a convex bulge in the posterior margin of the vertebra • The tumor is often distinguishable from the surrounding edema • Often asymmetric • Reduced diffusion coefficient.

Clinical Aspects

- **Typical presentation**
  Clinical symptoms are highly variable • Stable fractures can be asymptomatic • Osteoporotic fractures lead to increasing thoracic kyphosis.
- **Complications**
  Severe neurologic symptoms including paraplegia can occur, depending on the site of injury.
- **What does the clinician want to know?**
  Acute or chronic fracture? • Stable or unstable? • Osteoporotic or metastatic? • Which imaging modality should be used?
  Differentiating low-risk and high-risk-patients (Canadian nexus study):
  Radiologic examination is indicated in patients with:
  - Abnormal alertness.
  - Intoxication.
  - Neurologic deficit.
  - Bleeding in the brain.
  - Painful dorsal midline.
  - Distraction injury.
  - Multiple fractures continuation.

  Low-risk patients should fulfill all three low-risk criteria:
  - No high-risk factor (age > 50 years, high-risk trauma, paresthesia of extremities).
  - Presence of low-risk factors (minor car crash, sitting position, no pain in dorsal midline).
  - Active skull rotation > 45° is possible on both sides.

  High-risk patients are those who:
  - Have experienced high-energy trauma (velocity > 50 km/h; fall from a height of more than 3 m)
  - Are > 50 years of age.
  - Are unconsciousness.

  High-risk patients need a spiral CT exam!
- **Therapeutic options**
  Treatment depends on the neurologic symptoms and the severity of injury • Conservative therapy is indicated for stable fractures without neurologic symptoms • In all other cases, surgical management with appropriate stabilization of the spine is indicated • Alternatives include kyphectomy or vertebroplasty.

Selected References

Baur A., Dietrich O., Reiser M. Diffusion-weighted imaging of bone marrow: current status. Eur Radiol. 2003; 13: 1699–1708

Daffner RH. Radiologische Diagnostik der Wirbelsäule. Stuttgart: Thieme 2003

Definition

- **Epidemiology**

  Fractures of the dens account for 11–13% of all cervical spine injuries (in children up to 75%) • The most often diagnosed injury in the upper cervical spine.

- **Etiology, pathophysiology, pathogenesis**

  Caused by hyperextension, extreme flexion, or even lateral bending • Osteoporosis predisposes to type II fractures and subsequent nonunion of the fragments. Fracture types according to the Anderson and d'Alonzo classification:

  - Type I (8%): Oblique fracture through the superior tip of the dens with avulsion of the alar ligament—stable.
  - Type II (59%): Fracture at the base of the dens—unstable.
  - Type III (33%): The fracture extends into the axis body (actually a C2 fracture) and may be stable or unstable (horizontal fractures in the upper third are more stable than oblique fractures coursing anteriorly in the middle or lower third).

Imaging Signs

- **Modality of choice**

  Multislice spiral CT (where a dens fracture is suspected).
  MRI (where spinal cord or vascular injury is suspected).

- **Radiographic findings**

  Direct visualization of the fracture line • Demonstrates indirect signs such as displacement of the dens, especially posteriorly • Prevertebral soft tissue swelling is often the only sign of a dens fracture (relatively specific, not very sensitive).

- **CT findings**

  Axial multislice CT with thin slices (1 mm) • Reconstruction in a high-resolution bone window with sagittal and coronal slices • Fracture line • Degree of displacement.

- **MRI findings**

  T1-weighted (sagittal, coronal):

  - Visualization of the fracture and degree of displacement • Integrity of the ligaments (especially the alar ligaments).

  T1-weighted, STIR (sagittal):

  - Visualization of the bone marrow and soft tissue edema and/or injuries to the surrounding soft tissue • This distinguishes acute injury from chronic nonunion • MRI can also visualize pathology in the spinal cord (impinging edema, necrosis, bleeding, severed spinal cord) • Avulsion of the vertebral artery.

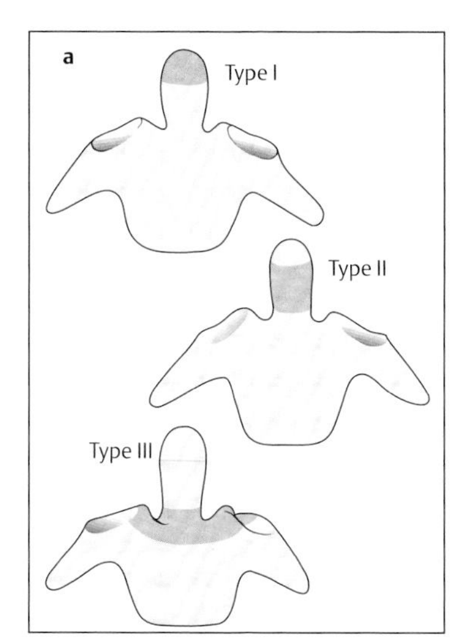

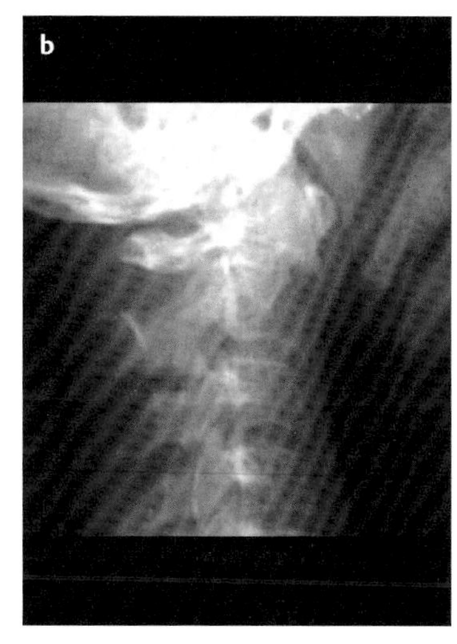

Fig. 2.6 a, b Dens fracture. Schematic diagram (**a**) of the Anderson and d'Alonzo classification: types I, II, and III. Conventional lateral radiograph (**b**). Dens fracture with severe anterior displacement.

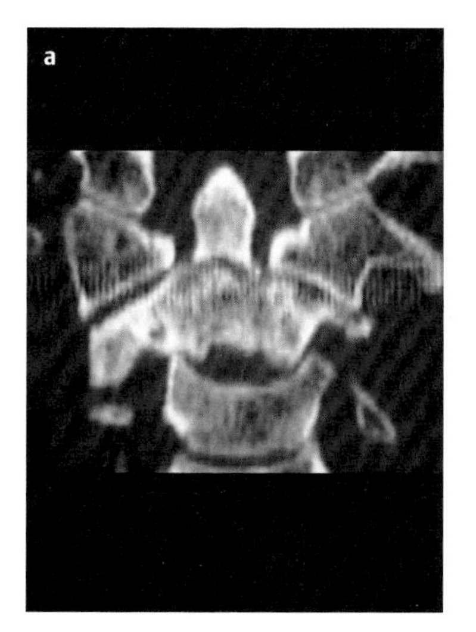

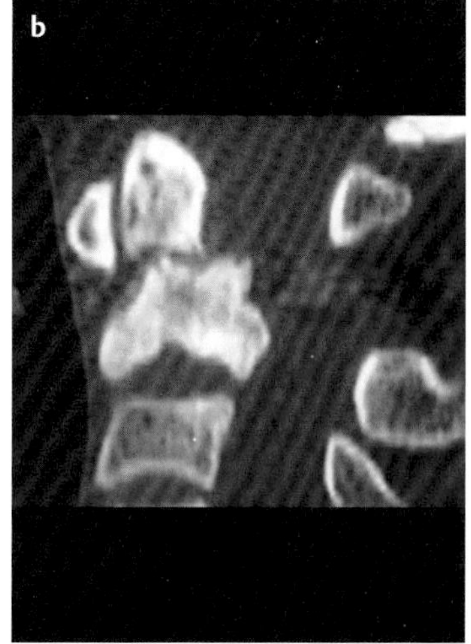

Fig. 2.7 a, b CT of C1–C2 (**a** coronal and **b** sagittal reconstructions): Displaced dens fracture (Anderson and d'Alonzo type II).

Clinical Aspects

▸ **Typical presentation**

Neck pain • Neurologic symptoms are rare • 41% of patients also have head, facial, or other injuries • Most patients cannot sit up from a supine position without using their hands.

▸ **Complications**

Compression of the vertebral artery with brainstem symptoms; very rarely spinal cord injuries from displaced comminuted fractures.

▸ **Therapeutic options**

- *Type I:* Four weeks of immobilization.
- *Type II:* Where the injury is unstable, primary fusion is indicated to avoid myelopathy.
- *Type III:* Stable injuries are immobilized with a halo brace and later a corset. Unstable injuries require surgical fixation.

Differential Diagnosis

Physiologic fusion at age 11–12	
Os odontoideum	– Failure of congenital fusion of the tip of the dens – No soft tissue swelling, typical round to oval configuration, smooth cortex – No history of trauma, absence of clinical signs
Subdural synostosis	– May persist until adolescence
Subluxation in rheumatoid arthritis	– Dens is destroyed by an arthritic process, leading to subluxation and possible instability – History
Pseudarthrosis secondary to chronic fracture	– Sclerotic halo

Selected References

Burke JT, Harris JH. Acute injuries of the axis vertebra. Skel Radiol 1989; 18: 335–446

Silberstein M, Hennessy O. Prevertebral swelling in cervical spine injury: identification of ligament injury with MRI. Clinical Radiology 1992; 46: 318–323

Definition

- **Epidemiology**
  Accounts for approximately 46% of cervical spine injuries.
- **Etiology, pathophysiology, pathogenesis**
  Results from maximum flexion of the cervical spine • Maximum extension of posterior vertebral elements and compression of anterior elements • Often associated with anterior disk herniation.
  The most important types of flexion fracture are:
  Anterior wedge fracture: Least severe form of flexion injury • Avulsion of a fragment from the anterior margin of the superior endplate with an intact posterior margin • Higher energy trauma will produce a wedge vertebra and may involve the posterior margin.
  Teardrop fracture: A triangular fragment resembling a teardrop is avulsed from the anteroinferior aspect of the vertebral body in flexion • This is usually combined with a tear in the posterior longitudinal ligament • Although the posterior margin is not affected, the injury is unstable • Often a cause of paraplegia • Occurs in the lower cervical spine (C5) in 70% of cases.
  Anterior subluxation or dislocation: Tearing of the posterior ligament complex or avulsion of the ligament from the vertebral body causes one vertebra within a segment to tilt anteriorly relative to the adjacent caudal vertebra • Stability depends on the severity of the angulation and translation.

Imaging Signs

- **Modality of choice**
  Multislice CT
  - Slice thickness in the cervical spine 1 mm to maximum 3 mm with sagittal reconstructions.
  - Where spinal cord injuries or injuries to the ligament complex are suspected.

  MRI.
- **Radiographic findings**
  Compression of the vertebral body • Disrupted alignment • Prevertebral soft tissue swelling (normal appearance of soft tissue does not exclude a fracture) • Avulsion of the anterior margin of the superior endplate in an anterior wedge fracture • Avulsion of the anterior margin of the inferior endplate in a teardrop fracture • In anterior subluxation or dislocation, one vertebral body is tilted anteriorly, opening a gap between the spinous processes and causing incomplete articulation of the facet joints. The subluxed vertebra may be displaced anteriorly.
- **CT findings**
  The signs seen on conventional radiographs are also visualized on CT, although with far greater sensitivity • Sagittal reformations are helpful.
- **MRI findings**
  T1-weighted, T2-weighted STIR: The fracture and degree of displacement are visualized • Integrity of the ligament complex can be evaluated • Spinal cord edema and/or bleeding are visualized.

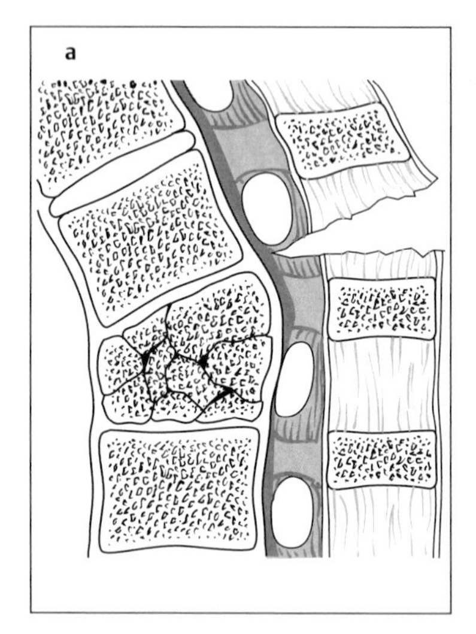

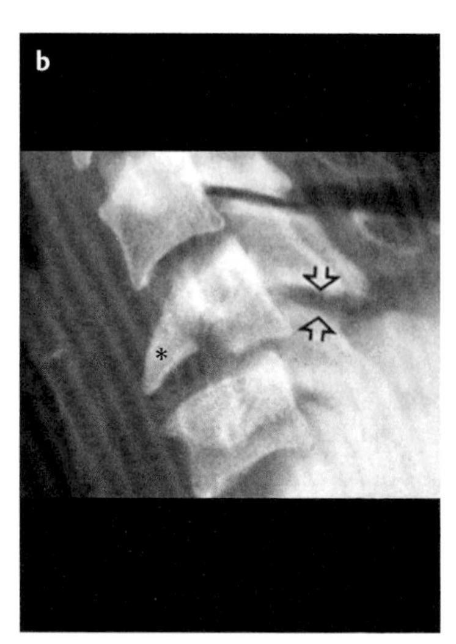

Fig. 2.8 a, b Schematic diagram (**a**). Anterior wedge fracture with rupture of the posterior longitudinal ligament, spinal canal stenosis, and spinal cord compression. Conventional lateral radiograph of the cervical spine (**b**). Teardrop fracture with widening of the facet joint space.

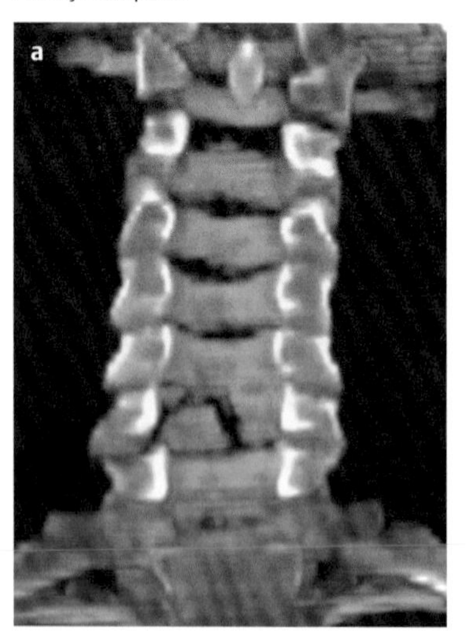

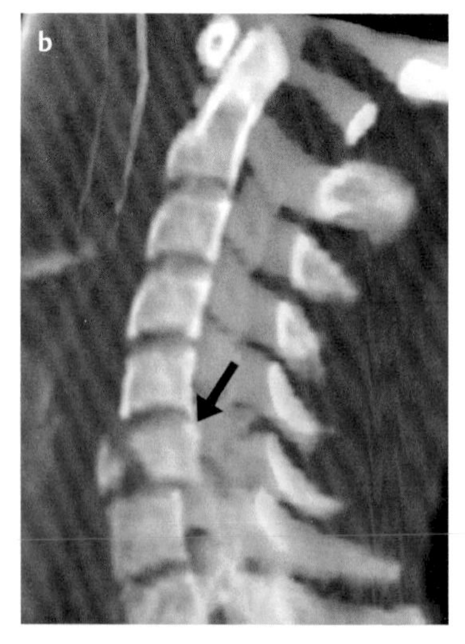

Fig. 2.9 a, b CT of the cervical spine (**a** coronal and **b** sagittal, volume-rendered). Teardrop fracture of C6 with posterior displacement of the vertebral body. To better visualize the injury, the respective slices anterior to the imaging plane have been cut away.

Clinical Aspects

- **Typical presentation**
  Trauma consistent with imaging findings • Severe neck pain • Neurologic symptoms may or may not be present.
- **Complications**
  Spinal cord injuries with distal neurologic symptoms.
- **Therapeutic options**
  Depends on the neurologic symptoms and degree of injury • Halo fixator is indicated in the absence of neurologic symptoms • Immediate decompression is indicated where neurologic symptoms and spinal cord compression are present.

Selected References

Burke JT, Harris JH. Acute injuries of the axis vertebra. Skel Radiol 1989; 18: 335–446

Galanski M, Wippermann B, Stamm G, Bazak N, Wafer A. Kompendium der traumatologischen Röntgendiagnostik. Berlin: Springer 1999

Definition

- **Epidemiology**
  Rare • Account for only 1.5 % of all spinal injuries.
- **Etiology, pathophysiology, pathogenesis**
  Caused by impaction with purely axial compression (as in a jump from a great height) • Localized largely in the thoracolumbar region, although such injuries may also occur in the lower thoracic spine • Neurologic symptoms occur where fragments are displaced into the spinal canal • Unstable when the posterior margin of the vertebra is also involved • Compression fracture.
  Fracture types:
  Incomplete burst fracture: Fracture involving primarily the anterior margin of the superior endplate and underlying portion of the vertebral body.
  Burst/fissure fracture: Invariably bisegmental, burst zones in the vertebral body are combined with fissure fractures of the other areas of the body.
  Complete burst fracture: Complete destruction of the entire vertebral body • Loss of axial load-bearing capability.

Imaging Signs

- **Modality of choice**
  Multislice CT: Primary modality in severe multiple trauma.
  In other cases, conventional radiographs in two planes will suffice.
  Where neurologic symptoms are present: Supplementary MRI.
- **Radiographic findings**
  Vertebral height is reduced • A vertical and/or horizontal fracture line may be directly visualized • Increased interpedicular distance • In the cervical spine, the traumatized segment may show slight extension or kyphosis on the lateral film • Partial or complete bulging of the posterior margin of the vertebra (often difficult to detect on a plain film).
- **CT findings**
  Axial multislice CT with thin slices (cervical spine: 1 mm; thoracic and lumbar spine: 3 mm) • Sagittal and coronal reconstructions in the soft tissue window and high-resolution window • Images show the same signs as conventional radiographs • The fracture line and the position of the posterior fragment relative to the spinal canal are better visualized • Bone fragments and epidural hematomas are visualized.
- **MRI findings**
  Sagittal and axial T1-weighted and T2-weighted STIR sequences • Indicated only where CT fails to demonstrate a correlate for neurologic symptoms • Signal intensity and height of vertebra are reduced on T1 images • Vertebra is hyperintense on the STIR sequence • Prevertebral hematoma • Blood in the spinal canal • Spinal cord contusion (edema and swelling).

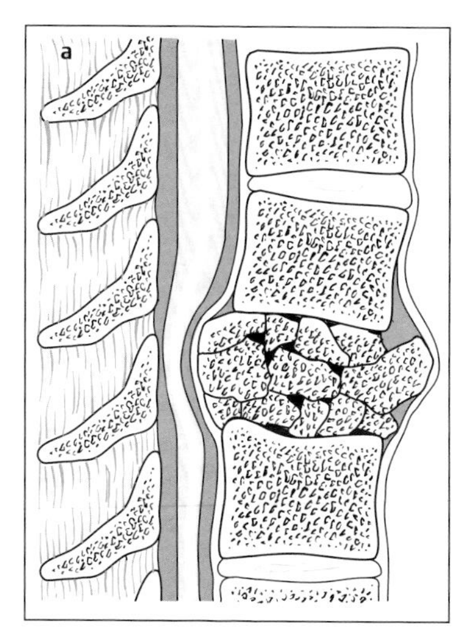

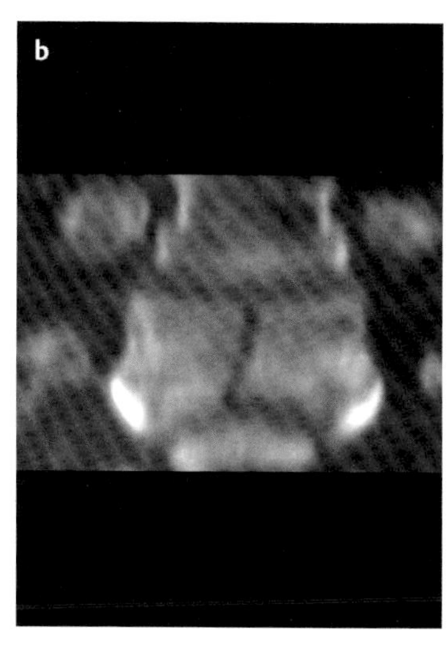

Fig. 2.10 a, b Schematic diagram of burst fracture (**a**). Conventional tomogram T12 (coronal; **b**). Vertical fracture line with bilateral lateral displacement. Impression fracture from the caudal vertebra.

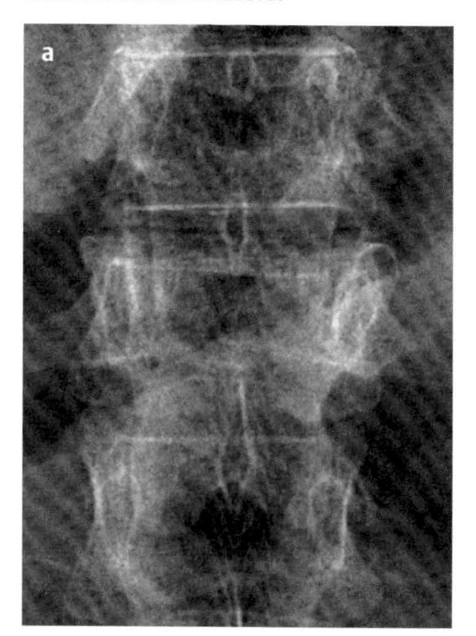

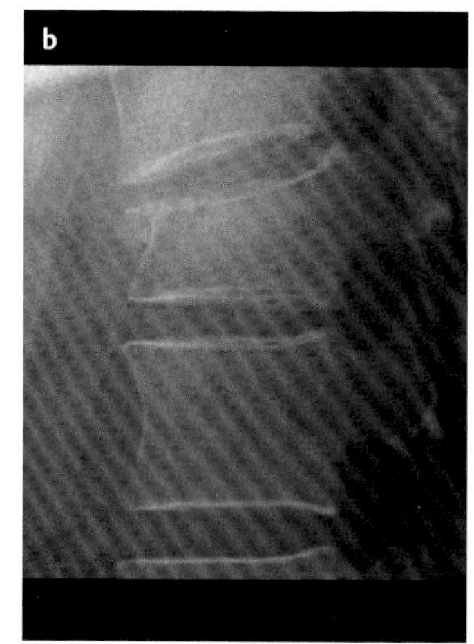

Fig. 2.11 a, b Conventional radiograph of the thoracolumbar junction (A-P, **a**). Complete burst fracture of vertebra L1. The height of the vertebral body is reduced and the interpedicular distance markedly widened. Conventional lateral radiograph (**b**). Significant reduction in anterior height with bulging of the posterior margin of the vertebra.

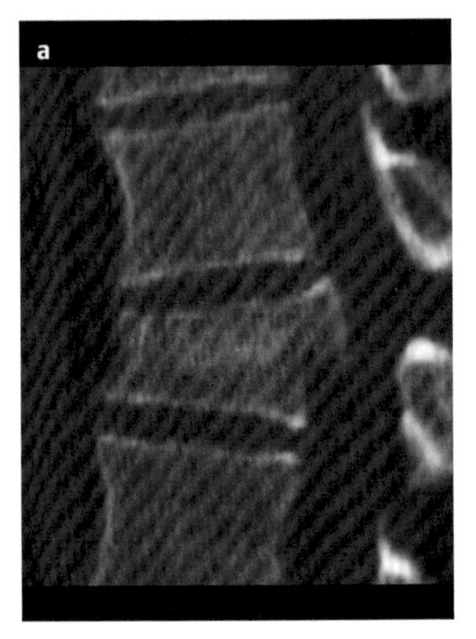

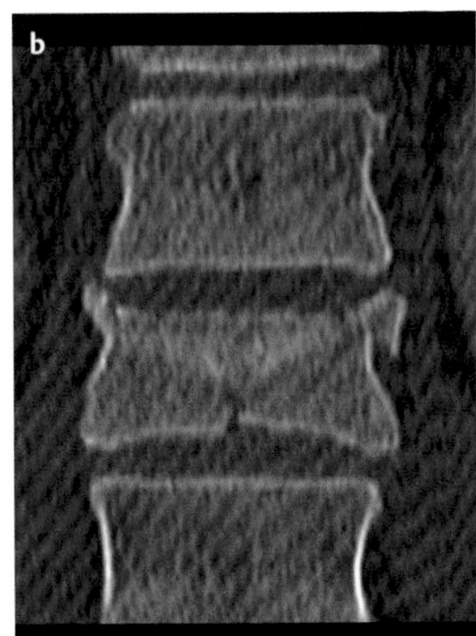

Fig. 2.12 a–c CT of T12 (sagittal reconstruction) (**a**). Complete burst fracture with compression of the dural sac. CT (**b** coronal and **c** axial). Fracture of the inferior endplate and marked spinal stenosis.

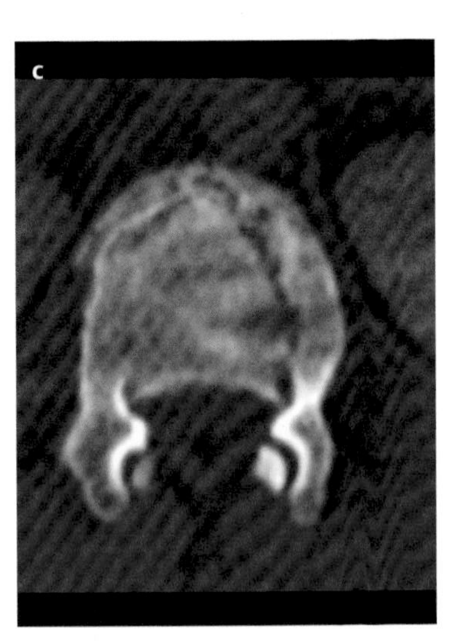

Clinical Aspects

- **Typical presentation**
  Highly variable depending on the severity of injury • History of trauma • Circumscribed back pain • Radiculopathy or myelopathy may be present.
- **Complications**
  Variable neurologic deficits including paraplegia.
- **What does the clinician want to know?**
  Relationship of vertebral fragments to spinal canal • Possible risks of secondary neurologic complications.
- **Therapeutic options**
  Conservative functional therapy for stable nondisplaced fractures • Surgical treatment for injuries with neurologic deficits, unstable injuries, and spinal fractures in ankylosing spondylitis • Direct screw fixation of fragments • Spinal fusion.

Selected References

Galanski M, Wippermann B, Stamm G, Bazak N, Wafer A. Kompendium der traumatologischen Röntgendiagnostik. Berlin: Springer 1999

Kinzl L, Arand M, Fleischmann W. Trauma der Wirbelsäule. In Kinzl L. Traumatologie, 2nd ed. Munich: Urban und Schwarzenberg 1993

Lomoschitz F. Bildgebung bei Wirbelsäulenverletzungen – Diagnostic Imaging. Wien Med Wochenschr 2001; 151: 502–505

Definition

- **Epidemiology**
  Less common than burst or compression fractures.
- **Etiology, pathophysiology, pathogenesis**
  Horizontal vertebral fracture and/or horizontal soft tissue laceration, especially at the thoracolumbar junction (T11–L3).
  Classic mechanism of injury (based on the Denis classification): Compression of the anterior column (anterior third of the vertebral body and anterior longitudinal ligament) and distraction of the middle column (posterior third of the vertebral body and posterior longitudinal ligament) and posterior column (vertebral arches, facet joints, spinous process, and transverse process) as a result of anterior hyperflexion over the lap belt in a car, which acts as a fulcrum.

Imaging Signs

- **Modality of choice**
  CT with sagittal and coronal reconstructions • Most reliable method of preoperative diagnosis and of differentiating a Chance fracture from a burst or compression fracture.
- **General**
  The distance between the spinous processes is increased or the spinous processes are fractured at the level of the main fracture • Often the fractured vertebra exhibits wedge deformation with a reduction in anterior height and secondary focal kyphosis.
- **Radiographic findings**
  Usually the initial imaging study. Radiographs in at least two planes should be obtained. Supplementary stress radiographs or oblique views are obtained where indicated.
- **CT findings**
  For better evaluating the extent of the fracture, especially in the posterior column.
- **MRI findings**
  For detecting discrete fractures (vertebral body edema and discrete fracture line) • For detecting ruptures of the longitudinal ligaments (the posterior longitudinal ligament in particular is often affected) and the interspinous ligaments • For detecting spinal cord contusions.

Clinical Aspects

- **Typical presentation**
  Low back pain secondary to high-speed trauma.
- **Therapeutic options**
  Surgical treatment is usually indicated.

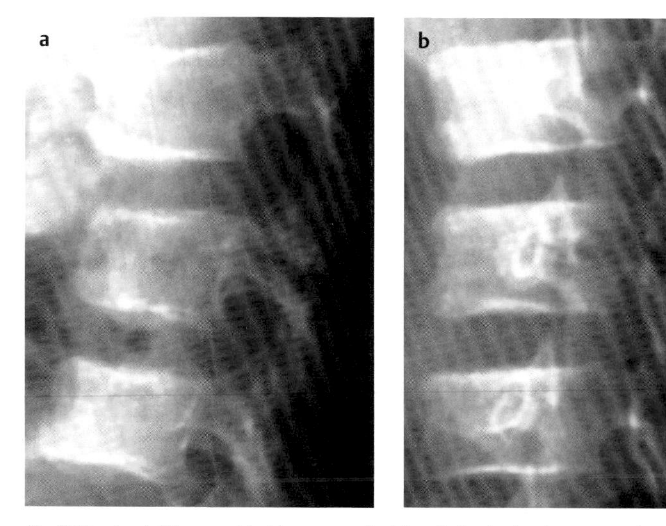

Fig. 2.13 a, b A 10-year-old girl presented with pain in the lumbar spine after a traffic accident 2 days previously. Conventional radiographs of the lumbar spine (**a** lateral, **b** oblique). Radiolucent line coursing horizontally through the spinous process, lamina, and posterior body of the third lumbar vertebra. The line narrows from posterior to anterior: Chance fracture of L3.

Differential Diagnosis

Compression fracture	– Results from axial forces with or without flexion; posttraumatic, osteoporotic, or tumor related
Burst fracture	– Results from axial forces; vertical fracture, normal distance between spinous processes
Shear fracture	– Results from transverse forces; all three columns are discontinuous, olisthesis
Distraction injury	– Results from vertical distraction or hyperextension; all three columns are discontinuous, distraction and/or olisthesis

Selected References

Ross JS, Brant-Zawadzki M, Moore KR. Diagnostic Imaging Spine. Salt Lake City: Amirsys 2004

Definition

▸ **Epidemiology**
C1 fractures: Account for approximately 6% of all spinal fractures.

▸ **Etiology, pathophysiology, pathogenesis**
Abnormal pressure of the occipital condyles on the atlas with the head extended • Compression fracture • Often occurs in combination with avulsion of the transverse ligament of the atlas • Unstable • Burst fracture of the atlas.
Classification of fractures of the atlas:
Type 1: Fracture of the anterior arch of the atlas • Extension fracture • Usually stable • Often combined with a dens fracture.
Type 2: Fracture of the posterior arch of the atlas • Typical extension fracture • The posterior arch of the atlas is compressed between the occiput and C2 and fractures • Stable fracture.
Type 3: Jefferson fracture • Fracture of the anterior and posterior arches of the atlas.

Imaging Signs

▸ **Modality of choice**
- Multislice CT: Primary modality in multiple trauma or where there is a strong suspicion of a fracture • Conventional radiographs of the cervical spine.
- MRI: Primary modality when ligament instability is suspected.
- Multislice CT is indicated where conventional radiographs are equivocal or suggest displacement of the lateral masses.

▸ **Radiographic findings**
The fracture lines are directly visualized • Displacement of the lateral masses of the atlas • Offset in the lateral atlantoaxial joints • The lateral film may show anterior soft tissue swelling.

▸ **CT findings**
Multislice CT with slice thickness of 1–2 mm • Bone and soft tissue windows • Precisely demonstrates fracture, exact location of injury, and signs of complications.

▸ **MRI findings**
Axial and coronal T1- and T2-weighted STIR sequences • Visualization of acute edema • Visualization of ligament injuries.

Clinical Aspects

▸ **Typical presentation**
Pain in the upper cervical spine.

▸ **Complications**
Simultaneous injuries to other cervical vertebrae are common • Ligament instability • Usually heals without complications • Recurrent displacement with widening of the C1 ring and posttraumatic degenerative joint disease can occasionally occur with purely conservative therapy.

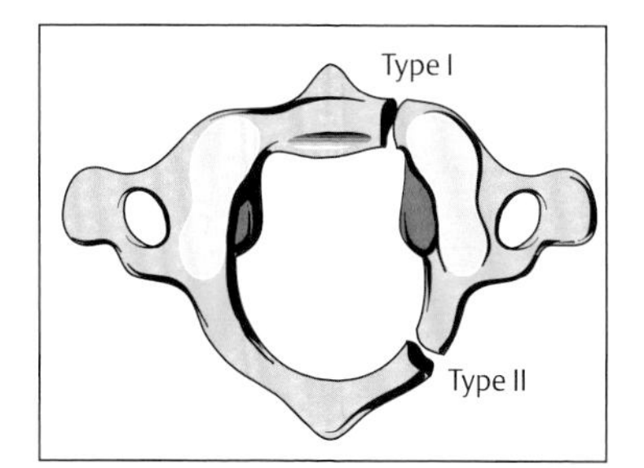

Fig. 2.14 Schematic diagram of atlas fractures.

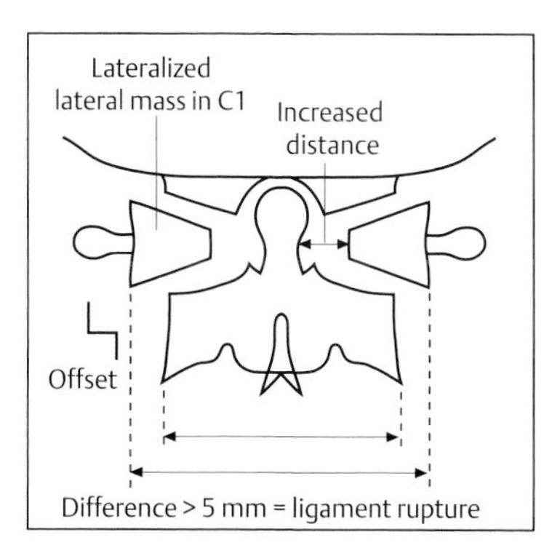

Fig. 2.15 Schematic diagram of radiographic signs in atlas fractures.

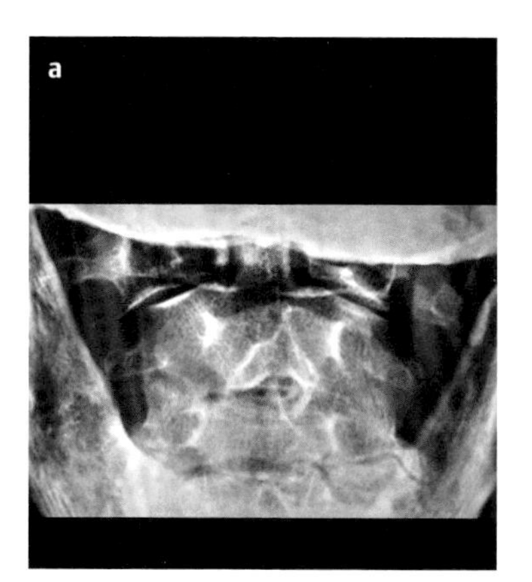

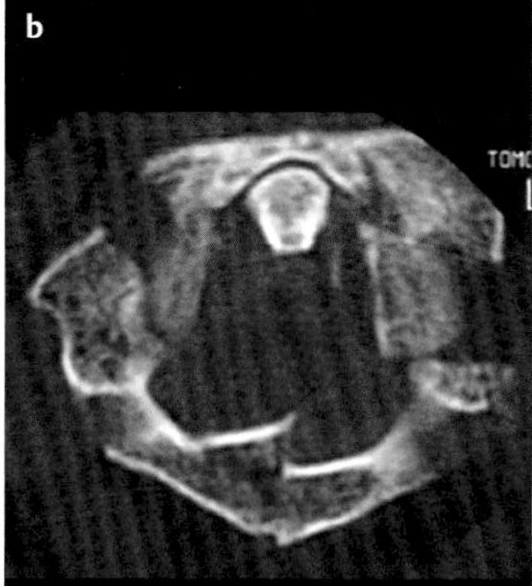

Fig. 2.16 a, b Conventional A-P radiograph (**a**). Severe cervical spine trauma, offset sign. Laterally displaced lateral masses. CT of C1–C2 (axial; **b**), Type 3 Jefferson fracture.

- **What does the clinician want to know?**
  Is the injury stable or unstable? • Are other vertebrae involved?
- **Therapeutic options**
  Types 1 and 2: Stable fractures • Immobilization in a neck collar for 4–6 weeks.
  Type 3: Usually immobilization with a halo brace for 10 weeks • Open reduction and internal fixation with plate and screws through an anterior or posterior approach may be indicated.

Differential Diagnosis

Apparent spreading apart of the lateral masses	– Findings are easily confused in children up to 4 years of age – Jefferson fractures are rare in children
Congenital variants	– Failure of fusion of the vertebral arch or other normal variants or anomalies – Pseudo "fracture lines" are less sharply defined and/or sclerotic

Selected References

Galanski M, Wippermann B, Stamm G, Bazak N, Wafer A. Kompendium der traumatologischen Röntgendiagnostik. Berlin: Springer 1999

Scharen S, Jeanneret B. Atlas fractures. Orthopäde. 1999; 28: 385–393

Definition

- **Epidemiology**
  Second most common injury to the cervical spine after the dens fracture (approximately 7% of injuries).
- **Etiology, pathophysiology, pathogenesis**
  Nowadays usually caused by head-on vehicle collision in which the forehead strikes the dashboard or steering wheel, and is immediately followed by extreme extension of the upper cervical spine (deceleration trauma) • Extreme extension alone results from a rear-end collision with the vehicle behind, and without a headrest • A high bending moment acts on the weak connections of the neural arch of the axis • Traumatic spondylolisthesis of C2 • Isthmus fracture • Pedicle fracture.
  Effendi classification:
  - Type 1: Bilateral nondisplaced arch fractures (potentially unstable).
  - Type 2: Diastasis in the arch with angulation between C2 and C3 > 10° (unstable).
  - Type 3: Distance between C2 and C3 exceeding 3.5 mm (unstable, complete disk tear and complete tears of the anterior and posterior longitudinal ligaments).

Imaging Signs

- **Modality of choice**
  - Spiral CT: Primary modality in multiple trauma or when there is strong clinical suspicion of a fracture • Conventional radiographs of the cervical spine.
  - MRI: Primary modality when ligament instability is suspected.
  - Spiral CT is indicated where conventional radiographs are equivocal.
- **Radiographic findings**
  The fracture plane courses obliquely from anteroinferior to posterosuperior • This makes nondisplaced fractures difficult to detect • Avulsed fragments from the anteroinferior margin of C2 or the anterosuperior margin of C3 indicate a tear in the anterior longitudinal ligament • Anterior slippage of C2 is a sign of instability from rupture of the fibrous connections between disk and ligament • "Fat C2 sign" (the inferior endplate of C2 appears elongated along the superior endplate of C3, an illusion created by a vertebral fragment remaining in situ as the rest of C2 displaces).
- **CT findings**
  Multislice CT with slice thickness of 1–2 mm • Bone and soft tissue windows • Multiplanar reconstructions • Fractures are readily demonstrated, as is any displacement, which is a sign of rupture of the fibrous connections between disk and ligament • Soft tissue swelling anterior to C2.
- **MRI findings**
  T1- and T2-weighted STIR sagittal, axial, and coronal where indicated • Useful mainly for visualizing ligament injuries • Edema sign on the STIR T2 sequences • The T1 sequence may show the fracture.

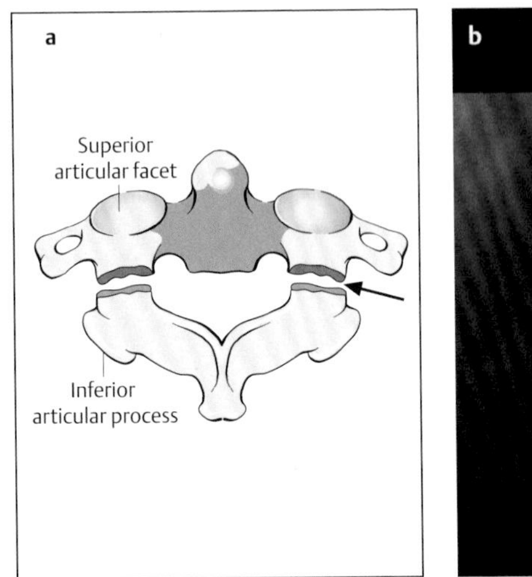

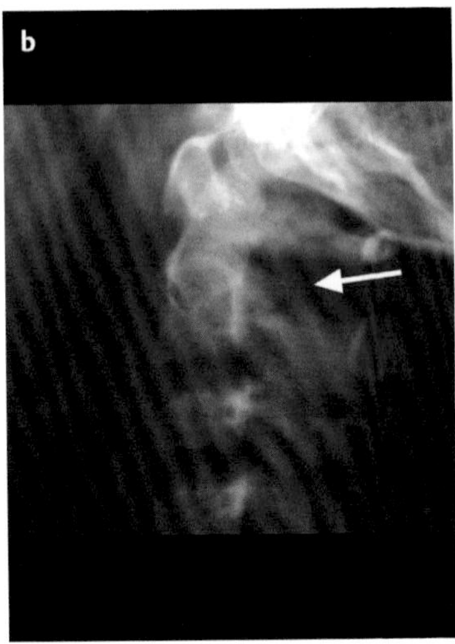

Fig. 2.17 a, b Schematic diagram of hangman's fracture (**a**). Conventional lateral radiograph (**b**). Type I C2 fracture in a 7-year-old girl.

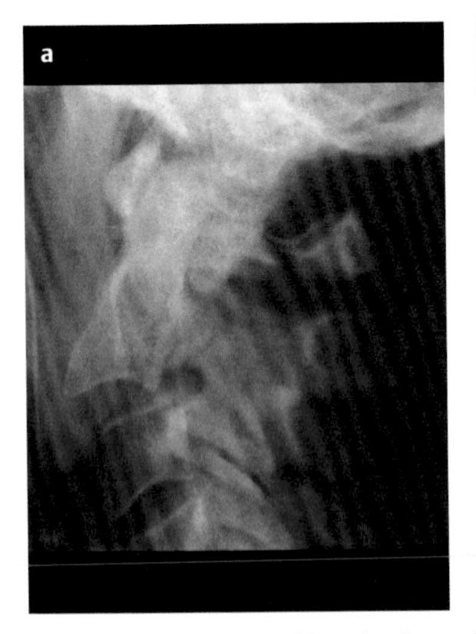

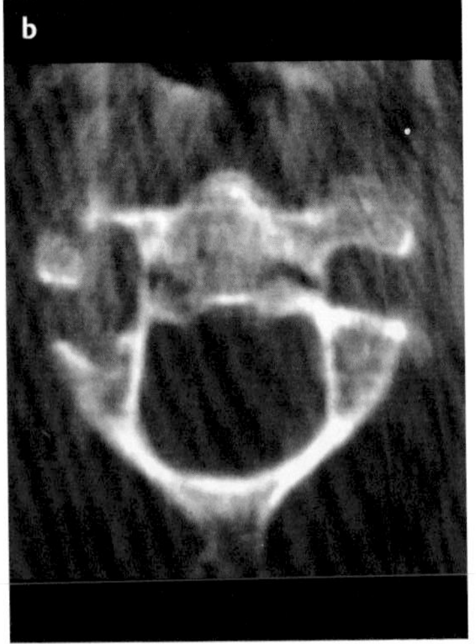

Fig. 2.18 a, b Conventional lateral radiograph (**a**). Type III hangman's fracture. C2 is anteriorly displaced and the C2–C3 interspace is widened anteriorly. The C2 pedicles are fractured. Posterior alignment is disrupted. The arch of the atlas is also fractured.
CT of C2 (axial, **b**). Hangman's fracture.

Clinical Aspects

- **Typical presentation**

  Appropriate history findings • Pain in the upper cervical spine region • Neurologic symptoms are rare (maximum of 25% of all cases) because the spinal canal is relatively wide in this region.
- **Complications**

  Simultaneous injury to C1 or injury to the vertebral artery • Undetected instability with late neurologic symptoms • Symptoms depend on neurologic damage • Secondary joint degeneration may occur.
- **What does the clinician want to know?**

  Is the injury stable or unstable?
- **Therapeutic options**

  Type 1: Six weeks of immobilization in a neck collar.

  Type 2: Selected cases may be immobilized for six weeks in a halo brace, otherwise direct Judet screw fixation of the arch of the axis is indicated.

  Type 3: Anterior (or anteroposterior) fusion of C2–C3 with an interposed bone graft and plate fixation.

Differential Diagnosis

Pseudosubluxation	– Approximately 20% of all children up to 8 years of age show physiologic anterior slippage of C2 or even C3 – Alignment of the spinous processes and laminae is preserved – No soft tissue swelling

Selected References

Effendi B, Roy D, Cornish B, Dussault RG, Laurin CA. Fractures of the ring of the axis. J Bone Joint Surg 1981; 63 B: 319–327

Galanski M, Wippermann B, Stamm G, Bazak N, Wafer A. Kompendium der traumatologischen Röntgendiagnostik. Berlin: Springer 1999

Samaha C et al. Hangman's fracture: the relationship between asymmetry and instability. J Bone Joint Surg [Br] 2000; 82: 1046–1052

Definition

- **Epidemiology**
  Damage to the spinal cord occurs in 10–30% of spinal injuries • In cervical spine trauma, purely soft tissue injuries without bony involvement predominate • Frequency of cervical spine injuries increases from cranial to caudal.
- **Etiology, pathophysiology, pathogenesis**
  Most cervical spine injuries involve ligament injuries and not bone or spinal cord. They lead to a posttraumatic reflex sympathetic dystrophy syndrome • Primary spinal cord injuries are directly related to the trauma • Secondary damage results from edema, circulatory disturbances, or late-onset hemorrhage • Spinal shock is seen relatively often in young athletes • Spinal shock results from a reversible complete loss of conduction with characteristic symptoms • No synonyms.
  Classification:
  - *Spinal shock = spinal concussion = neurapraxia:* Temporary, fully reversible loss of function in the spinal cord that may include complete cervical cord syndrome or anterior or posterior cord syndrome with characteristic symptoms, depending on the site of injury.
  - *Spinal contusion:* Transient compression of the spinal cord.
  - *Spinal cord compression:* Persistent impingement.

Imaging Signs

- **Modality of choice**
  MRI should be the primary study when a spinal cord injury is suspected (*Caution:* Clinical and imaging signs may appear several days after trauma!).
- **Radiographic findings**
  Not significant.
- **CT findings**
  Spiral CT of the cervical spine with maximum slice thickness of 2 mm • Reconstruction in sagittal and axial planes • Demonstrates directly bony injuries to the cervical spine and the possible cause of spinal cord damage • May demonstrate disk displacement.
- **MRI findings**
  Sagittal T1-, T2-weighted, STIR sequences • Axial T2 sequence in the affected segments • Precisely localization and visualization of spinal cord damage (edema, hemorrhage, disk displacement) • Demonstrates ligament injuries (edema sign on STIR an T1-weighted images) • In spinal shock, the spinal cord will occasionally appear slightly swollen and slightly hyperintense over a short distance • In a contusion, findings include a swollen, clearly edematous spinal cord (hyperintense on STIR images).

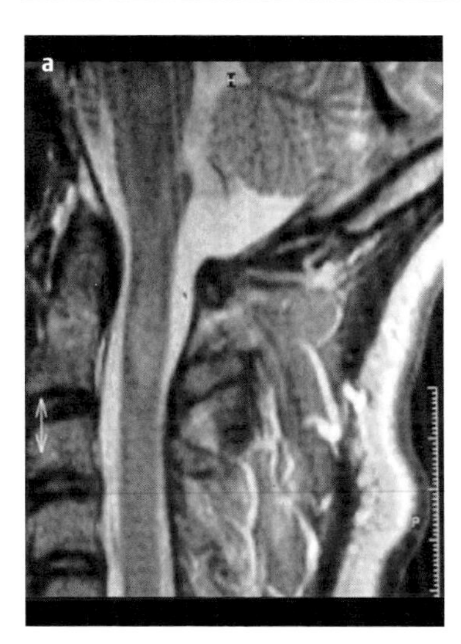

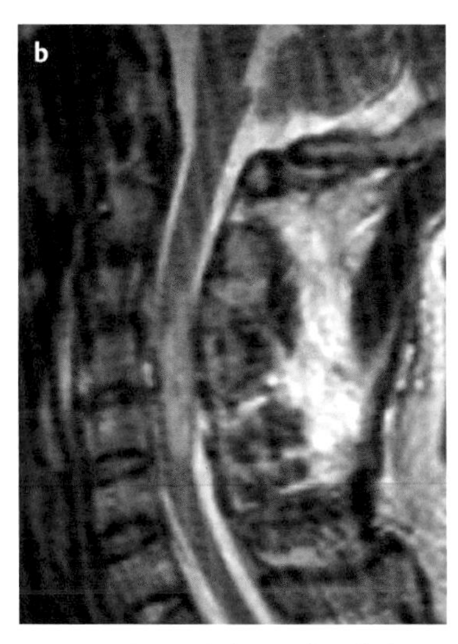

Fig. 2.19 a, b MR images of the cervical spine (**a**) (sagittal, T2). Slight spinal cord edema. Marked hyperintense signal alteration at the base of the dens. Type II dens fracture (**b**) (sagittal, T2). Hyperintense focal contusion in the spinal cord. Rupture of the anterior and posterior longitudinal ligaments.

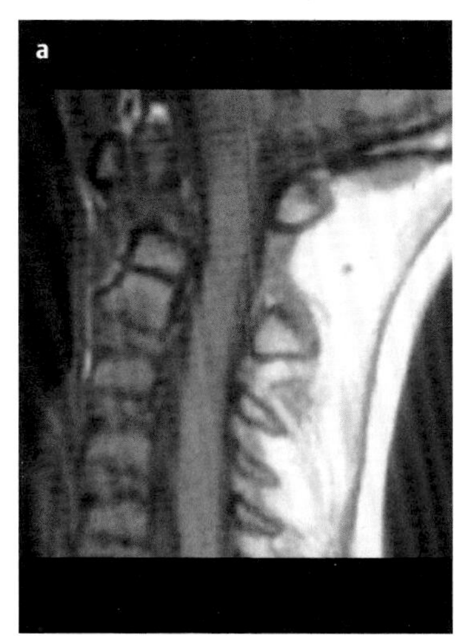

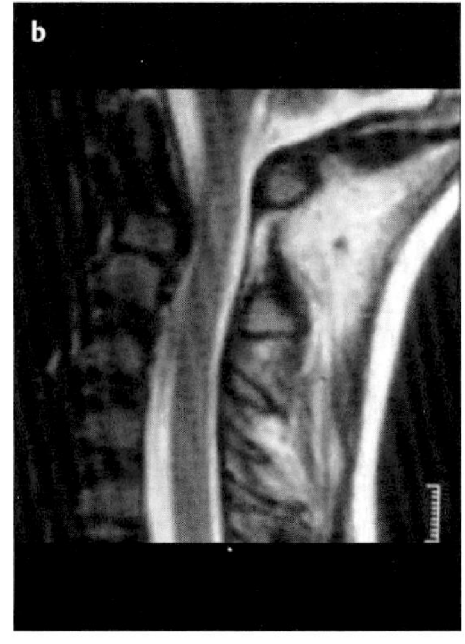

Fig. 2.20 a, b MR images of the cervical spine (**a**) (sagittal, T1). No bony destruction. Incidental findings include an os odontoideum (**b**) (sagittal, T2). Minimally hyperintense signal alteration in the spinal cord at the level of C1 consistent with a spinal cord contusion.

Clinical Aspects

- **Typical presentation**
  Variable • Sudden paralysis or paresis with variable sensory deficits • In many cases late onset of clinical symptoms (days after trauma) • Bladder dysfunction • Anterior cord syndrome involves flaccid paresis of the upper extremity • Posterior cord syndrome involves pain, hyperesthesia, and paresis in the arms and hands.
- **Complications**
  Loss of central regulation • Respiratory insufficiency • Paralytic ileus • Bladder atony • Permanent neurologic damage.
- **Therapeutic options**
  Stabilization of unstable injuries • Decompression of any focal stenosis • High-dose steroid therapy.
- **Prognosis**
  Spinal shock is completely reversible within 72 hours • Prognosis of spinal shock and compression is highly variable and depends on many factors • Late sequelae must be expected wherever symptoms fail to improve within four weeks.

Differential Diagnosis

Severed spinal cord	– Clinical and imaging findings
Spinal cord hemorrhage	– MRI can detect blood and its breakdown products, but only 24–36 hours after injury at the earliest! DWI may help

Selected References

Jörg, J, Menger H. Das Halswirbelsäulen- und Halsmarktrauma. Deutsches Ärzteblatt 1998; 21: 1307–1314

Definition

Intramedullary accumulation of cerebrospinal fluid resulting from dilation of the central canal (hydromyelia) or paracentral cavitation (syringomyelia); these conditions are often simultaneously present and indistinguishable • *Syringobulbia:* Spread into the medulla oblongata.

Communicating syringomyelia: Occurs in 14% of cases • Involvement of the fourth ventricle, associated with hydrocephalus.

- Congenital malformations: Chiari I malformation, encephalocele, Dandy-Walker syndrome, cysts.
- Meningitis.
- Intraspinal hemorrhage.

Noncommunicating syringomyelia: 65% ofcases • No communication with the fourth ventricle.

- Chiari I malformation.
- Spinal arachnoiditis.
- Tethered cord.
- Cystic degenerative tumors (ependymomas, astrocytomas).
- Atrophic syringomyelia (ex vacuo syringomyelia).
- Loss of parenchyma from spinal trauma or infarction.
- Equally common in both sexes • Peak age: 20–40 years.

Imaging Signs

- **Modality of choice**
  MRI.
- **Radiographic findings**
  Associated bony malformations of the spine: Atlantooccipital fusion, spina bifida, Klippel-Feil deformity • *Secondary bony changes:* Scoliosis, dilation of the spinal canal, degeneration, and/or destruction of the facet joints.
- **CT findings**
  Detailed visualization of bony changes • *CT myelography:* Where MRI is contraindicated • Widening of the spinal cord • Syrinx fills on late images.
- **MRI findings**
  General:
  - Sagittal and axial T1- and T2-weighted images.
  - CSF flow study (at the respective level or in the other CSF spaces).
  - Contrast studies are indicated in uncertain cases to exclude tumor.
  - *Complete spinal cord examination:* From the cervical spine including the foramen magnum (to exclude a Chiari malformation) to the lumbar spine.
  - Supplementary cerebral MRI to exclude a cerebral malformation.

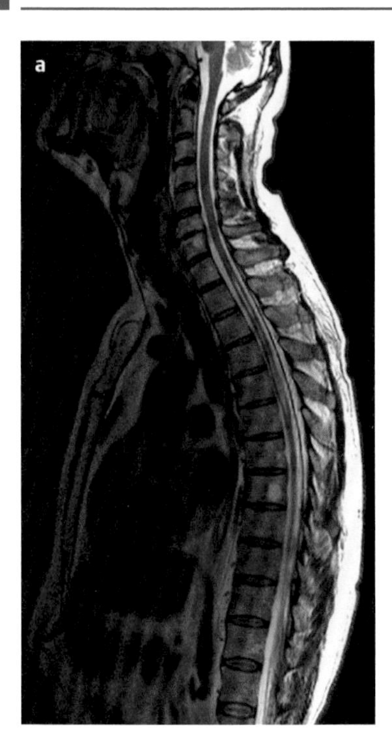

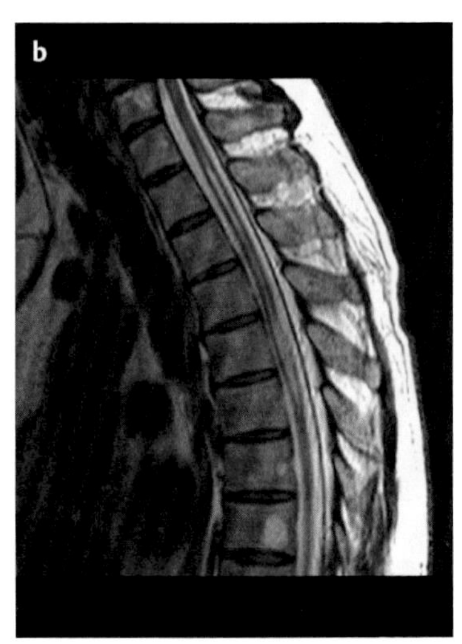

Fig. 2.21 a, b Spasticity, more pronounced on the left side, beginning several years after previous spinal trauma. MR image of cervicothoracic region (sagittal, T2). Intramedullary cavitation from T2 to T6, widest at T5 (detail, **b**).

T1:
Tubular to lobulated focal signal alteration in spinal cord, usually isointense to CSF, possibly partially septate.
- Signal is occasionally hyperintense to CSF due to increased protein content • Spinal cord may be distended.

T2:
- Focal signal alteration in the spinal cord, usually isointense to CSF.
- The pulsatile motion of the syrinx fluid produces flow voids, a finding of prognostic importance as these lesions usually respond well to creation of a shunt.

Clinical Aspects

▸ **Typical presentation**

Dissociated sensory deficits (often loss of sensitivity to pain and temperature) • Radicular pain • Weakness in the extremities, sensation of stiffness in the legs • Muscle atrophy in the upper extremities • Neurogenic arthropathy, progressive scoliosis • Brainstem symptoms where the lesion extends into the hindbrain.

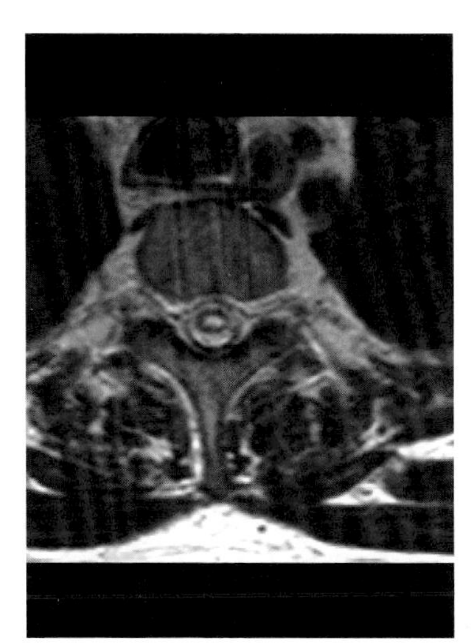

Fig. 2.22 MR image of T5 (axial, T2). Eccentric cavitation on the left side at the level of T5. A fine linear structure extends from the spinal cord to the dura: posttraumatic tethering.

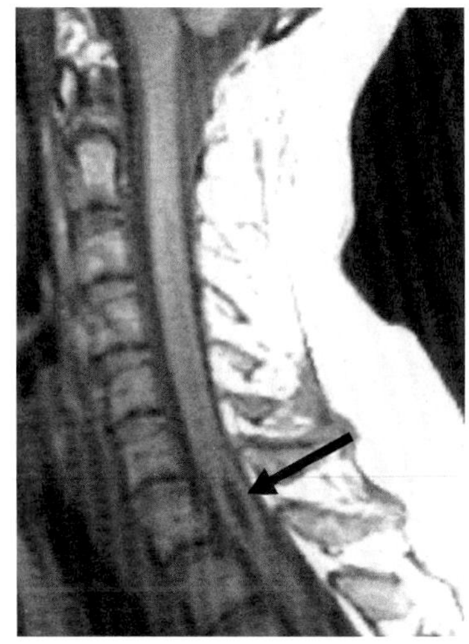

Fig. 2.23 MR image of the cervical spine (sagittal, T1) in an asymptomatic 27-year-old man. Hypointense longitudinal defect at C7.

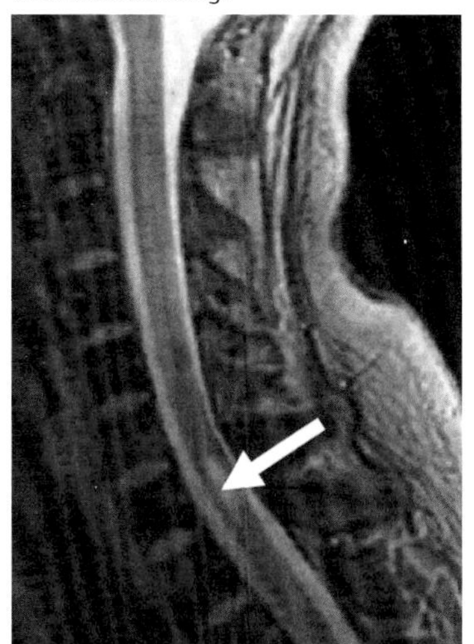

Fig. 2.24 Same patient as in Fig. 2.**23** (sagittal, T2). Hyperintense signal alteration.

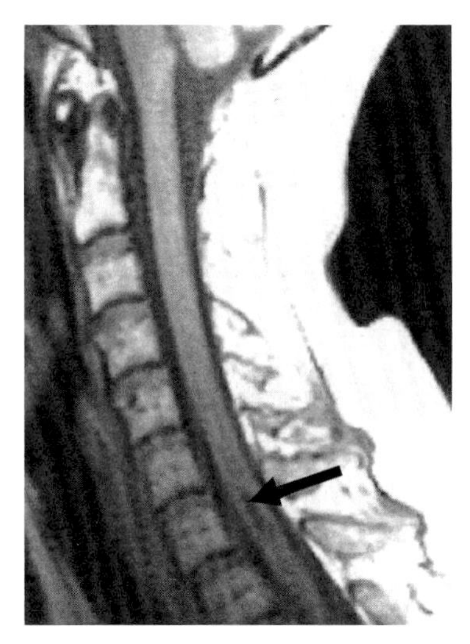

Fig. 2.25 Same patient as in Fig. 2.**23** (sagittal, T1 with contrast). No abnormal enhancement. No Chiari I malformation. Final diagnosis: typical syrinx.

▸ **Therapeutic options**
Treatment is indicated only for symptomatic syrinx • Decompressive laminectomy and syringotomy (posterolateral myelotomy to drain the syrinx into the subarachnoid space) • Syrinx shunting • Percutaneous needle aspiration (*Caution:* Syrinx may refill) • *Terminal ventriculostomy:* With a lumbar syrinx, the filum terminale is opened to create communication between the terminal ventricle and subarachnoid space • Patients with posttraumatic syrinx respond especially well to surgical treatment.

▸ **Prognosis**
This depends on the underlying cause and the severity of the neurologic deficit.

Differential Diagnosis

Cystic tumor or tumor component

Selected References

Brodbelt AR. Syringomyelia and the arachnoid web. Acta Neurochirurg (Wien) 2003; 145: 707–711

Brugieres P et al. CSF flow measurement in syringomyelia. AJNR Am J Neuroradiol 2000; 21: 1785–1792

Di Lorenzo N et al. Adult syringomyelia: classification, pathogenesis and therapeutic approaches. J Neurosurg Sci 2005; 49: 65–72

Definition

- **Epidemiology**
  Unilateral and bilateral facet joint dislocations accompany up to 50% of cervical spine injuries • Usually they occur at C4–C6 • Associated fracture is present in about 35% of all cases.
- **Etiology, pathophysiology, pathogenesis**
  Traumatic rupture of the posterior cervical ligament complex (primarily the interspinous ligaments and capsule, to a lesser extent the posterior longitudinal ligament) with or without an associated bony fracture • Anterior tilting of a vertebra relative to the next caudal vertebra, opening a gap between the spinous processes • Incomplete articulation of the facet joints ("jumped facet" usually unilaterally, in severe cases bilaterally with blockage) • Subluxed vertebra may be anteriorly displaced • Flexion and rotation.
  Classification:
  Unilateral facet dislocation: Hyperflexion and rotation • Rupture of the interspinous ligaments and capsule of the respective facet joint.
  Bilateral facet dislocation: Hyperflexion with distraction • Rupture of the interspinous ligaments • Rupture of both facet joint capsules • Rupture of the posterior longitudinal ligament • Rupture of the annulus fibrosus.

Imaging Signs

- **Modality of choice**
  Initial spiral CT is indicated with multiple trauma and extensive clinical symptoms • Otherwise conventional radiographs in two planes will suffice (not with the patient supine as this could mask signs) • MRI demonstrates ligament structures and possible spinal cord injuries.
- **Radiographic findings**
  Segmental hyperkyphosis (abrupt interruption of cervical lordosis) • Increased distance between the spinous processes ("fanning") • Focal malalignment of the facet joints in the lateral plane • Slight posterior widening or anterior narrowing of the affected disk interspace • Minimal anterior displacement may be present (1–3 mm).
- **CT findings**
  Spiral CT of the cervical spine (slice thickness 1 mm) • Sagittal reconstructions are very helpful • Direct visualization of facet dislocation • Anterior displacement of the articular process relative to the adjacent caudal one (double facet sign) • Visualization of bony injury.
- **MRI findings**
  T1- and T2-weighted STIR • Sagittal imaging plane • Demonstrates ligament injuries • Shows possible spinal cord injuries.

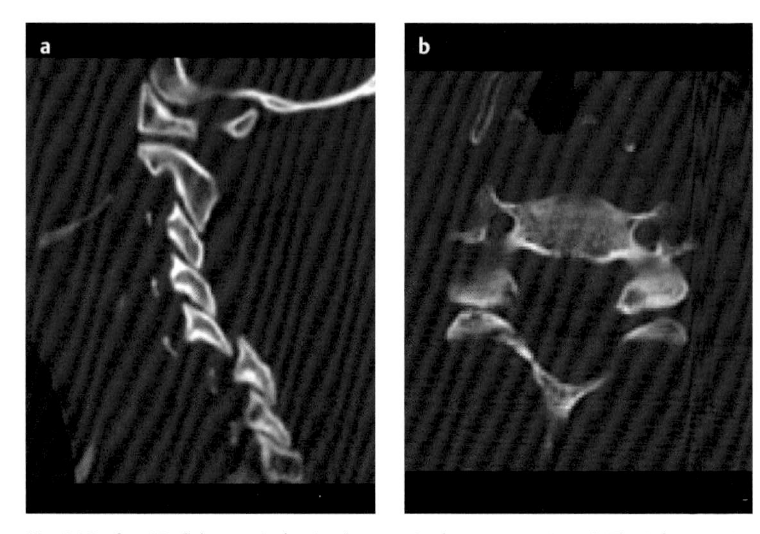

Fig. 2.26 a, b CT of the cervical spine (parasagittal reconstruction; **a**). The inferior articular processes of C5 lie anterior to the superior articular facets of C6. CT of C5–C6 (axial; **b**). Anterior subluxation with bilateral facet joint dislocation (double facet sign).

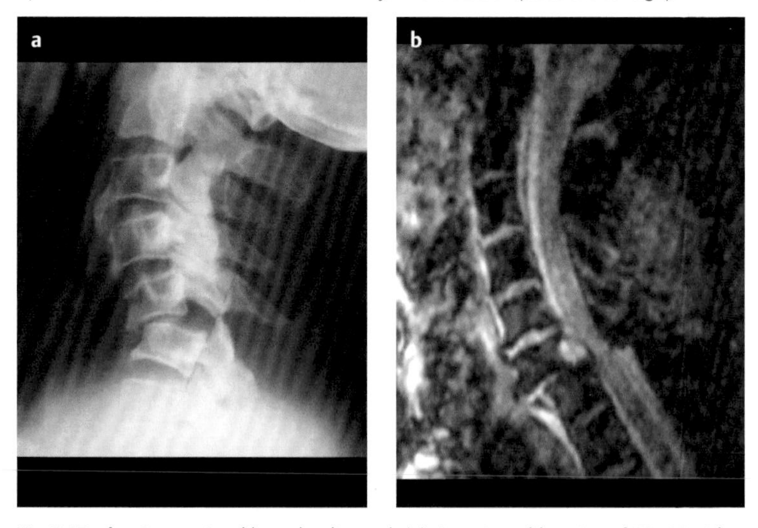

Fig. 2.27 a, b Conventional lateral radiograph (**a**). Anterior subluxation of C5–C6 with bilateral facet joint dislocation. Spinal cord compression. MR image of the cervical spine (sagittal, T2; **b**). Anterior subluxation of C6 relative to C7 with bilateral facet joint dislocation, severed spinal cord, and flaccid paralysis.

Clinical Aspects

- **Typical presentation**
  Severe neck pain • Restricted flexion and extension • Localized tenderness to palpation above the affected interspinous space • Neurologic symptoms are often present.
- **Complications**
  Nerve root injury occurs in 25% of cases of unilateral facet dislocation • Spinal cord injury occurs in 25% of cases • Bilateral facet dislocation often involves severe neurologic complications (quadriplegia in 72% of cases) • Spinal cord compression with edema, necrosis, hemorrhage, and/or severance.
- **What does the clinician want to know?**
  Unilateral or bilateral? • Spinal cord injuries? • Fracture?
- **Therapeutic options**
  Reduction may be attempted with halo traction (success rate approximately 50%) • Surgical decompression is indicated for neurologic complications • Fusion.
- **Prognosis**
  Late instability with recurrent dislocation is possible after conservative therapy • Slight spinal cord contusion is reversible • Other late neurologic sequelae can occur.

Selected References

Galanski M, Wippermann B, Stamm G, Bazak N, Wafer A. Kompendium der traumatologischen Röntgendiagnostik. Berlin: Springer 1999

Lomoschitz F. Bildgebung bei Wirbelsäulenverletzungen – Diagnostic Imaging. Wien Med Wochenschr 2001; 151: 502–505

Definition

- **Epidemiology**
  Relatively common in people with osteoporosis • Often occult.
- **Etiology, pathophysiology, pathogenesis**
  Sacral stress fracture • Relatively slight trauma or normal stresses act on deficient or abnormal bone • Predisposing factors include:
  - Osteoporosis.
  - Osteomalacia.
  - Rheumatoid arthritis.
  - Steroid therapy.
  - Pelvic irradiation.
  - Alcoholism.
  - Postoperative longstanding immobilization of the spine.

Imaging Signs

- **Modality of choice**
  MRI is suitable for diagnosing even minimal insufficiency fractures • CT is more suitable for directly imaging the fracture line • Bone scans can also provide valuable information although they often cannot clearly distinguish these fractures from sacroiliitis.
- **Radiographic findings**
  Up to 50% of all normal traumatic sacral fractures are missed • Most insufficiency fractures cannot be detected on conventional radiographs • In rare cases, a tiny fracture line will be visible • The fracture is typically located parallel to the sacroiliac joints.
- **CT findings**
  Axial thin-slice CT (maximum slice thickness 3 mm) • Coronal reconstructions • Direct visualization of the fracture line • Local destruction of cancellous bone without a fracture line is a sign of microtrauma • Osteopenic bone structure.
- **MRI findings**
  STIR (coronal) • T1 (axial, coronal) • Bone marrow edema is visualized on the STIR sequence • The fracture line is occasionally visualized on T1-weighted images • Other causes for clinical symptoms are visualized.

Clinical Aspects

- **Typical presentation**
  Low back pain • Radiates into buttocks or thigh • Neurologic deficits are rare • History includes only slight trauma or none at all.
- **What does the clinician want to know?**
  Exclude other possible causes of clinical symptoms.

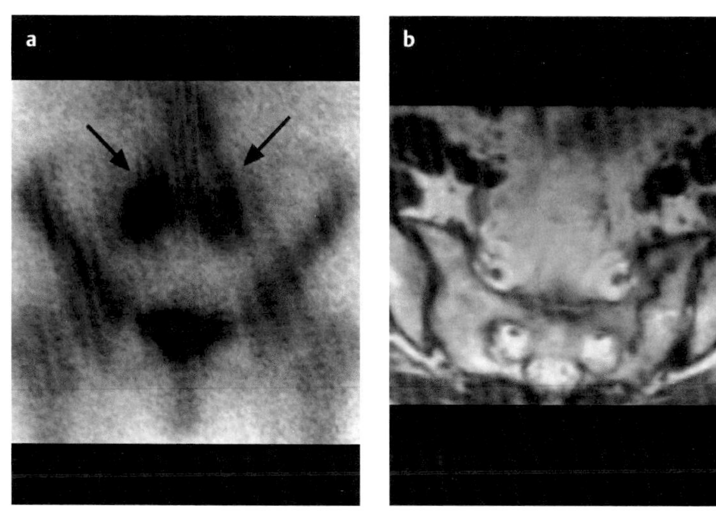

Fig. 2.28 a, b P-A bone scan of the pelvis and sacrum (**a**). Increased tracer uptake around both sacroiliac joints in typical butterfly pattern. MR image of the sacrum (axial, T1; **b**). Linear insufficiency fracture of the left sacrum.

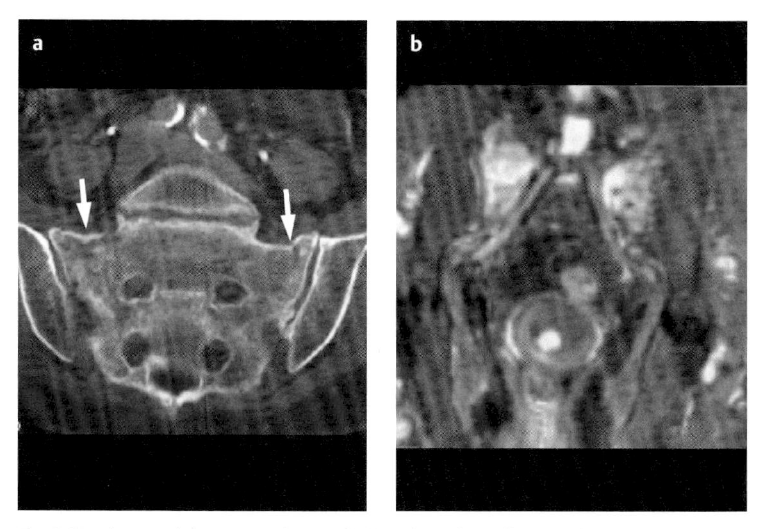

Fig. 2.29 a, b CT of the sacrum (coronal) (**a**). Bilateral insufficiency fractures of the sacrum. Cortical discontinuity with minimal local fracture of the cancellous bone. MR image of the sacrum (coronal, proton density fat-saturated; **b**). Diffuse bilateral bone marrow edema in the sacrum, an indirect sign of insufficiency fracture.

- **Therapeutic options**
  Treatment is invariably conservative • Bed rest and pain management are important in the initial phase • Later, the patient should be mobilized as quickly as possible (especially in osteoporosis) • Preventative osteoporosis therapy • Low dose of corticosteroids • Physical therapy.
- **Prognosis**
  Patients are usually free of pain within four weeks.

Differential Diagnosis

Metastases	– MRI or CT can directly visualize metastases – History of malignancy
Sacroiliitis	– Erosive changes in the sacroiliac joints
Lumbar radiculopathy	– Disk protrusion or extrusion – Spondylolisthesis

Selected References

König A. Insuffizienzfraktur des Os ileum und des Os sacrum. Z Rheumatol 2000; 59: 343–347

Weber M, Hasler P, Gerber H. Insufficiency fractures of the sacrum. Spine 1993; 18: 2507–2512

Definition (Spondylolysis, Spondylolisthesis)

▸ **Epidemiology**
Affects about 4.5% of children at 6 years of age • Affects about 6% in adulthood • Men are affected more often than women • In competitive athletes playing sport involving repetitive lordosis, the rate increases to about 50% • Predisposing disorders include Marfan syndrome, osteogenesis imperfecta, and osteopetrosis.

▸ **Etiology, pathophysiology, pathogenesis**
Stress reaction • Stress fracture = spondylolysis • Competitive sport at an early age involving repetitive reactions to stresses from muscle contraction, weight bearing, and rotational forces leads to a defect in the pars interarticularis • Spondylolysis can lead to slippage of the adjacent cranial vertebra (spondylolisthesis) • Unilateral (about 15% of cases) or bilateral spondylolysis.
Meyerding classification of spondylolisthesis:
- Grade I: Anterior slippage of the adjacent cranial vertebra by less than 25%.
- Grade II: Anterior slippage by 25–50%.
- Grade III: Anterior slippage by 50–75%.
- Grade IV: Anterior slippage by 75–100%.

Imaging Signs

▸ **Modality of choice**
Only MRI can demonstrate the stress reaction (cancellous fracture) • However, a stress fracture can be difficult to detect on MR images • Therefore, the modality of choice for imaging stress fractures is conventional radiography (oblique view) or, in uncertain cases, spiral CT • MRI alone is indicated in children and adolescents (to limit exposure to ionizing radiation).

▸ **Radiographic findings**
Spondylolysis is more readily detectable on oblique films than on lateral films • Visible as a defect in the “neck” of the “Scottie dog.”

▸ **CT findings**
CT with a maximum slice thickness of 2 mm • Sagittal reconstructions • Direct visualization of a fracture line • *Caution:* Findings can mimic an additional facet joint.

▸ **MRI findings**
Sagittal T1-weighted and STIR sequences • Additional axial sequences are indicated in the affected segments • Edema sign • Cancellous fracture line (no correlate on CT or conventional radiographs) • Axial slices show widening of the spinal canal • Reduction in the perineural fatty tissue at the nerve roots • Focal hypointensity in the pars interarticularis on axial T1- and T2-weighted sequences.

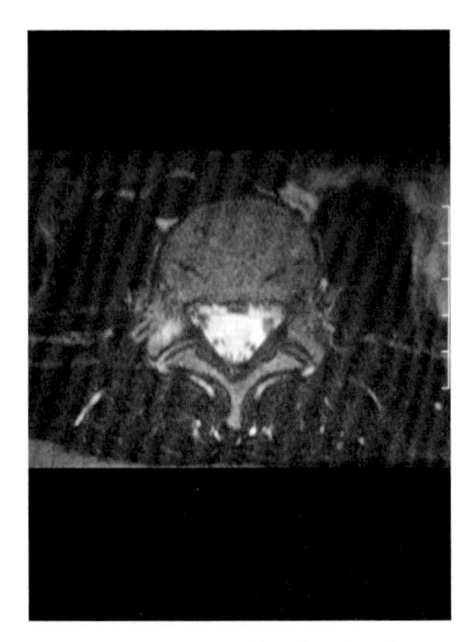

Fig. 2.30 MR image of L3 (axial, T2). Bone marrow edema in the right vertebral arch (chronic stress) with effusion in the facet joint (baseball player).

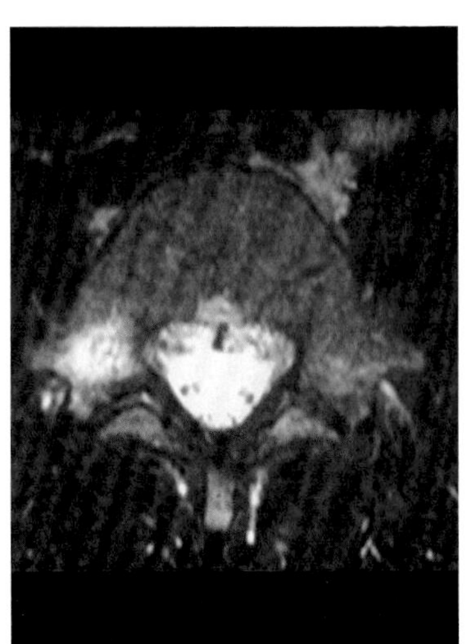

Fig. 2.31 MR image of L3 (axial, T2). Bone marrow edema in the right vertebral arch from chronic stress (baseball player).

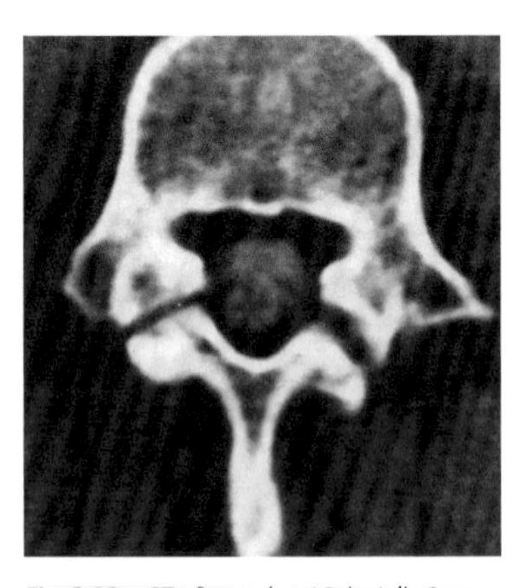

Fig. 2.32 CT of vertebra L3 (axial). Spondylolysis with visible asymmetrical defects in both laminae.

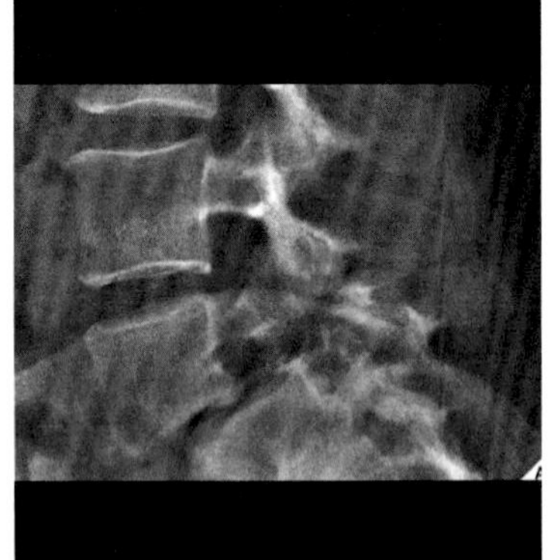

Fig. 2.33 Conventional lateral radiograph of the lower lumbar spine. Defect in the vertebral arch with anterior slippage of the vertebra (spondylolisthesis). Meyerding stage IV (= 50 %).

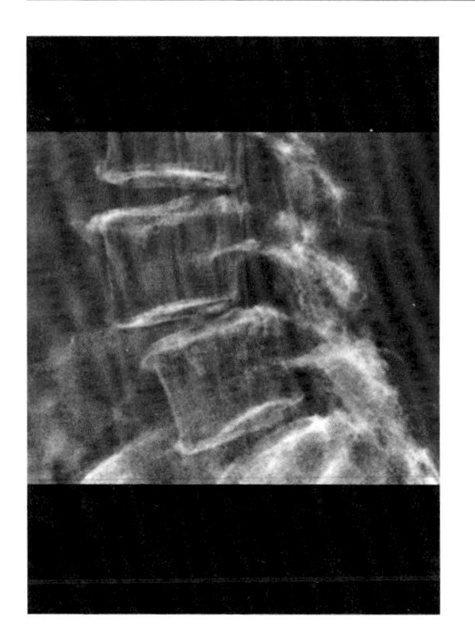

Fig. 2.34 Conventional lateral radiograph of the lumbar spine (detail). Pseudospondylolisthesis in disk degeneration.

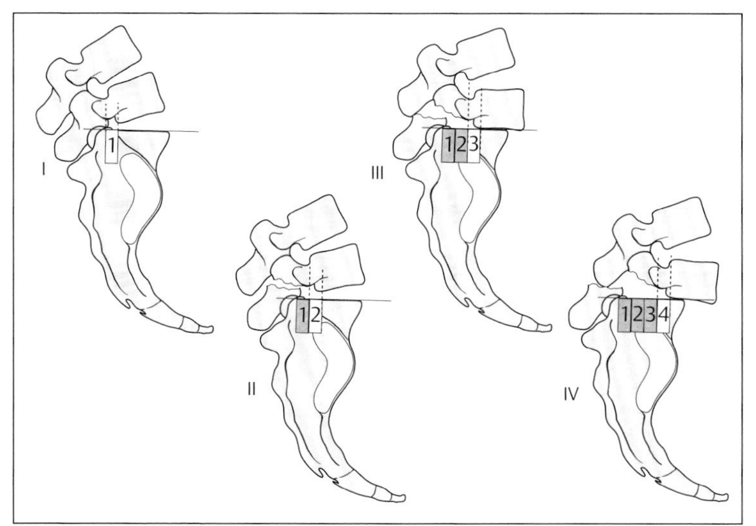

Fig. 2.35 Meyerding classification of spondylolisthesis.

Clinical Aspects

- **Typical presentation**
  Often asymptomatic in children • Later chronic low back pain is often present • Pain increases with exercise • Radiculopathy is present in higher grade spondylolisthesis.
- **Complications**
  Neurologic symptoms.
- **Therapeutic options**
  Treatment in most cases is conservative • Surgical treatment (posterolateral fusion) is indicated only in patients with spondylolisthesis of any grade where neurologic symptoms are present.
- **Prognosis**
  Conservative therapy has a success rate of up to 70% • Neurologic deficits persist in up to 10% of cases following spinal fusion.

Differential Diagnosis

Partial facetectomy	– History
Pseudospondylolisthesis	– Associated with marked degenerative changes in the lumbar spine
Osteogenic metastases (MRI)	– History of underlying malignant disorder
Healed spondylolysis (MRI)	– Signal loss in the pars interarticularis due to sclerosis – CT

Selected References

Brossmann J, Czerny Ch, Freyschmidt J. Grenzen des Normalen und Anfänge des Pathologischen in der Radiologie des kindlichen und erwachsenen Skeletts. Stuttgart: Thieme 2001

Cassas KJ, Cassettari-Wayhs A. Childhood and adolescent sports-related overuse injuries. Am Fam Physician 2006; 73: 1014–1022

Stäbler A, Paulus R, Steinborn M, Bosch R, Mathko N, Reiser M. Die Spondylolyse im Stadium der Entstehung: Diagnostischer Beitrag der MRT. RöFo 2000; 172: 33–37

Wilson JB et al. Spinal injuries in contact sports. Curr Sports Med Rep 2006; 5: 50–55

Wittenberg RH, Willbruger RE, Kramer J. Spondylolyse und Spondylolisthese. Diagnose und Therapie. Orthopäde 1998; 27: 51–63

Definition

The diskovertebral region is often affected (Andersson lesion of the noninflammatory type). Pseudarthrosis results where the fracture continues into the posterior elements and the ossified ligaments are discontinuous.

Imaging Signs

- **Modality of choice**
  Because of the low sensitivity of conventional radiography, multislice CT is indicated • MRI is indicated in the presence of neurologic symptoms to exclude spondylodiskitis.
- **Radiographic findings**
  Low sensitivity • Discontinuity of the ossified ligaments.
- **CT findings**
  Excellent visualization of bony structures • Visualization of the typical sclerosis at the pseudarthrosis.
- **MRI findings**
  In addition to purely bony changes, MRI also demonstrates the fibrous and fibrovascular tissue typical of pseudarthrosis, which is located primarily in the diskovertebral area and facet joints • Enhancement after contrast administration.

Clinical Aspects

- **Typical presentation**
  Ankylosing spondylitis • Back pain • Instability.
- **Therapeutic options**
  No consensus • Conservative or surgical • Spinal fusion involving several segments.

Differential Diagnosis

Spondylodiskitis	– Involvement of the posterior vertebral elements and integrity of the anterior longitudinal ligament suggest pseudarthrosis

Selected References

Rasker JJ, Prevo RL, Lanting PJ. Spondylodiscitis in ankylosing spondylitis, inflammation or trauma? A description of six cases. Scand J Rheumatol 1996; 25: 52–57

Shih TT, Chen PQ, Li YW, Hsu CY. Spinal fractures and pseudoarthrosis complicating ankylosing spondylitis: MRI manifestation and clinical significance. JCAT 2001; 25: 164–170

Trent G, Armstrong GW, O'Neil J. Thoracolumbar fractures in ankylosing spondylitis. High-risk injuries. Clin Orthop 1988; 227: 61–66

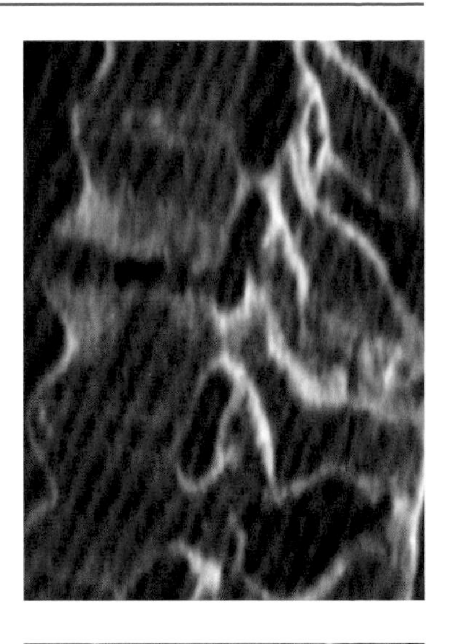

Fig. 2.36 CT reconstruction (sagittal). Pseudarthrosis from a stress fracture through all three columns in ankylosing spondylitis.

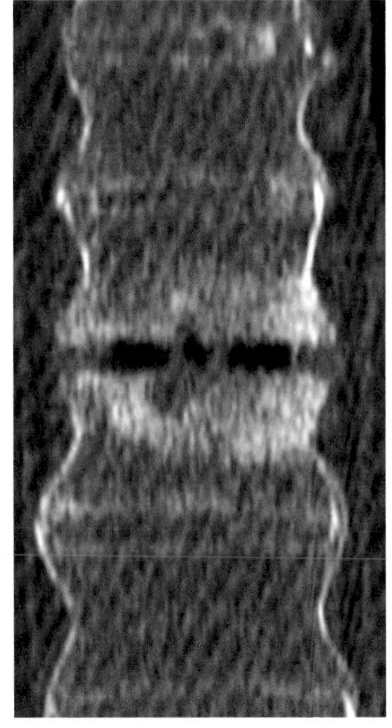

Fig. 2.37 CT reconstruction (coronal). The vertebral and disk components of the pseudarthrosis are visualized.

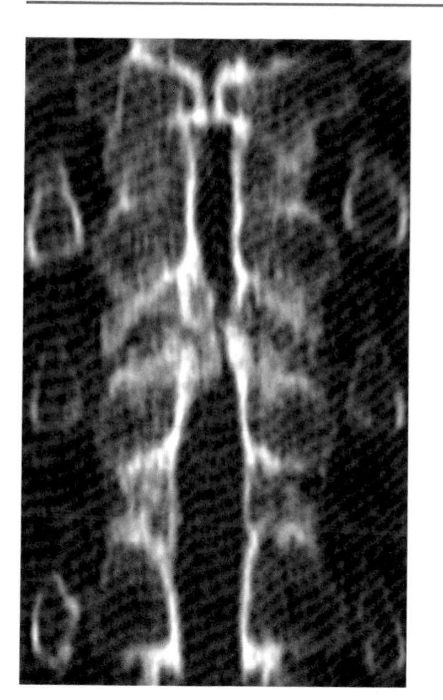

Fig. 2.38 CT reconstruction (coronal). Pseudarthrosis in the posterior spine is visualized.

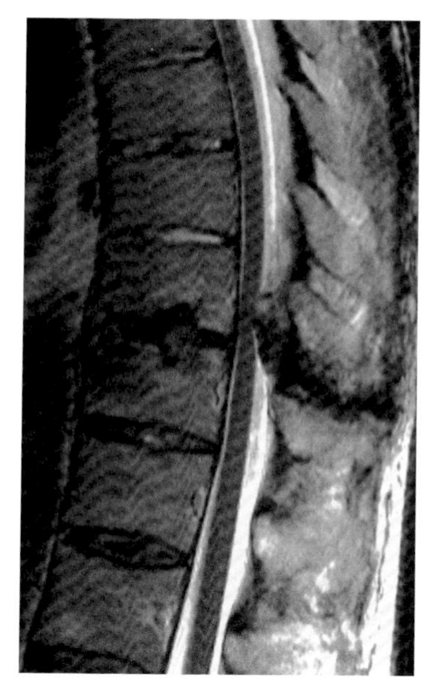

Fig. 2.39 MR image of the thoracic spine (sagittal, T2). Pseudarthrosis from a stress fracture in ankylosing spondylitis. Sclerosis in the fracture zones.

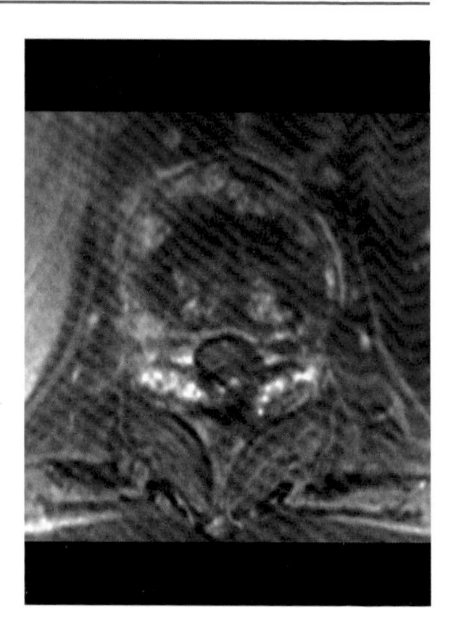

Fig. 2.40 MR image of the thoracic spine (T1 with contrast and spectral fat saturation). Axial view of the thoracic spine. Contrast uptake by the soft tissues.

Definition

- **Etiology, pathophysiology, pathogenesis**
  Wear resulting from aging and/or overuse, and other unknown causes • Associated with Scheuermann disease • There is dehydration with subsequent loss of function of the disk structures (primarily partial radial tears in the fibers of the annulus fibrosus, leading to broad-based disk bulge or protrusion) • Loss of height and deformation of the disk • Displacement of parts of the nucleus pulposus within the disk (T2 hyperintensity).
  Chronic overuse and abnormal stress results in wear and disturbs the supply of nutrients to the disk (loss of water and proteoglycans). This in turn leads to loss of tissue function and integrity (concentric and/or transverse fiber tears in the annulus fibrosis) and ultimately to disk deformation.
  Schmorl node: Circumscribed defect in the superior or inferior endplate leading to disk herniation. Etiology: Presumably osteonecrosis with insufficiency fracture.
  Nucleus pulposus: Gelatinous material with high water content in the center of the intervertebral disk.
  Annulus fibrosus: Consists mainly of fibrocartilaginous material and concentrically arranged collagen fibers.

Imaging Signs

- **Modality of choice**
  MRI (sagittal, T1 and T2) • Height reduction • Signal loss on water-sensitive sequences.
- **Radiographic findings**
  Height reduction in the disk interspace • *Schmorl nodes:* Defect in the vertebral body (close to the disk) with sclerosis.
- **CT findings**
  Height reduction • Deformation • *Schmorl nodes:* Sclerotic margin, normal trabecular structure.
- **MRI findings**
  Dehydration (T2 hypointensity) • Height reduction • Displacement of portions of the nucleus pulposus (T2 hyperintensity) into the annulus fibrosus (T2 hypointensity) • Deformation (broad, intraligamentous disk bulge; annulus fibrosus is intact) • *Schmorl nodes:*
  - Acute: Edematous halo.
  - Chronic: Sclerotic halo with conversion of fatty marrow.

Clinical Aspects

- **Typical presentation**
  Usually asymptomatic (75% of cases) • Nonspecific low back pain • Loss of function with limited motion in the spine • Degenerative disk disease.

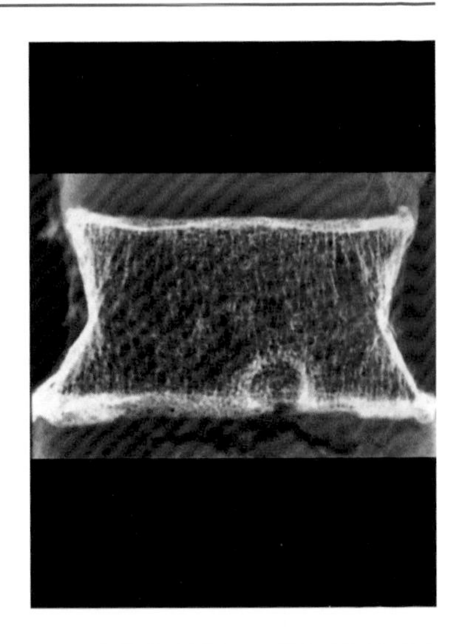

Fig. 3.1 Conventional radiograph (specimen). Schmorl node in the inferior endplate with fine marginal sclerosis (= chronic Schmorl node).

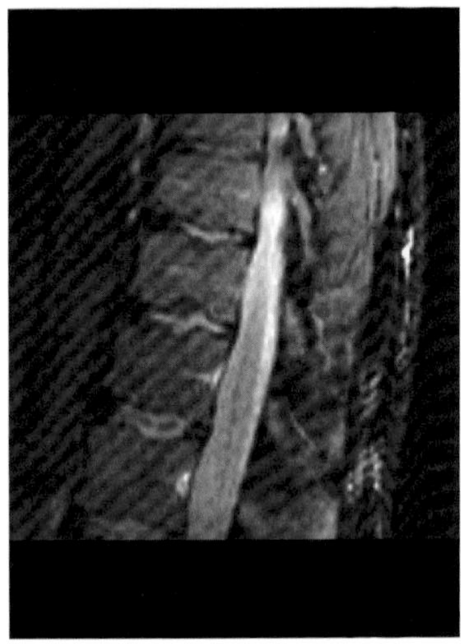

Fig. 3.2 MR image of thoracolumbar junction (STIR sagittal). Reduced disk height is indicative of degeneration. Circumscribed impression of the superior and inferior endplates of L1 and L2 with disk protrusion (Schmorl node).

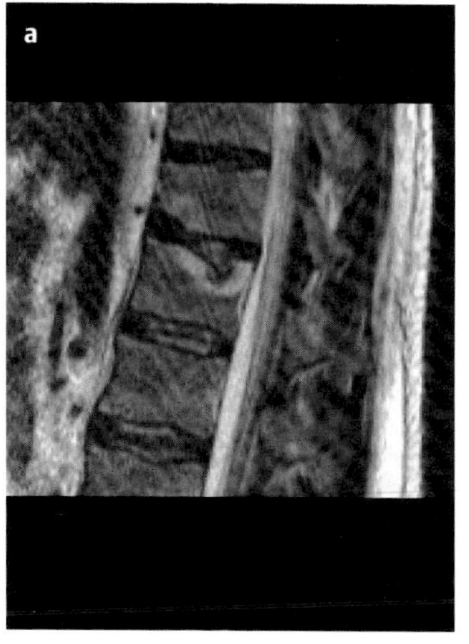

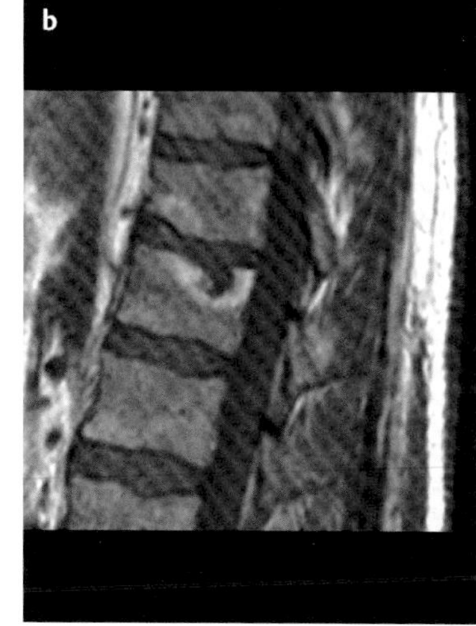

Fig. 3.3 a, b MR image of the lower thoracic and lumbar spine (sagittal, T2, T1). T1 and T2 showing a disk impression in the posterior half of the superior endplate and surrounding fatty marrow (= subacute Schmorl node).

▸ **Therapeutic options**

Acute low back pain: Analgesia • Physical therapy, specific back exercises • Correction of posture • Strengthening of the local musculature.

Differential Diagnosis

Nondiskogenic back pain	
Protrusion, extrusion, sequestration	
Diskitis, spondylodiskitis	
Schmorl node	– Osteoporotic or pathologic vertebral collapse
Chorda remnant	– Lying in dorsal part. No other degenerative changes!

Selected References

Bohndorf K, Imhof H. Radiologische Diagnostik der Knochen und Gelenke, 2nd ed. Stuttgart: Thieme 2006

Modic MT. Degenerative disc disease and back pain. Magn Reson Imaging Clin N Am 1999; 7: 481–491

Morgan S. MRI of the lumbar intervertebral disc. Clin Radiol. 1999; 54: 703–723

Schmorl G. Über Knorpelknötchen an den Wirbelbandscheiben. Fortschr Röntgenstr 1929; 38: 265

Vahlensieck M, Reiser M. MRT des Bewegungsapparates, 3rd ed. Stuttgart: Thieme 2006

Definition

- **Etiology, pathophysiology, pathogenesis**
  Initial stage of degenerative disk disease • Edema of the adjacent subcortical portions of the vertebral body in disk degeneration with decrease in fluid content and loss of disk height, usually in the lower cervical and lumbar spine • Pseudoinflammatory • Most likely a reactive change to abnormal stresses • Microangiopathy • Hyperemia • Endothelial damage • Fluid leakage, pseudoinflammatory or inflammatory reaction, ingrowth of fibrovascular tissue • General picture of edema.

Imaging Signs

- **Modality of choice**
  - Conventional A-P and lateral radiographs.
  - MRI (sagittal, STIR, T1, and axial to exclude disk herniation).
- **Radiographic findings**
  Loss of disk height • Postural deficiency.
- **MRI findings**
  Cancellous bone adjacent to the inferior and superior endplates of the affected segment appears hyperintense on T1-weighted images and hypointense on T2-weighted images, consistent with vasogenic bone marrow edema • Disk is darker on T2-weighted and STIR images, consistent with fluid loss.

Clinical Aspects

- **Typical presentation**
  Lumbago • Cervical spine pain • Painful edema • Often multiple spinal regions may be symptomatic, including symptoms of facet joint degeneration.
- **What does the clinician want to know?**
  Exclude spinal stenosis or stenosis of the neural foramina • Exclude spondylodiskitis • Exclude malignancy.
- **Therapeutic options**
  Conservative with physical therapy • Analgesia where indicated.
- **Prognosis**
  Progression to Modic II (often within 7–9 months).

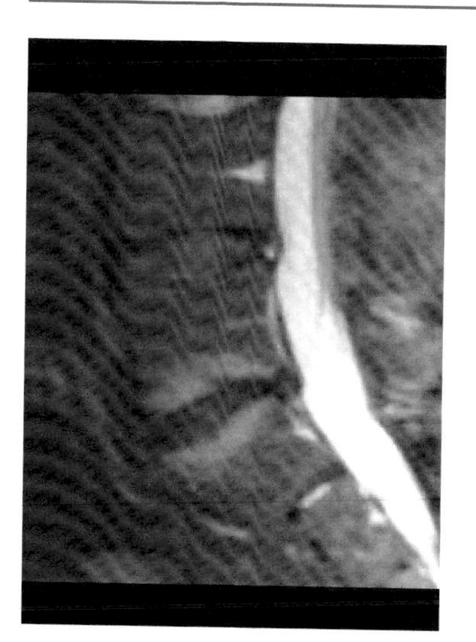

Fig. 3.4 MR image of the lumbar spine (sagittal, STIR). L5–S1 shows hyperintensity adjacent to the disk (edema). The disk is hypointense with reduced height. Posterior herniation with intact posterior longitudinal ligament.

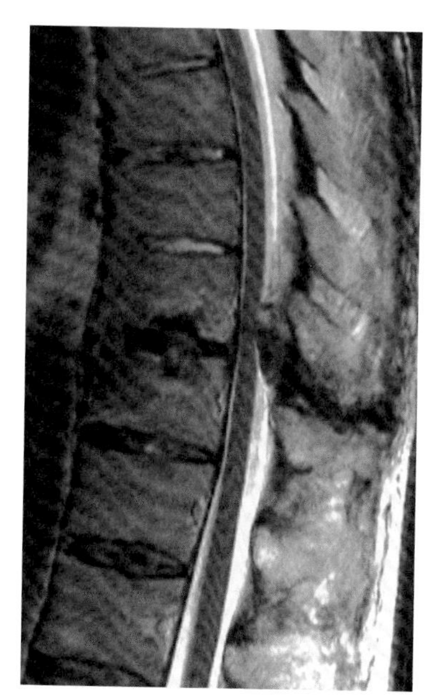

Fig. 3.5 Modic type I degenerative disk disease. MR image of the lumbar spine (sagittal, T2). Disk height is reduced. Posterior disk herniation. Subcortical hypointensity with fine hyperintense halo (edema and beginning fatty marrow conversion).

Differential Diagnosis

Diagnosis is obvious in most cases	
Spondylitis, spondylodiskitis	– History – Disk shows hyperintensity and may show increased volume – Irregularly demarcated from disk – Contrast administration
Atypical hemangioma	– Rarely confused – More central location – Tends to be round and limited to the affected vertebra – Also resembles edema – Increase in longitudinal trabeculae on plain radiographs and CT
Status post recent vertebral fracture	– History – May be difficult to differentiate after recent fracture – Height reduction in the vertebral body limited to the affected vertebra – Fluid signal in vertebra – Diffusion-weighted sequence

Selected References

Modic MT. Degenerative disc disease and back pain. MRI Clin N Am 1999; 7: 481

Modic MT, Steinberg PM, Ross JS, Masaryk TJ, Carter JR. Degenerative disc disease: assessment of changes in vertebral bone marrow with MR Imaging. Radiology 1988; 166: 193

Vahlensieck M, Reiser M. MRT des Bewegungsapparates, 3rd ed. Stuttgart: Thieme 2006

Definition

▸ **Etiology, pathophysiology, pathogenesis**

Degenerative disk disease with fatty degeneration of the cancellous bone adjacent to the endplates (stress-induced conversion of fatty marrow) • There is progressive fatty degeneration of the pseudoinflammatory area of the vertebra (Modic I) • Often occurs in the lower lumbar and lower cervical spine • See Modic I.

Imaging Signs

▸ **Modality of choice**

Conventional radiographs • MRI: sagittal (STIR, T1) and axial (T1).

▸ **Radiographic findings**

Reduced disk height • Postural deformity • Osteophytes may limit mobility on stress radiographs.

▸ **MRI findings**

There is a hyperintense area in the vertebral body adjacent to the disk on T1-weighted and T2-weighted images, appearing hypointense on the fat-suppressed sequence • Height reduction and increasing fluid loss in the disk, which appears hypointense on the T2-weighted and STIR sequences • Often associated with osteophytes, which occasionally mask bulging of the degenerative disk.

Clinical Aspects

▸ **Typical presentation**

Pain decreases as the Modic I edema recedes • This finding is pathognomonic.

▸ **Therapeutic options**

Physical therapy to strengthen the back musculature and stabilize the spine. *Surgical options:* Spinal fusion or prosthetic disk.

Differential Diagnosis

Posttraumatic vertebral fracture	– An older fracture may show fatty degeneration but not sclerosis – Limited to the affected vertebra – History
Hemangioma	– Typical hemangioma also shows fat-equivalent signal – Tends to be round and limited to the affected vertebra – Visible trabeculae on CT, occasionally on MRI as well
Liposarcoma	– Very rare

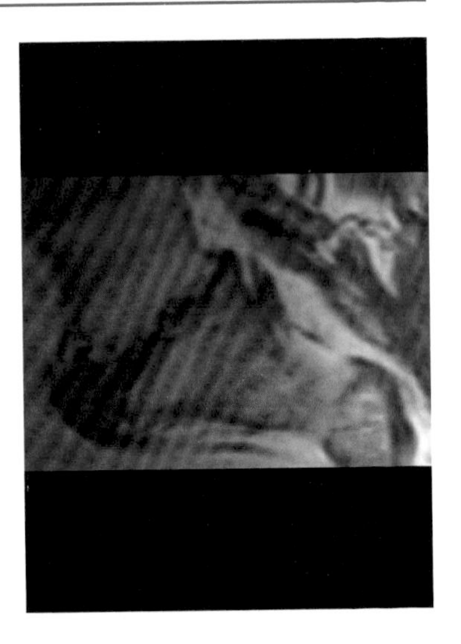

Fig. 3.6 MR image of the lumbosacral region (sagittal, T2). Markedly hyperintense subcortical band due to fatty marrow conversion.

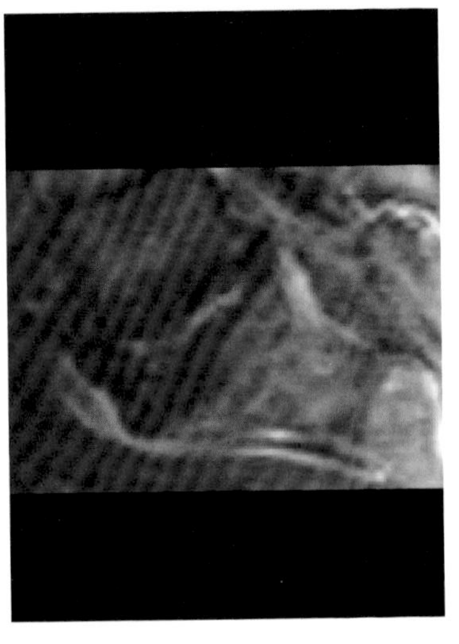

Fig. 3.7 MR image of the lumbosacral region (sagittal, STIR). Subcortical hyperintensity adjacent to the disk due to fatty marrow conversion. The disk is also hyperintense. The superior and inferior endplates are irregular, with tiny Schmorl nodes.

Selected References

Modic MT. Degenerative disc disease and back pain. MRI Clin N Am 1999; 7: 481

Modic MT, Steinberg PM, Ross JS, Masaryk TJ, Carter JR. Degenerative disc disease: assessment of changes in vertebral bone marrow with MR Imaging. Radiology 1988; 166: 193

Vahlensieck M, Reiser M. MRT des Bewegungsapparates, 3rd ed. Stuttgart: Thieme 2006

Definition

▶ **Epidemiology**

Reactive stiffening in the setting of spinal degeneration and abnormal mobility with increasing age (40–60 years) • More common in men than woman • More common with short pedicles • More pronounced on the concave side of scoliosis or asymmetry, more often on the right than left (probably due to the aorta) • Predilection for the lower lumbar spine, middle and lower cervical spine, and thoracolumbar junction.

▶ **Etiology, pathophysiology, pathogenesis**

Multisegmental osteophytes (horizontal, handlelike, etc.) • *Modic III:* Transformation of the Modic II fatty degeneration into subcortical sclerosis.

Reactive osteophytic proliferation in the setting of spinal degeneration (tension and compression, metabolic), creating functionally fused vertebrae • Outgrowths begin beneath the margin on the endplates, especially at the insertion of the anterior longitudinal ligament • *Maximal severity:* Bridging osteophytes.

Significance:
- Especially if posterior: Narrowing of the spinal canal.
- Lateral and posterolateral orientation: Narrowing of the neural foramina.
- With severe anterior osteophytes: Role in the development of aneurysms.

Imaging Signs

▶ **Modality of choice**
- Conventional A-P and lateral radiographs, stress radiographs where indicated.
- Where imaging findings are equivocal and conflict with clinical findings: supplementary MRI.

▶ **Radiographic findings**

Increased subchondral sclerosis • Osteophytes adjacent to the endplates • Bizarre configurations of proliferative and bridging osteophytes.

▶ **CT findings**

As on radiographs • Narrowing of the spinal canal and bony neural foramina is better visualized.

▶ **MRI findings**

Low subchondral bandlike intensity (= subchondral sclerosis) • Sagittal images often show multisegmental spinal osteophytes with obliteration of the subarachnoid space and perineural fatty tissue • The high soft tissue contrast is best for evaluating the overall situation, as the improved visualization of neural structures helps to identify secondary radiculopathy and myelopathy • Usually there are other signs of spinal degeneration • Significance of narrowing of the bony neural foramina and spinal canal is usually overestimated • For selected normal values of spinal canal width, see Disk Protrusion, p. 100.

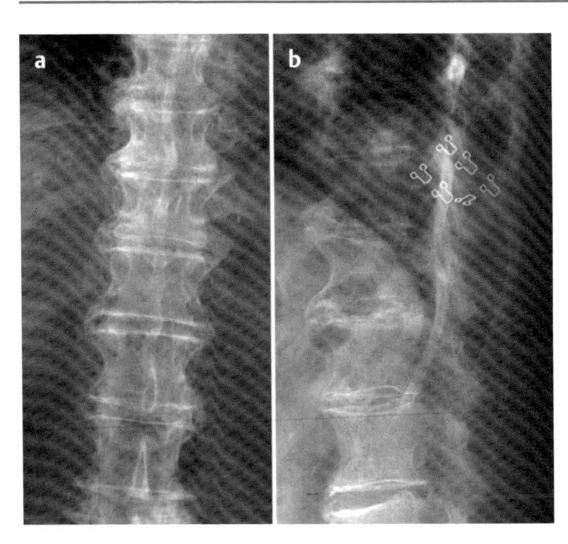

Fig. 3.8 a, b Conventional radiographs of the lumbosacral junction (A-P **a** and lateral **b**). Numerous lateral and anterior osteophytes, some growing in hairpin or beaklike shapes.

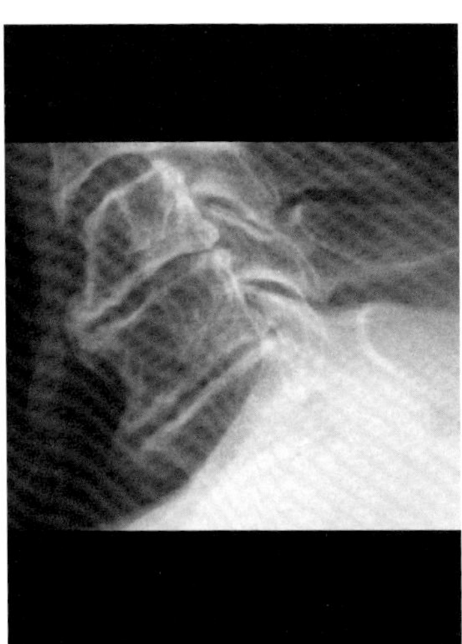

Fig. 3.9 Conventional lateral radiograph of the cervical spine. Marked bridging spondylosis deformans and degenerative disk disease, with reduced disk height and osteophytes. Modic III, with reduced disk height and subcortical sclerosis.

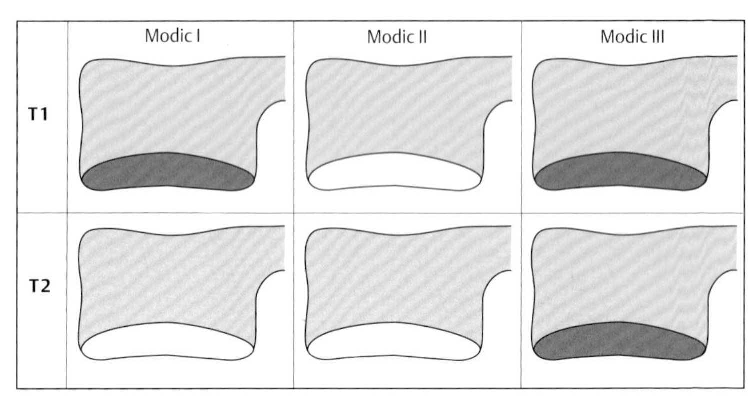

Fig. 3.10 Subchondral degenerative changes: Modic I = edema, Modic II = fatty marrow conversion, Modic III = sclerosis.

Fig. 3.11 Conventional lateral radiograph of L3–L4. Spondylosis with severe degenerative disk disease.

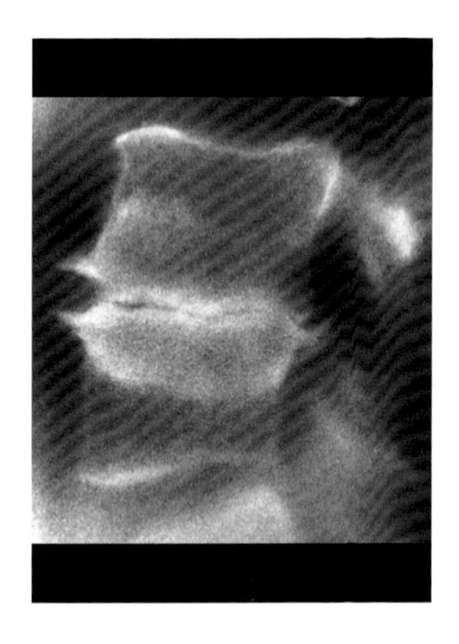

Clinical Aspects

- **Typical presentation**
  Ranges from asymptomatic to severe pain; rarely correlates with radiographic findings • Other disorders are often excluded based on radiographic findings • In particular, these include stenosis of the spinal canal and neural foramina, other degenerative spinal disorders such as spondylarthritis, synovial cysts, uncovertebral osteoarthritis of the cervical spine, disk displacement, abnormal mobility with pseudospondylolisthesis, and thickening of the ligamenta flava • Narrowing of the neural foramina will also involve segmental symptoms.
- **Therapeutic options**
  Lumbago is managed with analgesics and infiltration of pain relieving drugs • Physical therapy to strengthen the back musculature, etc. • Neurologic symptoms such as paraplegia and bladder paralysis require surgical decompression (foraminotomy, laminectomy, hemilaminectomy, fusion).

Differential Diagnosis

Syndesmophytes	– History – With progressive inflammatory disorders (especially ankylosing spondylitis) – Growth is vertical and initially thin
Parasyndesmophytes	– Occur in inflammatory disorders such as psoriasis and Reiter syndrome – Typically asymmetric, thicker than syndesmophytes, extend in an arc outward from vertebra
Vertebral collapse with displacement of anterior or posterior margin	– Osteopenic bone structure – Wedge or fishlike vertebrae
Ligament calcifications	– OPLL (ossified posterior longitudinal ligament) – DISH (diffuse idiopathic skeletal hyperostosis) – Rare

Selected References

Bohndorf K, Imhof H. Radiologische Diagnostik der Knochen und Gelenke, 2nd ed. Stuttgart: Thieme 2006

Dihlmann W. Joints and vertebral connections. Stuttgart: Thieme 1985

Möller T, Reif E. CT- und MRT-Normalbefunde. Stuttgart: Thieme 1998

Resnick, D, Niwayama G (eds.). Diagnosis of Bone and Joint disorders, 3rd ed. Philadelphia: Saunders 1995

Vahlensieck M, Reiser M. MRT des Bewegungsapparates, 3rd ed. Stuttgart: Thieme 2006

Definition (American Society of Neuroradiology)

Bulge: > 50% of the disk circumference (not a hernia).

Herniation: Bulging of disk material past the margins of the intervertebral space (< 50% of the disk circumference).

- Protrusion: Broad communication between hernia and disk ("broad-based" = 25–50%, "focal" = < 25%).
- Extrusion: Necklike (hourglass-shaped) communication between hernia and disk.
- Sequestration: Herniated disk material separated from the central disk. It can migrate cranially or caudally.

Caution: The term "prolapse" should no longer be used as it is not consistently defined.

Localization of the herniation:

Central • Central ipsilateral • Subarticular • Foraminal • Extraforaminal (axial image).

At disk level • Infrapedicular • Pedicular • Suprapedicular (lateral image).

Nucleus pulposus: Gelatinous material with high water content in the center of the intervertebral disk.

Annulus fibrosus: Composed mainly of fibrocartilaginous material and consists of concentrically arranged collagen fibers.

Chronic overuse and abnormal stress results in wear and disturbs the supply of nutrients to the disk (loss of water and proteoglycans). This in turn leads to loss of tissue function and integrity (concentric and/or transverse fiber tears in the annulus fibrosis) and ultimately to disk deformation • Increased risk of hernia or bulge.

Imaging Signs

- **Modality of choice**
  MRI.
- **Radiographic findings**
  Height reduction in the disk interspaces.
- **CT findings**
  Circumscribed bulging of disk material (isodense to soft tissue) • Disk material in the lateral recess (displacing the fatty tissue) • Sagittal reconstruction (multidetector CT) • Vacuum phenomenon.
- **MRI findings**
  Circumscribed disk deformation extending beyond the posterior longitudinal ligament • Displacement of parts of the nucleus pulposus within the disk (T2 hyperintensity) • Disk contour (axial and sagittal) • Relationship to dural sac (displacement, deformation, myelopathy), spinal stenosis • Relationship to the nerve roots (perineural fatty tissue, contact, displacement) • Neuropathy = nerve root thickening and signal alteration • Neural foramen stenosis • Vacuum phenomenon (T1 hypointensity, T2 hypointensity).

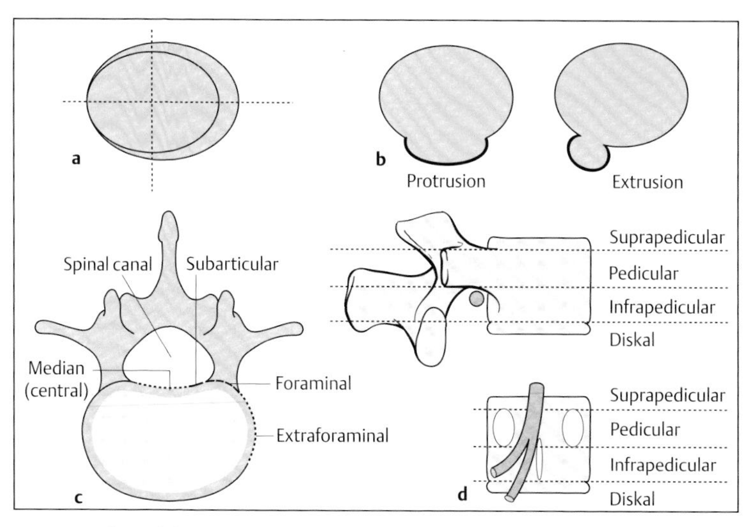

Fig. 3.12 a–d Disk herniation. Asymmetric "bulging" (**a**), protrusion and extrusion (**b**), anatomic position of disk hernias in the axial imaging plane (**c**) and sagittal plane (**d**).

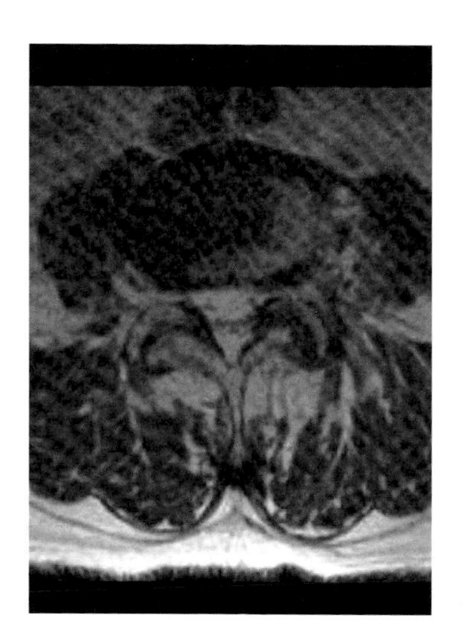

Fig. 3.13 MR image of T12 (axial, T2). Marked dehydration of the disks in the thoracolumbar junction with broad-based intraligamentous disk protrusions in the left lateral region (< 50 % of the circumference).

Clinical Aspects

- **Typical presentation**
  Usually asymptomatic • Nonspecific, nondiskogenic back pain • Typically, pain at the level of the disk, intensity of pain increased with coughing and pressing • Characteristic sensory and motor deficits.
- **Therapeutic options**
  Acute low back pain: Analgesia • Physical therapy, specific back exercises • Correction of posture • Strengthening of the local musculature • Surgery is indicated only if several attempts at conservative therapy are unsuccessful (except in the presence of distal neurologic deficits, or bladder or rectal paralysis).

Differential Diagnosis

Disk bulge	– > 50% of the circumference of the vertebra = disk bulge and not herniation
Nondiskogenic spinal stenosis or neural foraminal stenosis	– Osteophytes – Facet joint degeneration with marked proliferation of osteophytes and hypertrophy of the ligamenta flava
Diskitis	– Entire disk hyperintense on T2-weighted images – Associated bone marrow edema – Soft tissue component – Increased inflammatory markers (does not invariably occur)

Selected References

Bohndorf K, Imhof H. Radiologische Diagnostik der Knochen und Gelenke, 2nd ed. Stuttgart: Thieme 2006

Greenspan A. Orthopedic Radiology. A Practical Approach. 3rd ed. Philadelphia: Lippincott Williams and Wilkins 2000

Luoma K: Low back pain in relation to lumbar disc degeneration. Spine 2000; 25: 487–492

Milette PC. Differentiating lumbar disc protrusions, disc bulges, and discs with normal contour but abnormal signal intensity. Magnetic resonance imaging with discographic correlations. Spine 1999; 24: 44–53

Moulopoulos LA. MR prediction of benign and malignant vertebral compression fractures. J Magn Reson Imaging 1996; 6: 667–674

Pardon DF, Milette PC. Nomenclature and Classification of Lumbar Disc Pathology. Spine 2001; 26: E93–113

Vahlensieck M, Reiser M. MRT des Bewegungsapparates, 3rd ed. Stuttgart: Thieme 2006

Definition

- **Epidemiology**
  L5–S1 is most often affected • *Note:* Up to 50% of patients over 50 years may have asymptomatic disk protrusions and extrusions that often resolve within 9–12 months ("physiologic aging" of the disk).
- **Etiology, pathophysiology, pathogenesis**
  Rupture of the annulus fibrosus with circumscribed transligamentous bulging of the disk material (mainly portions of the nucleus pulposus, hyperintense on T1-weighted images).
  Extrusion: Disk material is primarily displaced posteriorly • The largest diameter of the displaced disk material is larger than its diameter where it exits the interspace, creating a "neck" of displaced material.
  Sequestration: Loss of continuity of the disk with displacement of portions of the nucleus pulposus, which migrate either through the ligament to lodge against the dura or within the ligament along the posterior margin of the vertebra • The migrating tissue has no connection with "mother" disk • Separation of disk material.

Imaging Signs

- **Modality of choice**
  - MRI (sagittal, axial).
  - CT (where MRI is not available or contraindicated).
- **Radiographic findings**
  Nonspecific (reduced height of disk interspaces) • Disk calcification (65% of cases) • Vacuum phenomenon.
- **CT findings**
  Bulging of disk material (isodense to soft tissue) • Disk material in the lateral recess (displacing the fatty tissue) or along the posterior margin of the vertebra, suggesting sequestration (sagittal reconstruction with multidetector CT) • Calcification • Vacuum phenomenon.
- **MRI findings**
  Position relative to posterior longitudinal ligament • Discontinuity of disk • Subligamentous or transligamentous bulging of disk material (isointense to soft tissue) • Position relative to dural sac (displacement, deformation, myelopathy), spinal stenosis • Position relative to nerve roots (contact with or displacement of perineural fatty tissue; neuropathy appears as thickening and signal alteration of the nerve root) • Neural foraminal stenosis • Separated disk material within the spine (sequestrum) • Marginal contrast enhancement • Accompanying vacuum phenomenon is proof of degeneration.
  Caution: Where spinal stenosis is present, CSF signal loss often occurs in the adjacent anatomy. This signal void due to flow turbulence can mimic a sequestrum • MRI findings should be correlated with the clinical findings.

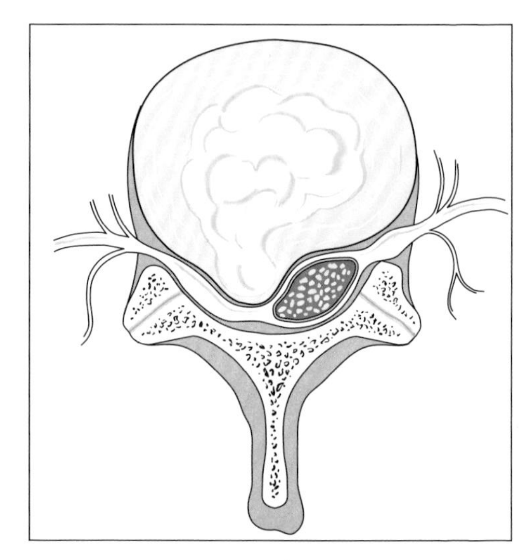

Fig. 3.14 Schematic diagram (axial). Broad-based protrusion of disk material. The outer part of the annulus fibrosus is torn, allowing the nucleus pulposus to protrude. Entrapment of the dural sac with displacement of the fibers of the cauda equina (protrusion).

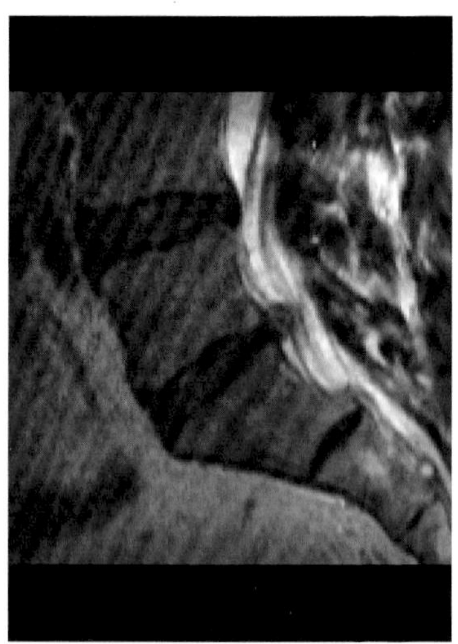

Fig. 3.15 MR image of the lumbosacral region (sagittal, T2). Posterior transligamentous disk herniation with a neck of displaced disk tissue (extrusion at the level of the disk).

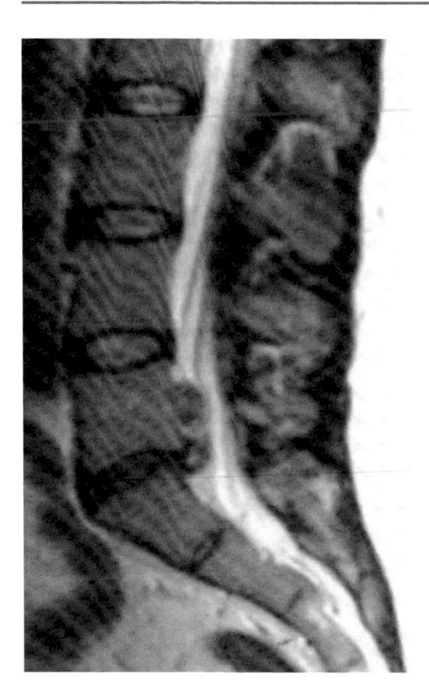

Fig. 3.16 MR image of the lumbar spine (sagittal, T2). Cranially displaced disk material (sequestration).

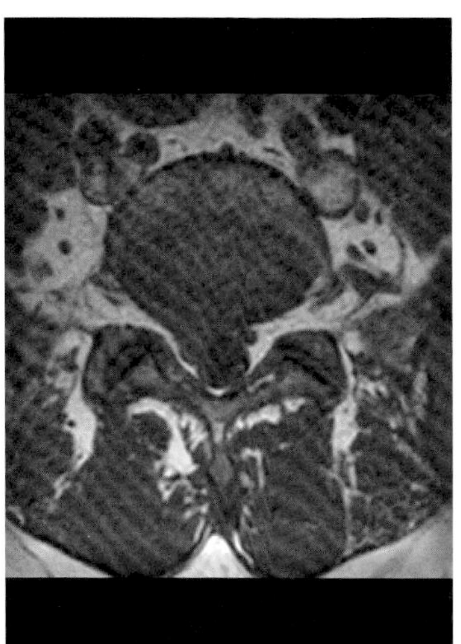

Fig. 3.17 MR image of the lumbar spine (axial, T1). Circumscribed right ipsilateral broad-based transligamentous disk herniation at L5 with displaced nucleus pulposus tissue in contact with the dural sac (disk protrusion).

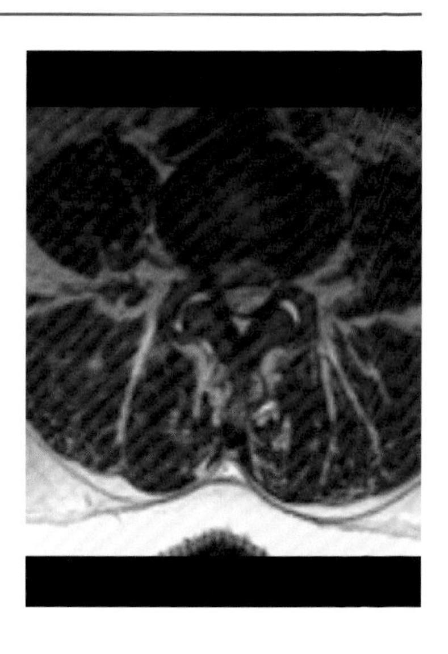

Fig. 3.18 MR image of L3 (axial, T2). Posterior sequestrum from L3.

Clinical Aspects

- **Typical presentation**
  Low back pain • Radicular pain • *Caution:* In the presence of motor deficits, bladder paralysis, and rectal paralysis a neurosurgeon or neurologist should be consulted about whether surgery is indicated.
- **Therapeutic options**
  This depends on the site of the extruded disk material (median, mediolateral, foraminal, or extraforaminal location) • In most cases (90%), symptoms disappear within 4–8 weeks • Like protrusion, disk extrusion in patients over 50 is mostly asymptomatic (reflecting physiologic aging of the disk) • Imaging findings should be correlated with clinical findings.
  Sequestration: Depends on clinical findings; sequestration can resolve spontaneously • *Acute low back pain:* Analgesia, NSAIDs, corticosteroids • Bed rest (controversial) • Physical therapy, specific back exercises • Correction of posture • Strengthening of the local musculature • Pain resistant to conservative therapy and/or neurologic deficits are treated by diskectomy, chemonucleolysis, or laminectomy.

Differential Diagnosis

Nondiskogenic spinal stenosis or neural foraminal stenosis	– Osteophytes – Facet joint degeneration with marked proliferation of osteophytes and hypertrophy of the ligamenta flava
Epidural fibrosis	– Postoperative – Homogeneous enhancement
Schwannoma	

Selected References

Bohndorf K, Imhof H. Radiologische Diagnostik der Knochen und Gelenke, 2nd ed. Stuttgart: Thieme 2006

Greenspan A. Orthopedic Radiology. A Practical Approach. 3rd ed. Philadelphia: Lippincott Williams and Wilkins 2000

Möller, Reif. CT- und MRT-Normalbefunde. Stuttgart: Thieme 1998

Pardon DF, Milette PC. Nomenclature and classification of lumbar disc pathology. Spine 2001; 26: E93–113

Vahlensieck M, Reiser M. MRT des Bewegungsapparates, 3rd ed. Stuttgart: Thieme 2006

Yasuma T. The histology of lumbar intervertebral disc herniation. The significance of small blood vessels in the extruded tissue. Spine 1993; 18: 1761–1765

Zollner J. Radiological assessment of loss of disk height in acute and chronic degenerative lumbar disk changes. Röfo 2001; 173: 187–190

Definition

- **Epidemiology**
  Disk displacement occurs in 5–6% of people aged over 50 years • Disk calcifications are more common in the thoracic spine. In children, they are not uncommon in the cervical spine (most likely a posttraumatic condition).
- **Etiology, pathophysiology, pathogenesis**
  Disk degeneration results in release of gas (nitrogen) from the disk material (vacuum phenomenon) • The vacuum phenomenon is pathognomonic of disk degeneration and occurs in the lower lumbar and cervical spine • Disk degeneration can also result in calcium deposits (hydroxylapatite, calcium pyrophosphate), usually in the annulus fibrosus, rarely in the nucleus pulposus.

Imaging Signs

- **Modality of choice**
  Conventional radiographs or CT
- **Radiographic findings**
  A-P and lateral • The vacuum phenomenon shows gas density and is mostly limited to the disk • Disk calcification appears as either spurlike or homogeneously dense calcification in the disk (usually the annulus fibrosus).
- **CT findings**
  The signs are the same as on conventional radiographs.
- **MRI findings**
  The gas is hypointense on T1 and T2 • The calcifications are typically hypointense on T1 and T2.

Clinical Aspects

- **Typical presentation**
  See p. 87 • Usually asymptomatic.
- **Therapeutic options**
  See p. 89.

Differential Diagnosis

Disk calcification	– Metabolic disorders (chronic pyrophosphate disease, hydroxylapatite, gout, diabetes, hyperparathyroidism, etc.) – Posttraumatic
Vacuum phenomenon	– Caution: bowel may be superimposed

Selected References

Bullough PC, Boachie-Adjei O. Atlas of Spinal Diseases. Philadelphia: JB Lippincott 1998

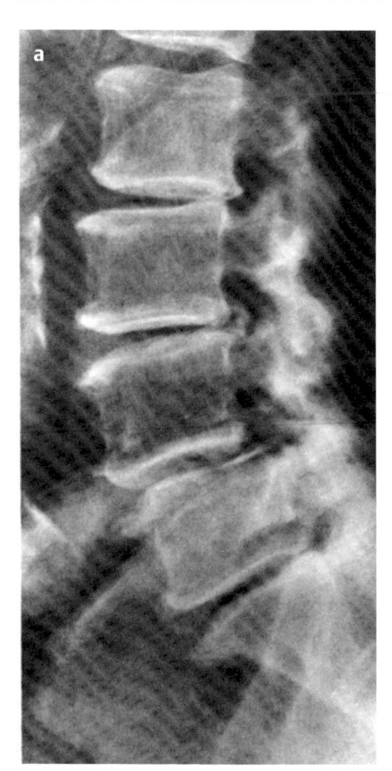

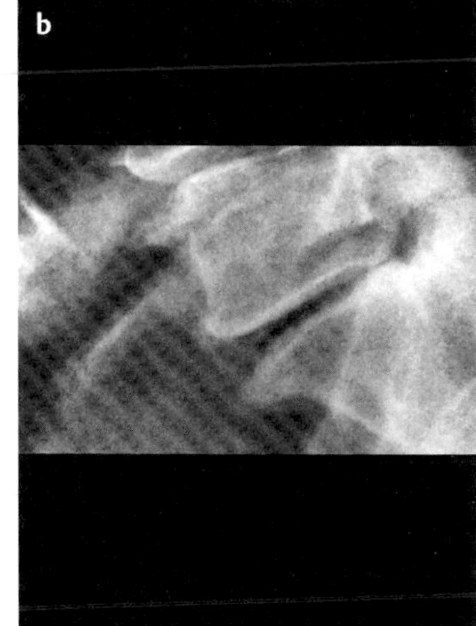

Fig. 3.19 ***a, b*** Conventional lateral radiographs of the lumbar spine. Reduced disk height at L2–S1 with vacuum phenomenon in each disk. Other findings include subchondral sclerosis (Modic III) and pseudospondylolisthesis at L4–L5 (Meyerding grade I) with osteophytes. Posterior osteophytes at L2–L3.

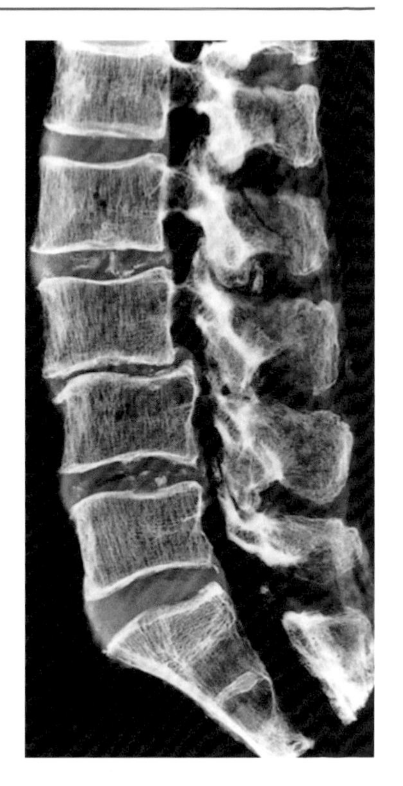

Fig. 3.20 Conventional lateral radiograph of the lumbar spine (specimen). Disk narrowing at L3–L4. Marked disk calcification is seen at L2–L3 and L4–L5. Pseudospondylolisthesis at L3–L4.

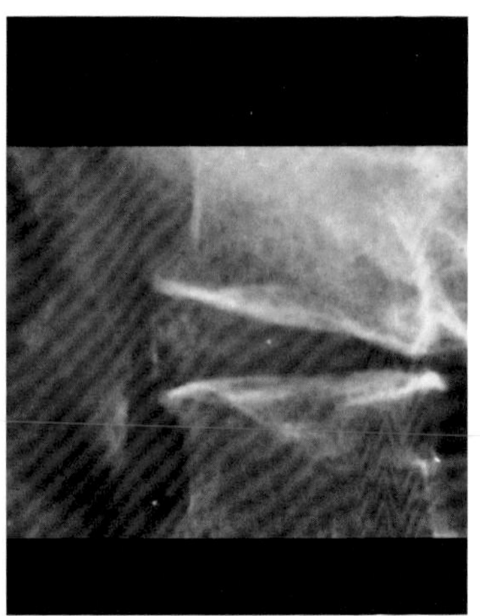

Fig. 3.21 Conventional lateral radiograph of L1–L2 (detail). Disk calcification. Schmorl nodes in the superior endplate of L2.

Definition (Spondylarthritis, Osteoarthritis of the Facet Joints)

- **Epidemiology**
  Occurs in the setting of degenerative spinal disease with increasing age (almost invariably present in people over 60 years of age).
- **Etiology, pathophysiology, pathogenesis**
  Facet joint degeneration, osteoarthritis of the facet joints • In the setting of degenerative spinal disease, reduced disk height and a consequent shift in the axis with disk degeneration lead to pseudospondylolisthesis and abnormal stresses that in turn cause facet joint degeneration • Scoliosis and asymmetry also influence facet joint degeneration, and vice versa.

Imaging Signs

- **Modality of choice**
  Conventional A-P, lateral, and oblique radiographs • MRI or CT indicated when radicular symptoms are present.
- **Radiographic findings**
  Typical signs of osteoarthritis of a synovial joint with joint space narrowing, marginal osteophytes, subchondral sclerosis and cysts, deformation, and synovial cysts • The stress view shows functionally fused vertebrae and increased mobility in adjacent segments.
- **CT findings**
  Typical signs of osteoarthritis of a synovial joint with joint space narrowing, occasional vacuum phenomenon, marginal osteophytes, subchondral sclerosis, subchondral cysts, and deformation.
- **MRI findings**
  Typical signs of osteoarthritis of a synovial joint with joint space narrowing, cartilage damage, marginal osteophytes, subchondral sclerosis, and occasionally effusion (or a synovial cyst), subchondral cysts, and deformation • Lateral recess > 4–5 mm.

Clinical Aspects

- **Typical presentation**
  Pain, and segmental symptoms where there is constriction of the neural foramina (see Prolapse) • Progressive as in osteoarthritis.
- **Therapeutic options**
  Lumbago is treated with analgesics and infiltration of pain relieving drugs where indicated • Physical therapy • Radicular symptoms may require foraminotomy, posterior spacers, or spinal fusion.

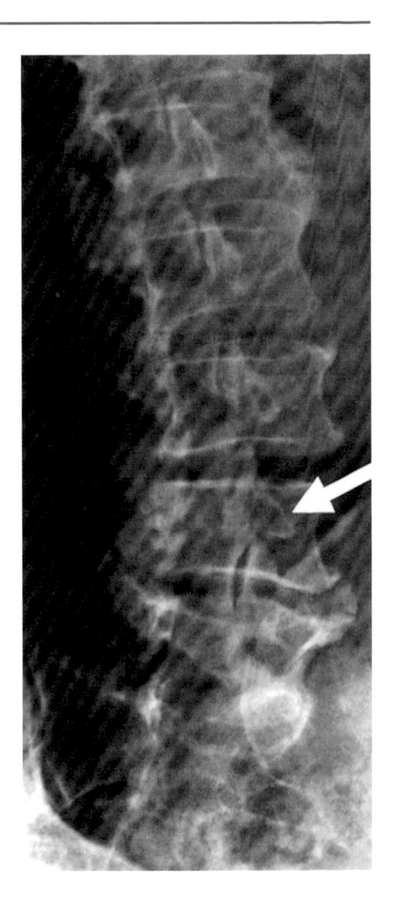

Fig. 3.22 Conventional oblique radiographs of the lumbar spine. Marked spondylarthritis with joint space narrowing, subchondral sclerosis, and marginal osteophytes.

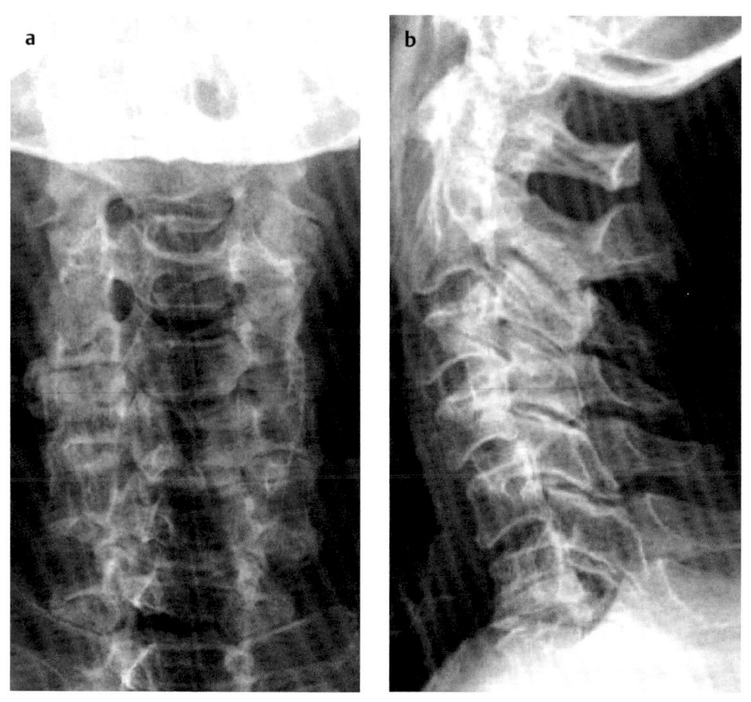

Fig. 3.23 a, b Conventional A-P and lateral radiographs of the cervical spine. Sclerosis in the facet joints with significant thickening and joint space narrowing.

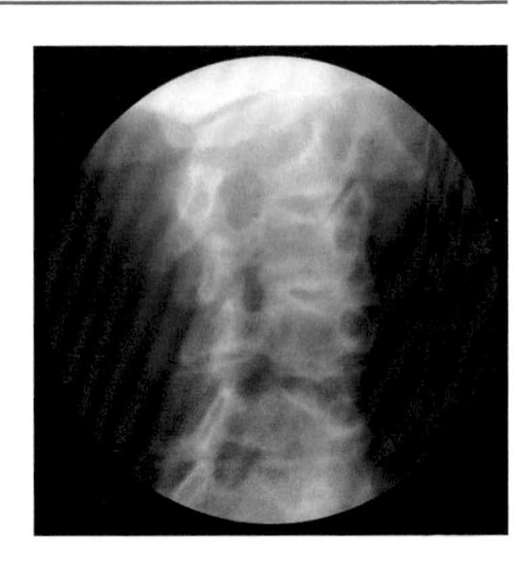

Fig. 3.24 Conventional oblique radiograph of the cervical spine. Marked foraminal stenosis at C3–C4 in spondylarthritis.

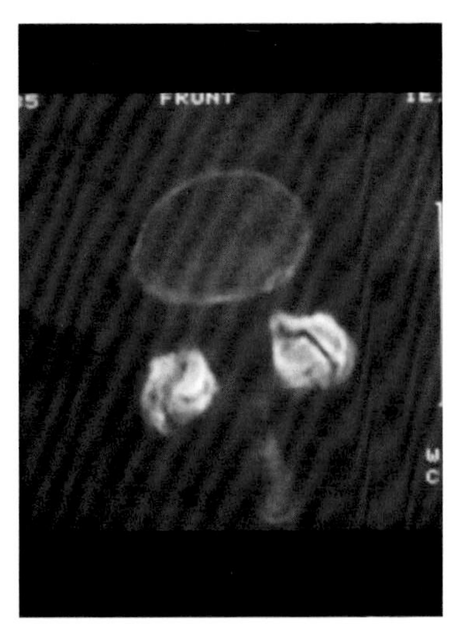

Fig. 3.25 CT of L3 (axial, bone window). Markedly irregular demarcated facet joints with subchondral sclerosis, joint space narrowing, and marginal osteophytes consistent with spondylarthritis.

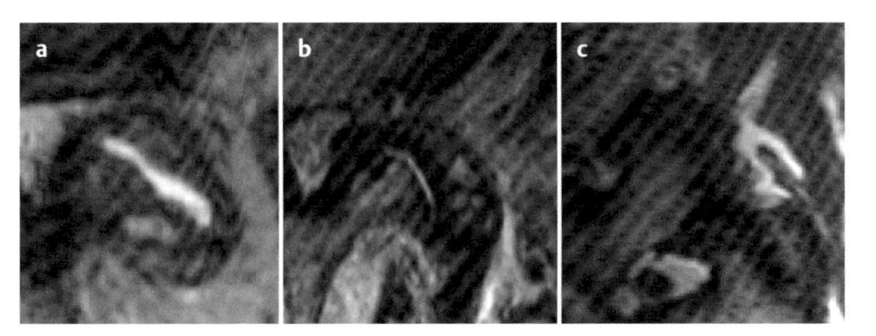

Fig. 3.26 a–c MR image of the lumbar spine (detail **a**; axial **b**; sagittal **c**; T2). Effusion, subchondral sclerosis, osteophytes, deformation.

Differential Diagnosis

Inflammation	– History – Erosion – Other changes typical of inflammation or infection – Possibly synovitis
Fracture	– CT is often better – History

Selected References

Bohndorf K, Imhof H. Radiologische Diagnostik der Knochen und Gelenke, 2nd ed. Stuttgart: Thieme 2006

Resnick, D, Niwayama G (eds.). Diagnosis of Bone and Joint Disorders. 3rd ed. Philadelphia: Saunders 1995

Tournade A, Patay Z, Krupa P, Tajahmady T, Millon S, Braun M. A comparative study of the anatomical, radiological and therapeutic features of the lumbar facet joints. Neuroradiology 1992; 34: 257

Vahlensieck M, Reiser M. MRT des Bewegungsapparates, 3rd ed. Stuttgart: Thieme 2006

Definition

- **Epidemiology**
  Occurs in the setting of degenerative spinal disease with increasing age.
- **Etiology, pathophysiology, pathogenesis**
  Proliferation of osteophytes along the posterolateral margins of the cervical disk interspaces • Uncovertebral "spondylosis" • Posttraumatic • Typically there is no disk material along the margins of the disk interspaces in the cervical spine • Loss of disk height leads to local irritation with compression and traction • This stimulates bone remodeling • Subsequent osteoarthritic changes, which are also influenced by scoliosis and asymmetry.

Imaging Signs

- **Modality of choice**
  - Conventional A-P, lateral, and oblique radiographs.
  - CT and/or MRI are indicated for radicular symptoms.
- **Radiographic findings**
  In the cervical spine, the posterolateral vertebral margins appear jagged with proliferation of osteophytes and narrowing of the disk interspaces • Subchondral sclerosis • Deformation.
- **CT findings**
  Signs of osteoarthritis in a pseudarthrosis with joint space narrowing • Marginal osteophytes • Sclerosis • Deformation.
- **MRI findings**
  Degenerative changes in a pseudarthrosis with marginal osteophytes • Joint space narrowing • Bone marrow changes • Edema • Fatty degeneration • Sclerosis • Deformation.

Clinical Aspects

- **Typical presentation**
  Pain especially in rotation • Narrowing the neural foramina will also produce segmental symptoms.
- **Therapeutic options**
  In cervical pain syndrome, analgesics, corticoids, and/or infiltration of pain relieving drugs may be indicated • Physical therapy • Manual therapy • Surgery (foraminotomy) may be indicated for radicular symptoms.

Differential Diagnosis

Congenital vertebral deformity

Selected References

Bohndorf K, Imhof H. Radiologische Diagnostik der Knochen und Gelenke, 2nd ed. Stuttgart: Thieme 2006

Dihlmann W. Joints and Vertebral Connections. Stuttgart: Thieme 1985

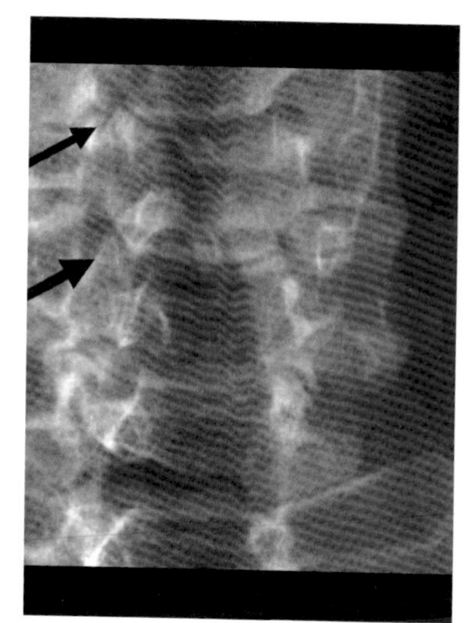

Fig. 3.27 Conventional A-P radiograph. The uncovertebral joints are seen (some vertebral rotation is present due to degenerative abnormal mobility). The margins appear jagged and the joint space narrowed with increased sclerosis in the superior segment (arrow); the uncovertebral joint in the inferior segment (arrow) appears normal.

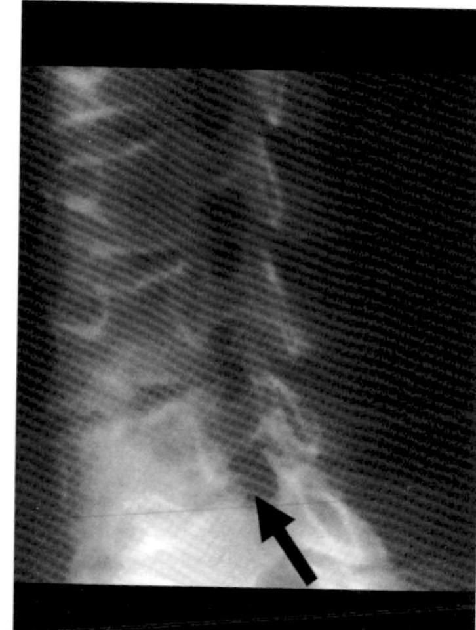

Fig. 3.28 Conventional oblique radiograph. Large osteophytes in the uncovertebral region consistent with uncovertebral "joint osteoarthritis."

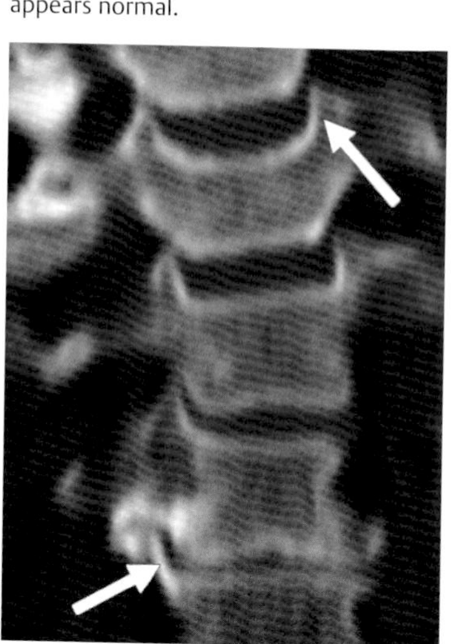

Fig. 3.29 CT (coronal reconstruction). The uncovertebral "joints" appear thickened and jagged with narrowing of the joint spaces and subchondral sclerosis.

Definition

- **Epidemiology**
  Occurs in the setting of facet joint degeneration with increasing age • Lower lumbar spine • More common in men than women • Peak age 40–60 years.
- **Etiology, pathophysiology, pathogenesis**
  Synovial cyst of the facet joint in spondylarthritis (synovial irritation with effusion) • No synonyms • Degenerative synovial cyst in the setting of spondylarthritis and synovial irritation and synovitis.

Imaging Signs

- **Modality of choice**
  MRI: Sagittal, axial (STIR, T2).
- **CT findings**
  Difficult to detect because of the poor soft tissue contrast • Osteoarthritis of the facet joints is visualized and synovial enhancement is seen with contrast administration • Hemorrhagic contents and calcification are visualized.
- **MRI findings**
  Synovial cyst (epidural posterolateral lesion) is visualized adjacent to the degenerative facet joint • Signal intensity varies according to whether the contents are isointense to fluid, have a high protein content, or are hemorrhagic • The facet synovium may be thickened; enhancement after contrast administration is a sign of synovitis (= synovialitis).

Clinical Aspects

- **Typical presentation**
  Spondylarthritis is often symptomatic • Lumbago is present, as are segmental symptoms in the presence of spinal stenosis or narrowed neural foramina • Symptoms of degenerative spinal disease.
- **Therapeutic options**
  Infiltration of pain relieving drugs may be indicated for lumbago • Radicular symptoms require surgery (cyst removal with laminectomy or hemilaminectomy).
- **Course and Prognosis**
  Typical course of osteoarthritis • Good success rate.

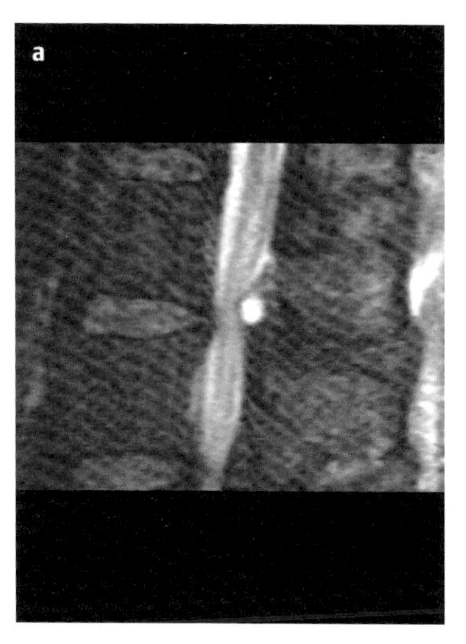

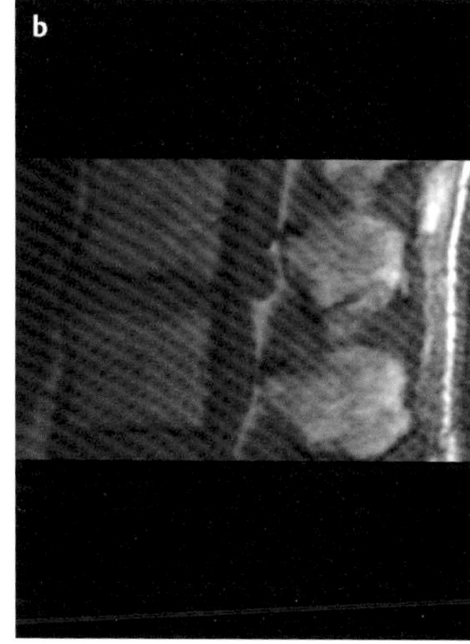

Fig. 3.30 a, b MR image of the lumbar spine (sagittal, STIR, T1). Synovial cyst isointense to fluid with significant compression of the dural sac.

Differential Diagnosis

Root canal cyst	– Communicates with the subarachnoid space, isointense to CSF – Root courses within the cyst
Disk herniation	– Continuous with and often isointense to the disk – Rarely posterolateral – Not always identifiable

Selected References

Bohndorf K, Imhof H. Radiologische Diagnostik der Knochen und Gelenke, 2nd ed. Stuttgart: Thieme 2006

Vahlensieck M, Reiser M. MRT des Bewegungsapparates, 3rd ed. Stuttgart: Thieme 2006

Definition

Thickening of the ligamenta flava in excess of 6 mm in the setting of degenerative spinal disease • Often due to muscular insufficiency • Often incipient degenerative spinal or disk disease • Shift in the axis and resulting abnormal stresses place excessive loads on the ligaments • Scoliosis and asymmetry also influence this disorder • Predilection for the lumbar spine.

Imaging Signs

- **Modality of choice**
  MRI: axial, T1.
- **MRI findings**
  Thickening of the ligamenta flava in excess of 6 mm.

Clinical Aspects

- **Typical presentation**
  Most cases are asymptomatic, although pain may occur • With spinal stenosis there may also be segmental symptoms (see also Spinal Stenosis, p. 126).
- **Therapeutic options**
  See also Spinal Stenosis, p. 126.

Differential Diagnosis

Ligament ossification	– Ossification of the ligamentum flavum, middle cervical and lower thoracic spine – Rare

Selected References

Vahlensieck M, Reiser M. MRT des Bewegungsapparates, 3rd ed. Stuttgart: Thieme 2006

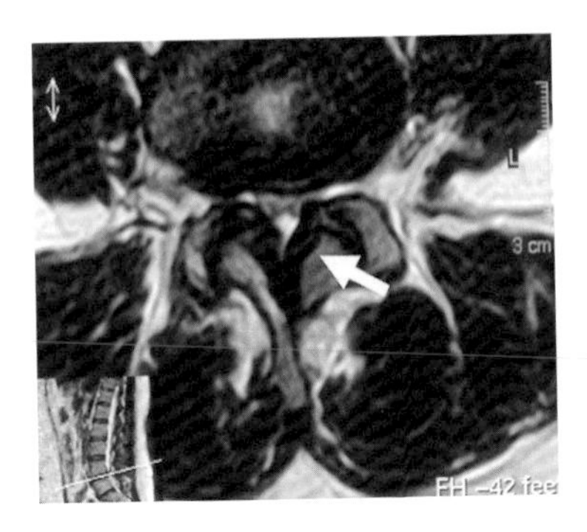

Fig. 3.31 MR image (axial, T1). Spinal stenosis with marked thickening of the ligamenta flava.

Definition

Interspinous pseudarthrosis • "Kissing spine" • In the setting of increased lordosis, reactive cartilage and bone formation occurs in the spinous processes • This in turn leads to calcifications in the supraspinous and interspinous ligaments, also rarely in the ligamentum flavum • The height of the disk interspaces is often reduced • In the terminal stage this leads to thickening of the spinous processes • Most commonly occurs in the lumbar spine • In rare cases, the cervical spine may also be affected.

Imaging Signs

- **Modality of choice**
  Conventional radiographs with supplementary stress views.
- **Radiographic findings**
  Sufficient in nearly all cases • A-P and lateral • Additional flexion and extension views may be needed to confirm the diagnosis • Abnormal contact between adjacent spinous processes with increased sclerosis.
- **MRI findings**
  - Calcification of the ligaments (hypointense on T1- and T2-weighted images)
  - Cystoid ligament degeneration (hyperintense on T2-weighted images).

Clinical Aspects

- **Typical presentation**
  Middle-aged and elderly patients complain of chronic lumbago • Symptoms are aggravated by activity requiring prolonged stooped posture (spinal flexion) • Affected areas are tender on palpation and painful when tapped • Very rarely, the discomfort can also radiate to the legs.
- **Therapeutic options**
  Physical therapy with muscle strengthening and muscle relaxing exercises • Heat therapy • Ergotherapy • Acute symptoms may require a brief course of analgesics or local infiltration of pain relieving drugs.

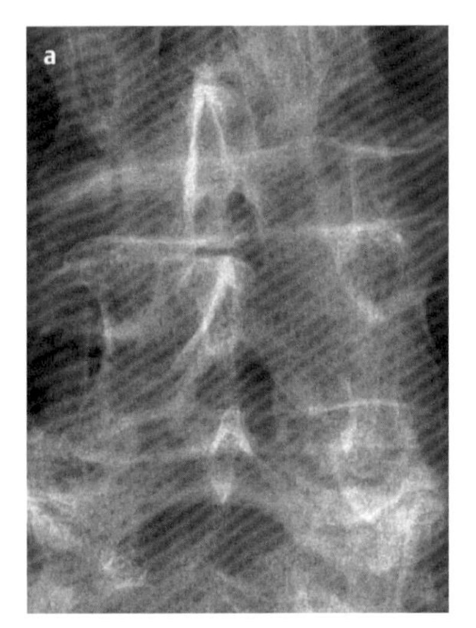

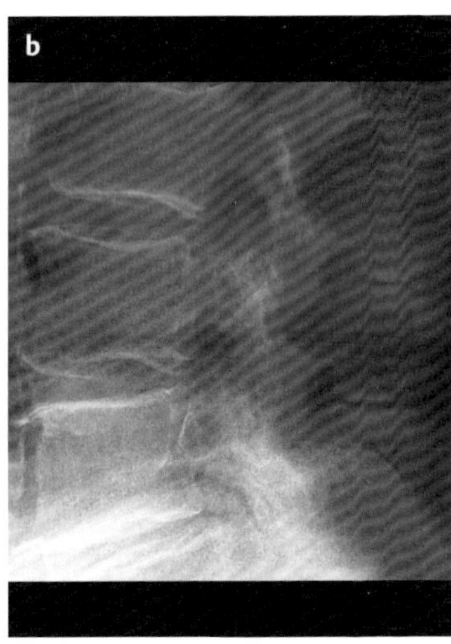

Fig. 3.32 a, b Baastrup disease. Conventional radiographs of L2–L4 (A-P and lateral, detail). Thickening of the spinous processes with “kissing spine.”

Differential Diagnosis

Scoliosis	– Severe deviation from normal axis – Peak age from birth to age 20
Trauma	– Fracture of the spinous process is extremely rare – Bony bridging in the fracture region – Ossification in the surrounding soft tissue mantle – Often accompanied by degenerative disk disease and osteoarthritis in the adjacent joints
Disk herniation	– Sensory deficits or loss of strength in the extremities
Calcium pyrophosphate disease (CPPD)	– Sclerosis occurs only in the ligamenta flava; the interspinous ligaments are not involved

Selected References

Josenhans G. Kreuzschmerzen bei Dornfortsatzveränderungen: Eine Studie zur Baastrupschen Krankheit. Z Rheumaforsch 1954; 13: 361

Resnick D. Degenerative diseases of the vertebral column. Radiology 1985; 156: 3

Definition

- **Epidemiology**
  L4 or L5 is involved in 90% of all cases • Spondylolisthesis is usually diagnosed during childhood or adolescence • Pseudospondylolisthesis usually occurs after 40 years of age • Predisposing factors for spondylolisthesis include Marfan syndrome, osteoporosis, osteogenesis imperfecta, hereditary factors, and sport such as wrestling, weight lifting, and soccer.
- **Etiology, pathophysiology, pathogenesis**
  "Genuine or apparent" vertebral slippage • Spondylolisthesis.
  - *Spondylolisthesis:* Anterior subluxation of a vertebra with a defect in the pedicle and/or pars interarticularis. This occurs in the setting of either spondylolysis or pars interarticularis dysplasia (the spinous process is in a normal position whereas the vertebral body is anteriorly displaced).
  - *Pseudospondylolisthesis:* Anterior subluxation of a vertebra with interruption of posterior continuity of the spine (i.e., the entire vertebra is anteriorly displaced). Causes include degenerative disk changes and/or facet joint degeneration.

  The Meyerding classification has four grades: 1–4 (displacement of < 25%, < 50%, < 75%, and 100%) (see also Fig. 2.**35**, p. 81).

Imaging Signs

- **Modality of choice**
  Conventional oblique and stress radiographs are sufficient in most cases • CT or MRI may be indicated where extensive clinical symptoms are present (spinal stenosis).
- **Radiographic findings**
  Anterior displacement of a vertebra relative to the adjacent caudal vertebra • In spondylolysis, a typical "collar" can be observed on the "Scotty dog" figure on the oblique films.
  Stress radiographs: Evaluation of stability (degree of maximal anterior and lateral displacement) in flexion, extension, and lateral bending.
- **CT findings**
  - Used for detailed evaluation of spondylolysis, as incomplete ring following a fracture or spinal stenosis can be precisely visualized.
  - Evaluation of degenerative changes causing pseudospondylolisthesis.
- **MRI findings**
  T1- and T2-weighted images show reduced signal intensity in the pars interarticularis in spondylolisthesis • In pseudospondylolisthesis, findings include degenerative changes (reduced disk height, a hypointense disk, Modic sign, and osteoarthritis of the facet joints).
  Early spondylolysis: Vertebral arch shows edema with linear interruptions.
  Spondylolisthesis: Only the vertebral body displaces anteriorly (spinous process remains in its normal position).

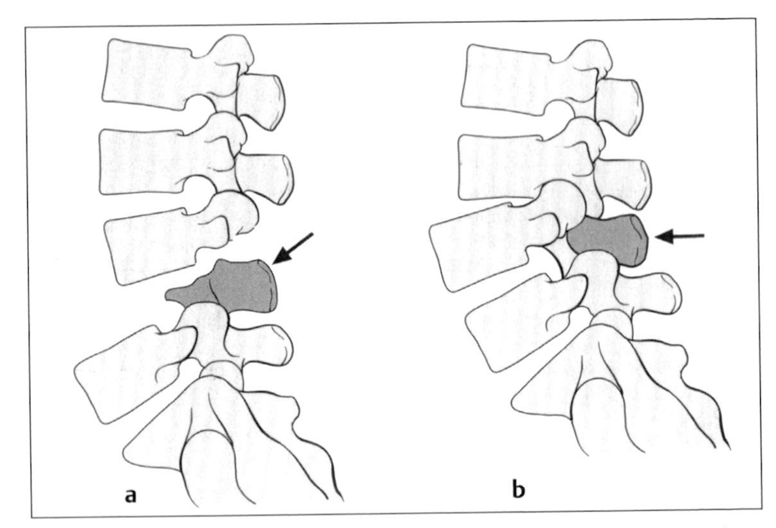

Fig. 3.33 a, b Lateral view of lumbar spine. Spondylolisthesis with defect (**a**), Pseudospondylolisthesis without defect (**b**).

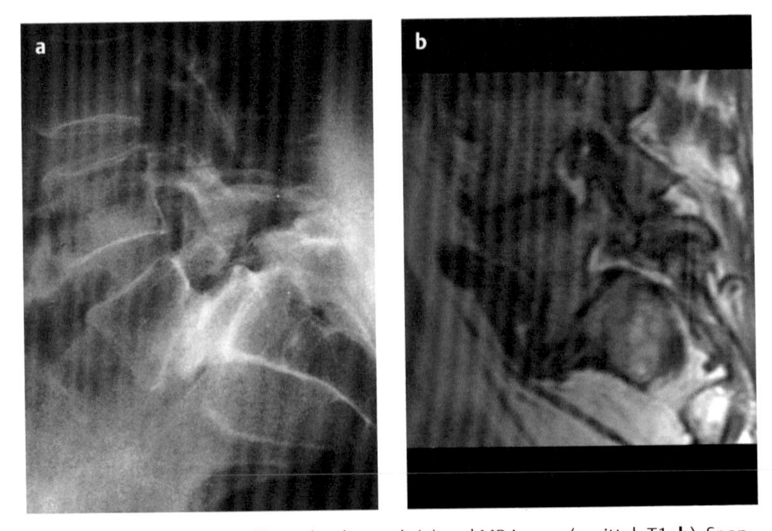

Fig. 3.34 a, b Conventional lateral radiograph (**a**) and MR image (sagittal, T1; **b**). Spondylolisthesis with anterior slippage at L5–S1, spondylolysis in the vertebral arch of L5.

Pseudospondylolisthesis: Entire vertebral displaces anteriorly (including the spinous process) • The spinal canal and/or neural foramina may be narrowed (spinal stenosis) • Loss of fatty tissue around the nerve root.

Clinical Aspects

- **Typical presentation**
  Often asymptomatic in younger patients • Chronic back pain that increases with strenuous activity • Higher-grade spondylolisthesis is often also associated with radicular symptoms, gait abnormalities, paresthesias, or signs of spinal stenosis with bladder and rectal dysfunction.
- **Therapeutic options**
  Grades 1 and 2: Conservative therapy with a corset, restriction of physical activity, and physical therapy.
  Grades 3 and 4 (also applies to any symptomatic form): Posterolateral fusion or cast treatment • Analgesics may be prescribed for a short period of time when acute symptoms are present.

Differential Diagnosis

Partial facetectomy or sclerotic neck of the pars interarticularis	– Can mimic spondylolysis
Trauma with fracture	
Post laminectomy	
Spondylitis	

Selected References

Coughlin WF, McMurdo SK. CT diagnosis of spodylolysis of the axis vertebra. AJR 1989; 153: 195

Lee J-H, Ehara S, Tamakawa Y et al. Spondylolysis of the upper lumbar spine: Radiological features. Clin Imag 1999; 23: 389

Shipley JA, Beukes CA. The nature of the spondylolytic defect: Demonstration of a communicating synovial pseudarthrosis in the pars interarticularis. J Bone and Joint Surg Br 1998; 80: 662

Definition

Narrowing of the spinal canal from all sides due to numerous changes that reinforce each other in the setting of degenerative spinal disease • Spinal stenosis resulting from several components of degenerative spinal disease:
- Spondylosis deformans.
- Disk displacement.
- Osteoarthritis of the facet joints.
- Synovial cysts.
- Uncovertebral osteoarthritis.
- Thickening of the ligamenta flava.
- Subsequent abnormal mobility in the spine with degenerative pseudospondylolisthesis, which itself is conducive to the pathology described above.

Imaging Signs

- **Modality of choice**
  - Conventional radiographs: A-P, lateral, and stress radiographs.
  - CT: coronal, axial • Bony stenosis.
  - MRI: coronal, axial, T1, T2 • Neural structures.
- **Radiographic findings**

  An initial radiograph will provide an overview of axial deformities and of the severity and distribution of overall pathology. Stress view obtained with patient standing (or sitting). Other stress views (flexion, extension, lateral bending) to quantify degenerative instability. Exclusion of other severe pathology.

  Stress views are obtained in maximal flexion, extension, and/or lateral bending. Normally the individual vertebrae overlap one another like roof shingles in flexion, while the disk interspaces show uniform anterior expansion in extension. Look for any segmental blocks, motion in the opposite direction, or vertebral displacement. Motion must invariably progress uniformly, with the angle of motion increasing continuously from C2 to C7.
- **CT findings**

  Demonstrates the width of the spinal canal and also the width of the neural foramina.
- **MRI findings**

  This modality allows the best evaluation of the overall situation with high soft tissue contrast and good visualization of the neural structures with any secondary radiculopathy or myelopathy.

  There may be atrophy of the paravertebral musculature.

  Width of the spinal canal: Interpedicular distance < 16 mm (gray area above this). Transverse diameter < 20–21 mm, L5 < 24 mm, lateral recess < 4–5 mm. It is crucial to obtain a semiquantitative evaluation by comparing findings with unaffected sections. The severity of degenerative spondylolisthesis is graded according to the Meyerding classification (see Spondylolisthesis and Fig. 2.**35**, p. 81).

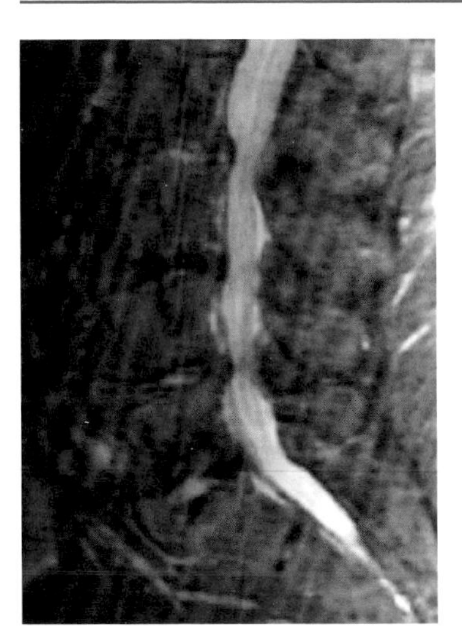

Fig. 3.35 MR image of the lumbar spine (sagittal, T2). Multisegmental stenosis of the spinal canal from posterior osteophytes.

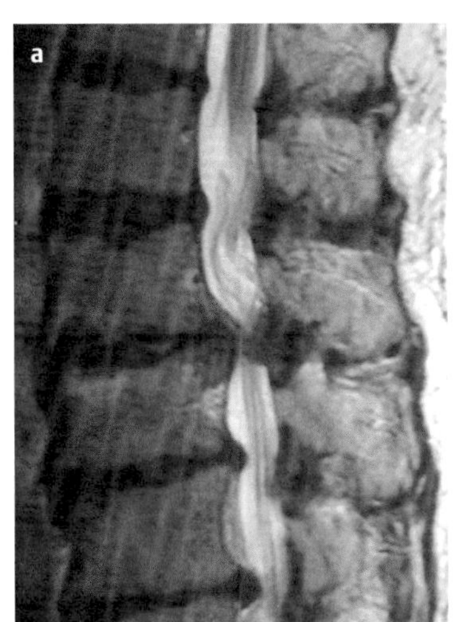

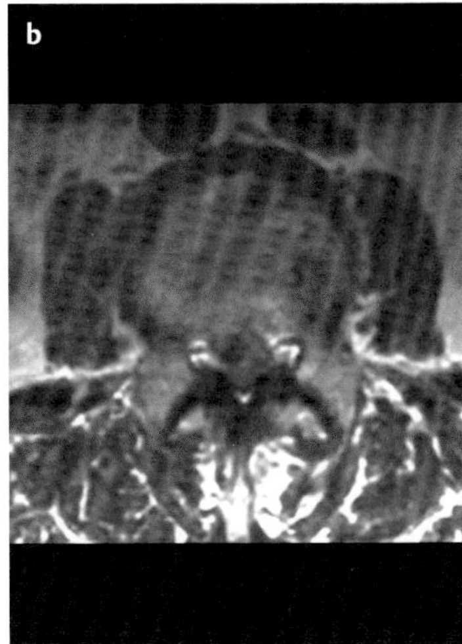

Fig. 3.36 a, b MR image of the thoracolumbar spine (**a** sagittal, **b** axial; T2). Multisegmental stenosis with maximal severity at L2–L3, where there is median disk protrusion. Hypertrophy of the ligamenta flava. Elongated course of the fibers of the cauda equina. Modic II disk degeneration with Schmorl nodes.

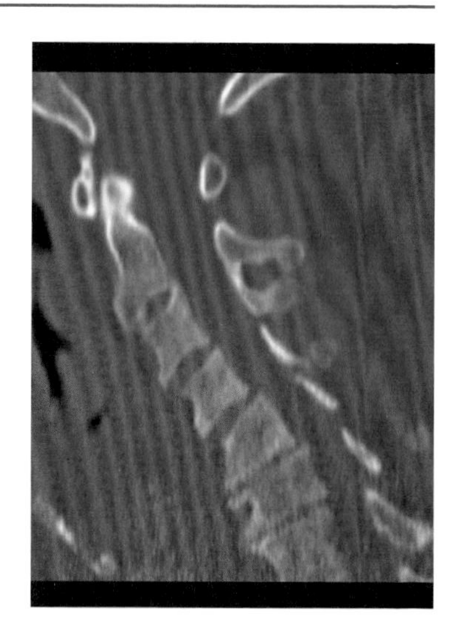

Fig. 3.37 CT of the cervical spine (coronal reconstruction). Pronounced extension with marked paradoxical kyphosis C5–C7. Posterior pseudospondylolisthesis with spinal stenosis in the presence of severe degenerative disk disease at levels C5–C7.

Clinical Aspects

- **Typical presentation**

  Symptoms range from none to severe pain (usually pseudoradicular or segmental pain).

  Sensory or motor deficits may occur. These will depend on the level of the pathology; cauda equina syndrome involves bladder and rectal dysfunction and "saddle" anesthesia. Simultaneous narrowing of the neural foramina will also produce segmental symptoms (see Herniation). Progressive clinical symptoms suggest primary bone pathology.

- **Therapeutic options**

  Treatment is conservative, although neurologic symptoms may require surgical decompression (laminectomy, hemilaminectomy, fusion). Diskogenic symptoms often resolve spontaneously, especially in older patients.

Differential Diagnosis

Inflammatory	– Pannus in rheumatic disorders – Abscess in bacterial infection
Tumorous conditions	– Such as ependymoma, bone tumors

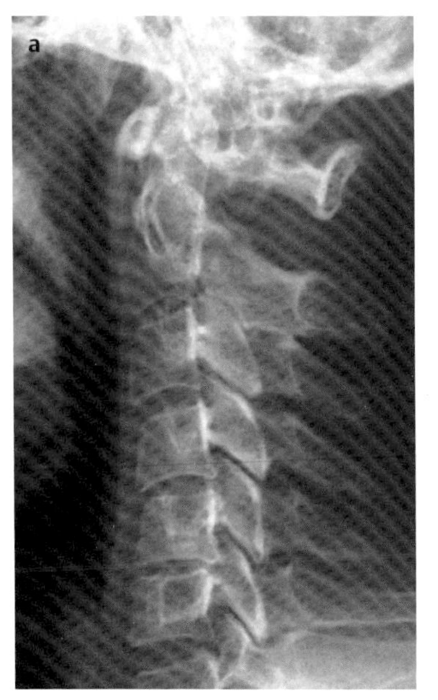

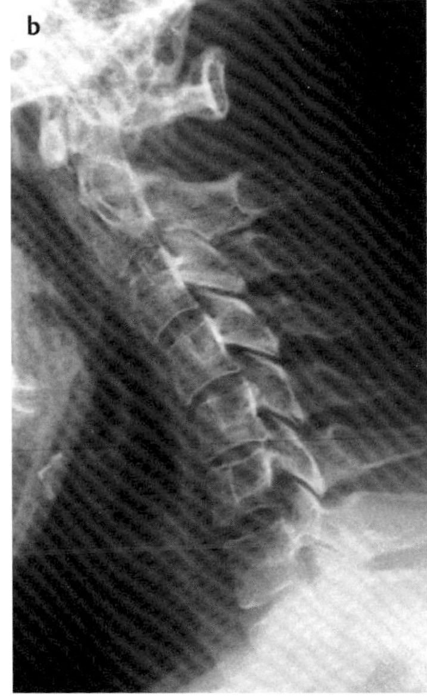

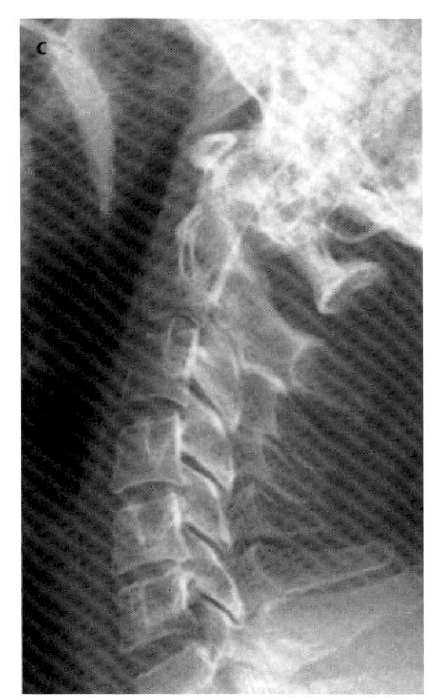

Fig. 3.38 a–c Lateral stress radiographs of the cervical spine. Extension with slight kyphosis at levels C4–C6 and moderate degenerative disk disease. The shingle-like anterior displacement is absent in C5–C7, especially in flexion. Functionally fused vertebrae at C5–C6.

Selected References

Bohndorf K, Imhof H. Radiologische Diagnostik der Knochen und Gelenke, 2nd ed. Stuttgart: Thieme 2006

Dihlmann W. Joints and vertebral connections. Stuttgart: Thieme 1985

Greenspan A. Orthopedic Radiology. A Practical Approach. 3rd ed. Philadelphia: Lippincott Williams and Wilkins 2000

Möller T, Reif E. CT- und MRT-Normalbefunde. Stuttgart: Thieme 1998

Vahlensieck M, Reiser M. MRT des Bewegungsapparates, 3rd ed. Stuttgart: Thieme 2006

Definition

- **Epidemiology**
  Present in 6–12% of people over 40 years • Thoracic: 100%, cervical: 65–80%, lumbar: 70–90% • Twice as common in men than women.
- **Etiology, pathophysiology, pathogenesis**
  Etiology: unclear; presumably there is some relation to diabetes mellitus, hypoglycemia, and hyperuricemia.
  Synonyms: Forestier disease, ankylosing hyperostosis • "Flowing" ossification of the anterior longitudinal ligament • The height of the disk interspaces is normal • The facet joints appear normal. Combined with enthesis ("whiskering") of the iliac crest, ischial tuberosity, and greater trochanter.

Imaging Signs

- **Modality of choice**
  Conventional radiographs.
- **General**
  Broad-based, "flowing" ossifications on the anterior spine, extending across at least four vertebrae • Slight associated degenerative changes • The facet joints and sacroiliac joints are normal! • The disks are largely intact.
- **Radiographic findings**
  Bone remodeling on the anterior aspect of the vertebral bodies • Rarely occurs in combination with ossified posterior longitudinal ligament (OPLL).
- **CT findings**
  Thick ossification anterior to the vertebral bodies. Initially, there is a typical gap between the ossification and the vertebral bodies • Ossification is more pronounced in the right lateral than left lateral region.
- **MRI findings**
  Bone marrow present in ossifications • Spinal stenosis with ossified posterior longitudinal ligament.

Clinical Aspects

- **Typical presentation**
  Restricted mobility • Rarely difficulties swallowing • Usually asymptomatic.
- **Therapeutic options**
  Mostly none • In severe cases with clinical symptoms, surgery with removal of the calcifications.

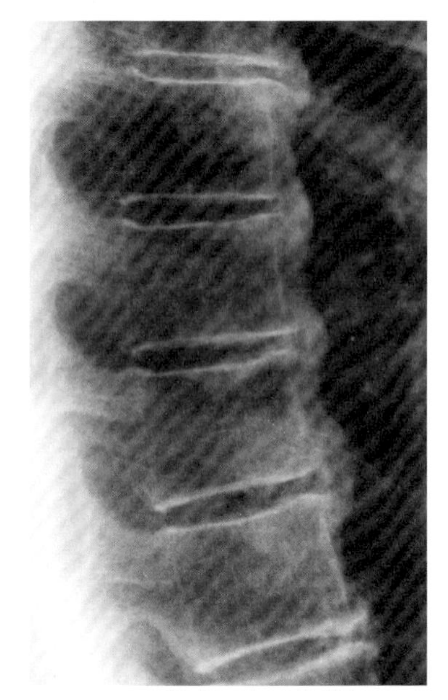

Fig. 3.39 Conventional lateral radiograph of the thoracic spine. "Flowing" hyperostosis along the anterior margins of the vertebrae (= typical DISH).

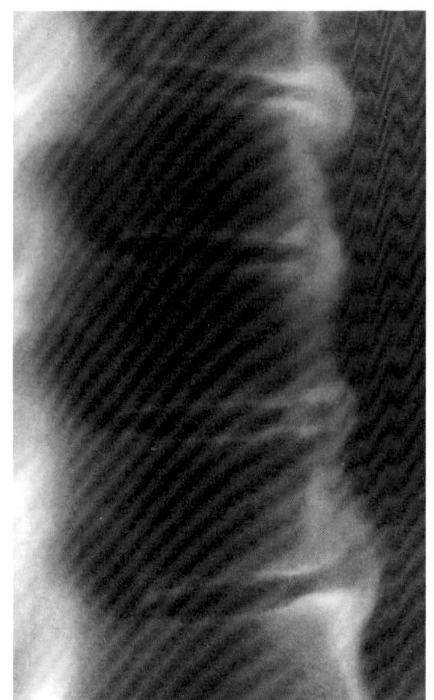

Fig. 3.40 Conventional lateral tomograph of the thoracic spine. "Flowing" anterior hyperostosis; disks are of normal height (= typical DISH).

Differential Diagnosis

Spondylosis	– Osteophyte formation – Rarely extends over several segments – Additional degenerative signs
Ankylosing spondylitis	– Sacroiliac and facet joints are also involved – Syndesmophytes ("bamboo" sign)

Selected References

Brossmann J, Czerny Chr, Freyschmidt J. Grenzen des Normalen und Anfänge des Pathologischen in der Radiologie des kindlichen und erwachsenen Skeletts. Stuttgart: Thieme 2001

Resnick D et al. Association of diffuse idiopathic skeletal hyperostosis (DISH). AJR 1978; 131: 1049–1053

Definition

- **Epidemiology**
  The disorder affects 0.5–1.0% of the population. • Annual incidence is 12.0–24.5/100 000 in men and 23.9–54/100 000 in women. • More common in men than in women (1:2–3).
- **Etiology, pathophysiology, pathogenesis**
  Chronic systemic disorder affecting mainly the synovial tissue • Autoimmune disease • *Synonym:* chronic polyarthritis (obsolete term) • *Multifactorial:* Genetic susceptibility, association with HLA-DR4, environmental factors, Epstein–Barr virus infection, and certain strains of *Escherichia coli* • Synovitis (= synovialitis), pannus (= fibrovascular scar tissue), erosion, destruction, deformity.
  Diagnosis: According to the 1987 criteria of the American College of Rheumatology (formerly American Rheumatism Association):
  - Morning stiffness.
  - Joint swelling (more than three joints).
  - Swelling in the wrist, metacarpophalangeal, and proximal interphalangeal joints.
  - Symmetrical joint swelling.
  - Radiologic abnormalities in the hand (swelling, erosion).
  - Subcutaneous rheumatoid nodules.

Imaging Signs

- **Modality of choice**
  Conventional cervical spine radiographs including stress views • Conventional radiographs of the peripheral joints of interest in the hands • MRI of the cervical spine including contrast series, paying special attention to the atlantoaxial joint.
- **General**
  Primarily peripheral joints are affected • In the spine, the disorder shows a predilection for the atlantooccipital, atlantoaxial, and facet joints (the latter especially in the cervical spine) • Rarely, unilateral asymmetric sacroiliitis occurs.
- **Radiographic findings**
  Most important sign: Anterior atlantoaxial subluxation (occurring in 26% of cases), defined as an atlantodental interval in the sagittal plane exceeding 2.5 mm • Lateral atlantoaxial subluxation (occurs in 14% of cases) • It is important to note that subluxation is occasionally detectable only on stress films • Deformities • Blurred cortex, and erosion of the dens and facet joints • Inflammatory destruction of the diskovertebral region (rare).
- **CT findings**
  CT is superior to conventional radiographs for visualizing bony changes • Useful in preoperative diagnostics, prior to surgical stabilization.

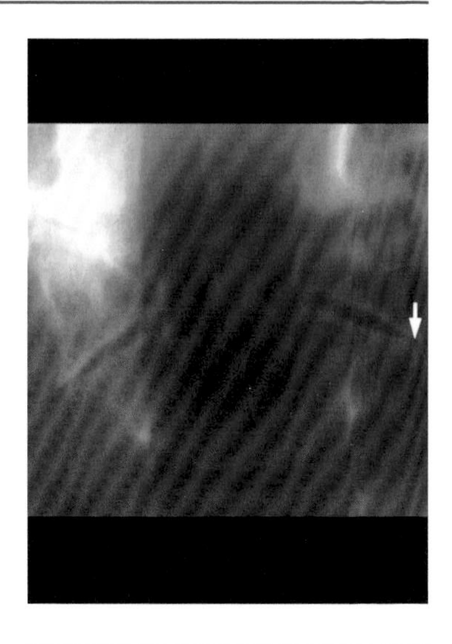

Fig. 4.1 Conventional tomogram of the dens axis (A-P). Erosion of the dens. Minor erosion in the left lateral atlantoaxial joint (arrow).

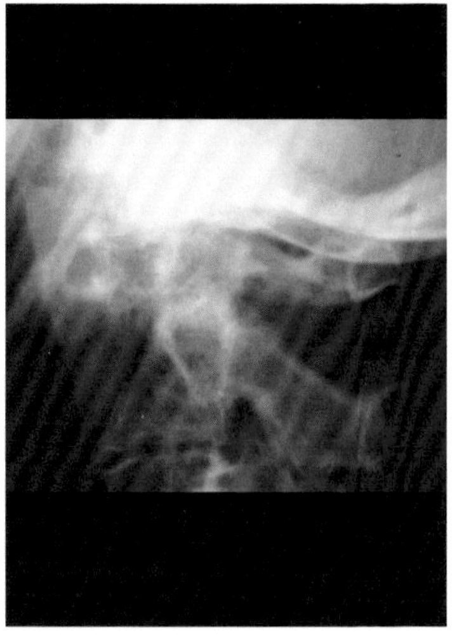

Fig. 4.2 Conventional lateral radiograph of the cervical spine (detail, extension view). Atlantodental subluxation due to inflammatory destruction of the ligament complex and capsule.

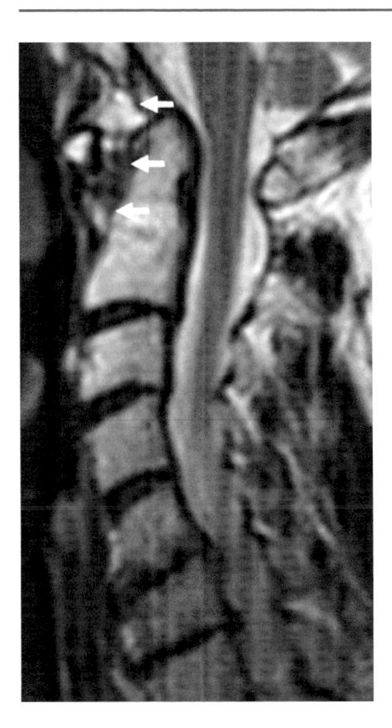

Fig. 4.3 MR image of the cervical spine (sagittal, T2). Atlantodental subluxation. Pannus (arrows).

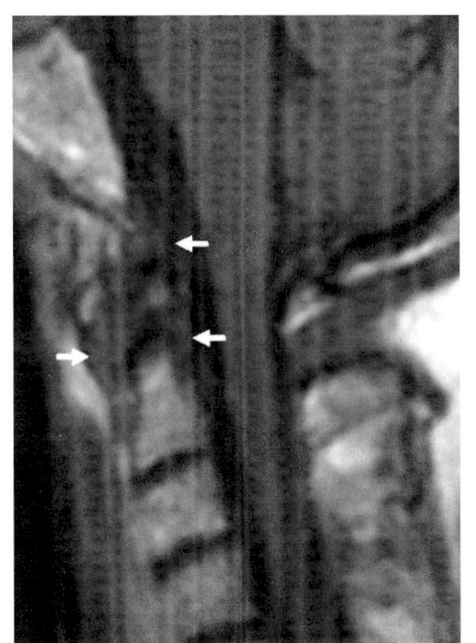

Fig. 4.4 MR image of the cervical spine (sagittal, T1, detail). Dens destruction from extensive pannus tissue (arrows).

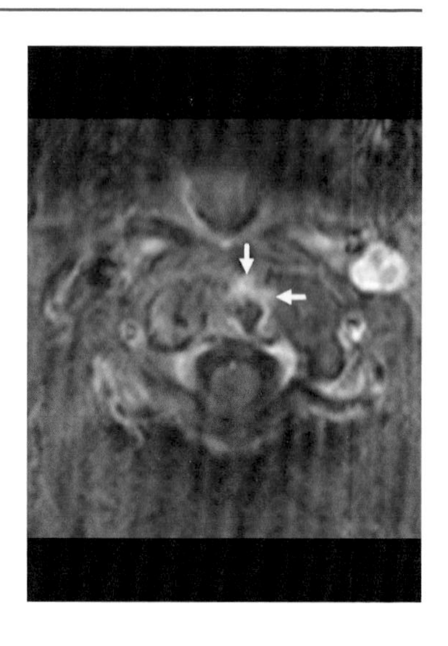

Fig. 4.5 Axial MR image of the atlanto-dental joint (axial fat-saturated T1-weighted image with contrast). Hypervascularized pannus tissue (arrows). Dens destruction.

▸ **MRI findings**

Shows bony changes and the inflammatory process • Pannus is hypointense on T1-weighted images, heterogeneous on T2-weighted images, and enhances proportionally to inflammatory activity • Identifies reactive, inflammatory, and stress-related bone marrow edema (hypointense on T1-weighted images, hyperintense on T2-weighted and STIR images, enhances with contrast administration) • Effusion into the facet joints (hypointense on T1-weighted images, hyperintense on T2-weighted images, contrast diffusion) • For evaluating spinal canal, spinal cord, and spinal nerves • Early identification of fractures and stress lesions.

Clinical Aspects

▸ **Typical presentation**

Peripheral joint symptoms • Back pain • Morning stiffness • Neurologic symptoms.

C-reactive protein is elevated • Rheumatoid factor is elevated • Hereditary factors • Rheumatoid nodules.

▸ **Therapeutic options**

Physical therapy • *Medical therapy:* Nonsteroidal antiinflammatory agents, sulfasalazine, methotrexate, corticosteroids, anti-TNF • Surgical treatment to achieve stabilization and/or decompression of the spinal canal.

Differential Diagnosis

Seronegative spondyloarthropathy	– Syndesmophytes – Squaring of the vertebral bodies – Pronounced proliferative component – Predilection for thoracic spine, lumbar spine, and sacroiliac joints
Degenerative changes in the spine	– Osteophytes, sclerosis, joint space narrowing
Juvenile rheumatoid arthritis	– Cervical subluxation, fused vertebrae, occurs in children (below 18 years) – Symptoms in Still disease also include fever, anemia, and hepatosplenomegaly
Infection	– Predilection for thoracic and lumbar spine – Clinical aspects

Selected References

Arnett FC, Edwotzhy SM, Bloch DA, et al. The American Rheumatism Association 1987 revised criteria for the classification of rheumatoid arthritis. Arthritis Rheum 1988; 31: 315–324

Gabriel SE. The epidemiology of rheumatoid arthritis. Rheum Dis Clin North Am 2001; 27: 269–281

Resnick D. Rheumatoid arthritis. In: Resnick D, ed. Bone and Joint Imaging. 2nd ed. Philadelphia: Saunders 1996: 211–234

Definition

- **Epidemiology**
  Anterior atlantoaxial subluxation: 26% of affected people • Lateral atlantoaxial subluxation: 14% of affected people • Pathology mimicking basilar impression: approximately 5.5% of affected people.
- **Etiology, pathophysiology, pathogenesis**
  Minor trauma or physiologic stresses on tissue damaged and weakened by inflammation and poor quality bone.
  Insufficiency fracture: Slight trauma or physiologic stresses on poor-quality or osteoporotic bone.

Imaging Signs

- **Modality of choice**
  - Conventional radiographs.
  - CT to evaluate complex fractures and to demonstrate spondylolysis.
  - MRI to evaluate ligaments, joint capsules, inflammatory tissue, and neurologic symptoms.
- **Radiographic findings**
  Anterior atlantoaxial subluxation: Atlantodental interval in the sagittal plane exceeding 2.5 mm • Interval of 2.5–4 mm results from compromised transverse ligament • Interval > 4 mm results from other compromised ligaments, capsule, and bone.
  Lateral atlantoaxial subluxation: Asymmetric width of the lateral joint spaces.
  Pathology mimicking basilar impression: Apex of the dens > 3 mm over the McGregor line.
  Insufficiency fracture: Volume loss in the affected vertebra, vertebra plana, wedge-shaped vertebra, fish vertebrae, reduced bone density • Spondylolysis in fractures of the pars interarticularis.
- **CT findings**
  Multislice CT with multiplanar reconstructions • Demonstrates fractures and displacement.
- **MRI findings**
  Visualization of inflammatory tissue: Hypointense on T1-weighted, heterogeneous on T2-weighted images, enhances with contrast • Permits evaluation of ligaments and capsules • Bone marrow edema: Hypointense on T1-weighted, hyperintense on T2-weighted and STIR images, enhances with contrast • *Osteoporosis:* Strongly hyperintense bone marrow signal on T1- and T2-weighted images • T1-weighted images are well suited for demonstrating fractures.

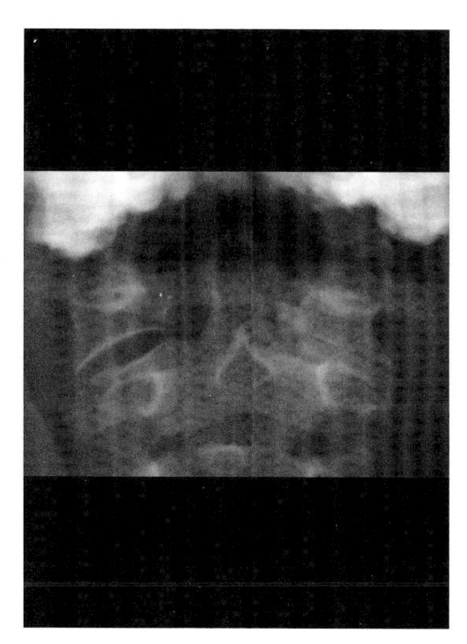

Fig. 4.6 Conventional A-P radiograph of the atlantoaxial joint. Lateral atlantoaxial dislocation with inflammatory erosive changes in the left lateral region in rheumatoid arthritis.

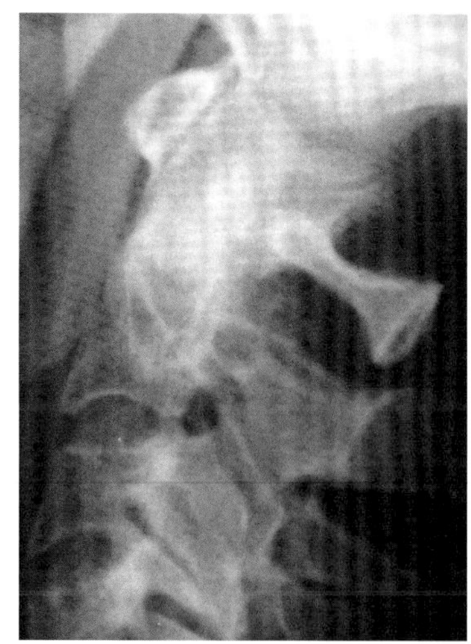

Fig. 4.7 Conventional lateral radiograph of the cervical spine (detail). Normal atlantodental interval.

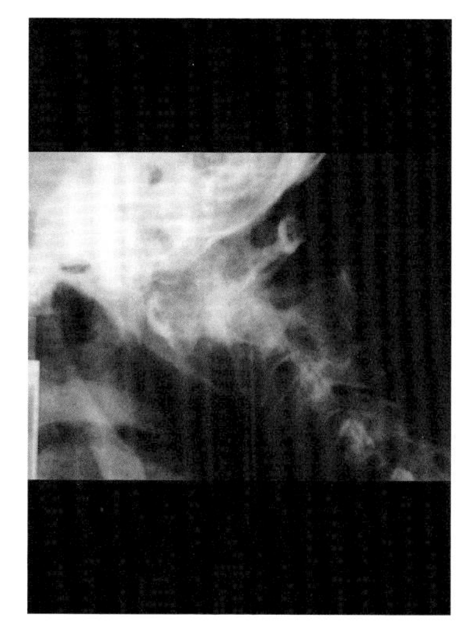

Fig. 4.8 Conventional lateral radiograph of the cervical spine in flexion (detail). Widened atlantodental interval in rheumatoid arthritis.

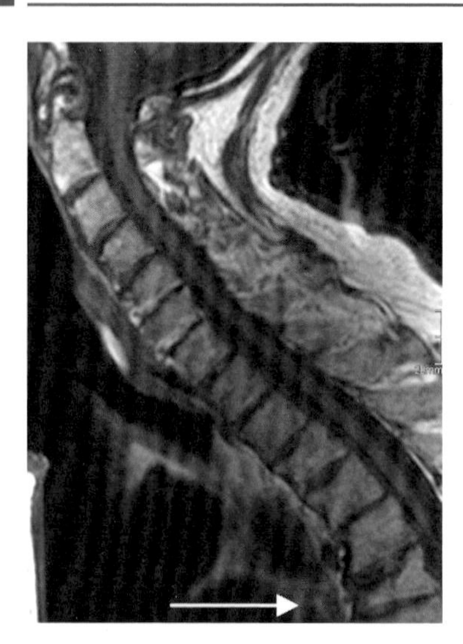

Fig. 4.9 MR image of the cervical spine (sagittal, T1). Compression fracture of vertebra T6, osteoporotic fish vertebra T3. Degenerative changes in the spine.

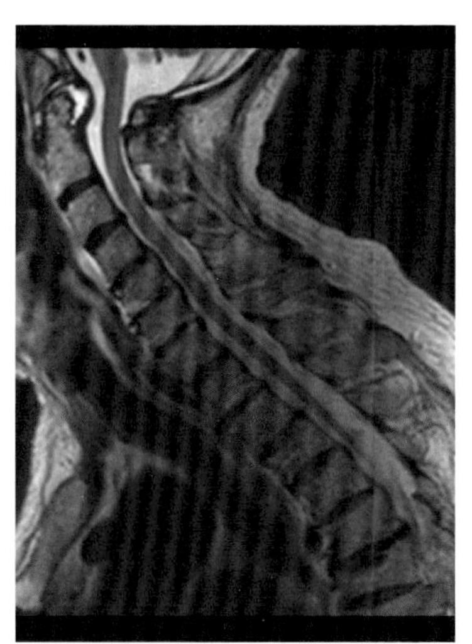

Fig. 4.10 MR image of the cervical and upper thoracic spine (sagittal, T2). Insufficiency fracture of vertebra T6 with multisegmental loss of vertebral height in osteoporosis (T1- and T2-weighted images, markedly hyperintense bone marrow signal). Patient with rheumatoid arthritis on long-term corticoid therapy. Pannus around the dens.

Clinical Aspects

- **Typical presentation**
  Usually asymptomatic or with only minor symptoms • Neurologic deficits are occasionally present.
- **Therapeutic options**
  Depend on the symptoms • Conservative or surgical (stabilization, decompression where indicated) • Management of osteoporosis.

Differential Diagnosis

Traumatic subluxation	– No inflammatory pathology such as erosion or pannus

Selected References

Freyschmidt J. Rheumatoide Arthritis. In: Freyschmidt J. Skeletterkrankungen. Klinisch-radiologische Diagnose und Differenzialdiagnose. Berlin: Springer 1997: 669–685

Definition

- **Epidemiology**
  Approximately 7% of patients with psoriasis develop arthropathy; spinal involvement usually occurs only in HLA-B27–positive patients • In 15–30%, joint pathology develops even decades before skin manifestations • Predilection for the hands and feet • The sacroiliac joints and spine (especially the thoracic and lumbar spine) are involved in up to 50% of cases.
- **Etiology, pathophysiology, pathogenesis**
  Erosive destructive seronegative polyarthritis with proliferation in bone.

Imaging Signs

- **Modality of choice**
  - Conventional radiographs: These are usually sufficient for the spine and sacroiliac joints.
  - CT and MRI: Where there are neurologic symptoms, complications (trauma, stress lesions), and equivocal findings.
- **Radiographic findings**
  Squaring of the vertebral bodies (anterior spondylitis produces a straight anterior margin) • Ossification of the paraspinal ligaments and syndesmophytes (ossification of the outer fibers of the annulus fibrosis) • Proliferative osteoarthritis (especially in the facet joints) • Asymmetric unilateral or bilateral sacroiliitis with destruction, subchondral sclerosis, and ankylosis.
- **CT findings**
  Multislice CT with multiplanar reconstruction is especially suitable for optimally visualizing destructive and proliferative changes in the facet joints and sacroiliac joints.
- **MRI findings**
  T1-weighted (with and without contrast administration), T2-weighted, and STIR sequences, sagittal and axial • Demonstrates active inflammatory processes (synovitis, abnormal bone marrow signal) in the spine and sacroiliac region • Early identification of stress lesions due to the pathologic bone marrow signal (hypointense on T1-weighted images, hyperintense on T2-weighted images, enhancing with contrast) • Identifies vertebral and foraminal stenoses • In up to 38% of cases, radiologic findings are identical to those in rheumatoid arthritis • In up to 30% of cases, radiologic signs of psoriatic spondyloarthropathy coexist with those of rheumatoid arthritis.

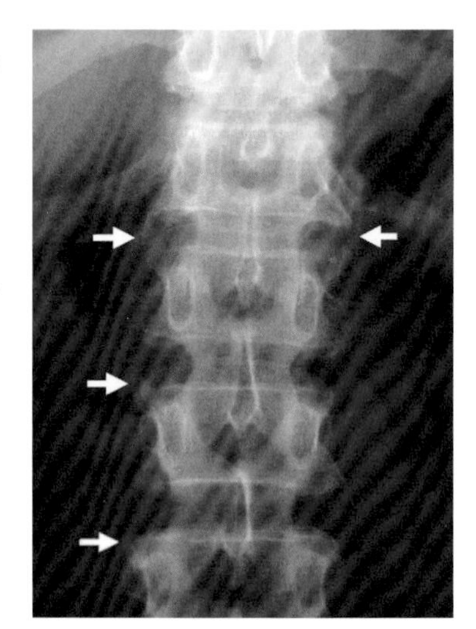

Fig. 4.11 Conventional A-P radiograph of the thoracolumbar junction. Ossification of the paraspinal ligaments (arrows) in a patient with psoriasis.

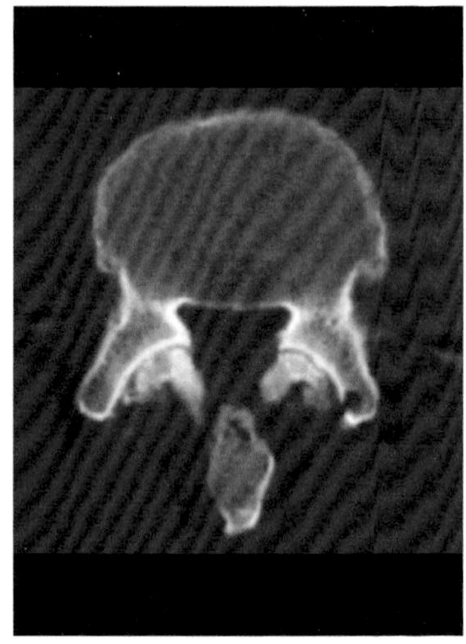

Fig. 4.12 Axial CT of the lumbar spine (detail). Erosive and markedly proliferative arthritis of the facet joints.

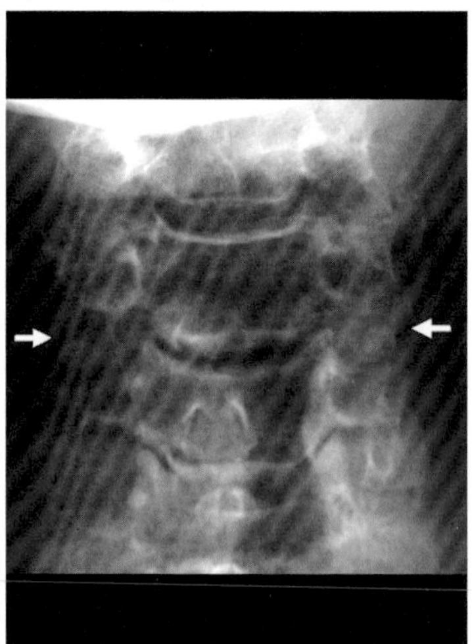

Fig. 4.13 Conventional A-P radiograph of the cervical spine (detail). Facet joint arthritis at C4–C5 (arrows) in a psoriasis patient.

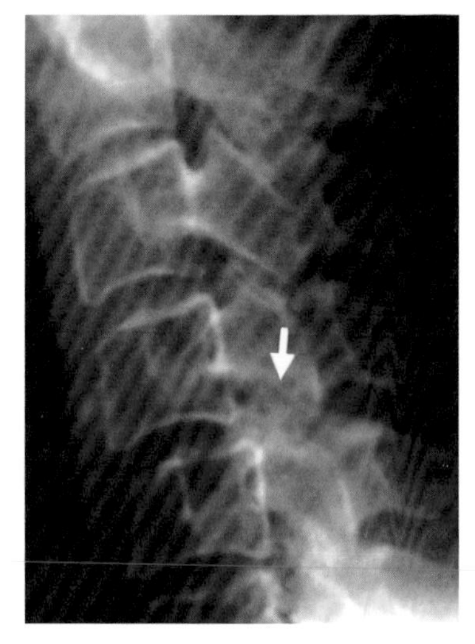

Fig. 4.14 Conventional lateral radiograph of the cervical spine (detail). Facet joint arthritis at C4–C5 (arrow) in a patient with psoriasis and spondylolisthesis.

Clinical Aspects

▸ **Typical presentation**
Begins with joint pain in one or several joints • In up to 85% of cases, there is skin pathology • Sacroiliitis is present with low back pain, especially at night.

▸ **Therapeutic options**
Physical therapy • *Medical therapy:* NSAIDs, corticosteroids, retinoids, methotrexate, sulfasalazine, ciclosporin, TNF-α blockers.

Differential Diagnosis

Rheumatoid arthritis	– Predilection for the cervical spine – Erosive and destructive disease components outweigh proliferation – Sacroiliitis is rare (no ankylosis) – Ankylosis is rare
Ankylosing spondylitis	– No skin changes – Symmetric bilateral sacroiliitis
Forestier disease (DISH)	– Ossification of the longitudinal ligaments – Normal sacroiliac joints

Selected References

Freyschmidt J. Psoriasisarthritis. In: Freyschmidt J. Skeletterkrankungen. Klinisch-radiologische Diagnose und Differenzialdiagnose. Berlin: Springer 1997: 711–718

Stern RS. Psoriasis. Lancet 1997; 350: 349–353

Queiro R, Belzunegui J, Gonzalez C, et al. Clinically asymptomatic axial disease in psoriatic spondylarthropathy. A retrospective study. Clin Rheumatol 2002; 21: 10–13

Definition

- **Epidemiology**
  Morbidity: 0.01% of the population • Occurs more often in men than women (estimated ratio 9:1) secondary to venereal infection and equally often (1:1) secondary to enteric infection.
- **Etiology, pathophysiology, pathogenesis**
  Reactive postinfectious seronegative arthritis • *Reiter syndrome:* Severe arthritis involving the axial skeleton, skin, mucosa, and eyes (uveitis); urethritis • Autoimmune process secondary to gastrointestinal and venereal disease • Associated with HLA-B27 (70–90% of cases).
  Predilection for:
  - Joints in the lower extremity and heel region.
  - Sacroiliac joints (in at least 20% of cases).

  Rarely in the spine (especially in the lower thoracic and lumbar spine).

Imaging Signs

- **Modality of choice**
  Conventional radiographs are usually sufficient.
  CT and MRI when there are negative radiographic and positive clinical findings.
  CT for precise evaluation of bony structures.
- **Radiographic findings**
  No oblique views • Coexisting bony destruction and proliferation • Full radiologic picture of sacroiliitis with destruction, subchondral sclerosis, and ankylosis, often asymmetric • Ossification of the paraspinal ligaments • Syndesmophytes (ossification of the peripheral fibers of the annulus fibrosus) • Erosion of the vertebral endplates and narrowing disk interspaces • Rarely atlantoaxial dislocation • Bony ankylosis.
- **CT findings**
  High sensitivity for detecting sacroiliac changes • Early detection of erosion in the endplates.
- **MRI findings**
  Early identification of sacroiliitis: Bone marrow edema and synovitis (hypointense on T1-weighted images, hyperintense on T2-weighted and STIR images, enhancing with contrast).

Clinical Aspects

- **Typical presentation**
  Onset up to 60 days after venereal or gastrointestinal infection • Acute occurrence of arthralgia, joint effusion, and inflammation, especially in the lower extremity • *Reiter's triad:* Arthritis, uveitis, and urethritis • Mucocutaneous symptoms • Conjunctivitis • Occasionally fever • Course is usually self-limiting, occasionally chronic.

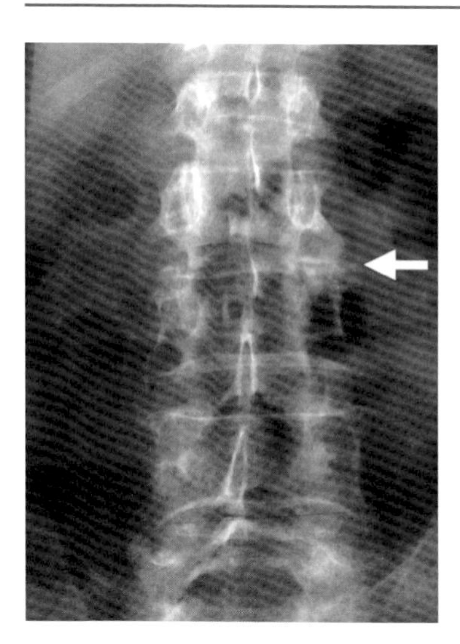

Fig. 4.15 Conventional A-P radiograph of the lumbar spine. Marginal erosive changes and narrowing of disk space at L2–L3 (arrow) in Reiter syndrome. Coexisting degenerative changes.

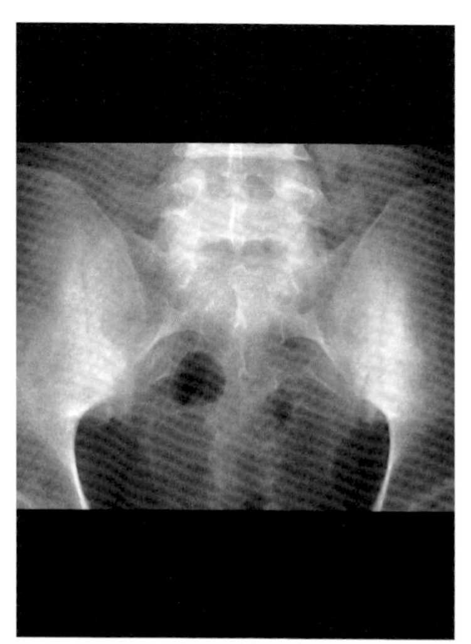

Fig. 4.16 Conventional A-P radiograph of the sacroiliac joints. Bilateral symmetric sacroiliitis with erosions, sclerosis, and joint space narrowing.

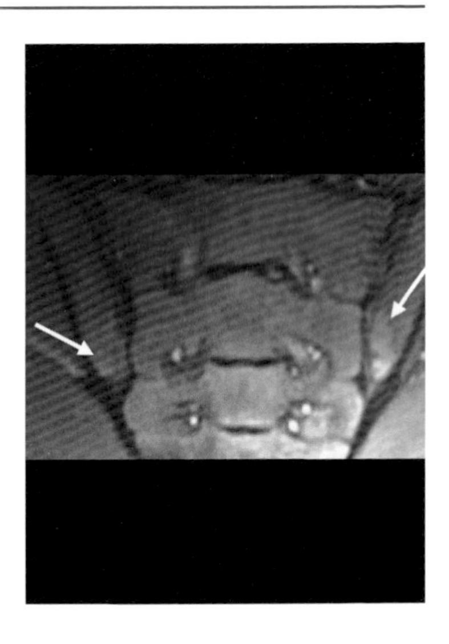

Fig. 4.17 MR image of the sacroiliac joints (semiaxial, T2). Bone marrow edema and slight joint effusion in Reiter syndrome.

▸ **Therapeutic options**
Physical therapy • *Medical therapy:* NSAIDs, antibiotics (tetracyclines), sulfasalazine.

Differential Diagnosis

Ankylosing spondylitis	– No mucocutaneous changes
Psoriasis	– Joints in the upper and lower extremities are involved – Typical skin changes
Rheumatoid arthritis	– Bony destruction without proliferation – Osteoporosis – Appearance and pattern of involvement (hands and feet)

Selected References

Freyschmidt J. Reiter-Syndrom. In: Freyschmidt J. Skeletterkrankungen. Klinisch-radiologische Diagnose und Differenzialdiagnose. Berlin: Springer 1997: 706–711

Hellmann DB, Stone JH. Reiter's syndrome. In: Tierney LM, McPhee SJ, Papadakis MA, eds. Current Medical Diagnosis and Treatment. Stamford: Appleton & Lange 1999: 827–828

Martel W, Braunstein EM, Borlaza G, et al. Radiologic features of Reiter disease. Radiology 1979; 132: 10

Mohana-Borges AV et al. Monoarticular arthritis. Radiol Clin North Am 2004; 42: 135–149

Definition

▸ **Epidemiology**

Onset: Age 20–40 years • More common in men than women (range 3:1 to 10:1) • *Prevalence:* 0.2–1.6%.

▸ **Etiology, pathophysiology, pathogenesis**

Autoimmune disorder • 96% of affected people are HLA-B-27 carriers (chromosome 6) • *Synonym:* Bechterew disease • Chronic inflammatory disorder with predilection for the spine • Seronegative spondyloarthropathy • Affected structures include (a) diskovertebral region, (b) ligamentous insertions, (c) facet joints, (d) costovertebral joints • Peripheral skeletal involvement is seen in 10–20% of cases.

Associated with:

- Ulcerative colitis
- Iritis
- Aortic insufficiency and atrioventricular conduction disturbance
- Pulmonary fibrosis

Imaging Signs

▸ **Modality of choice**

Conventional radiographs in two planes • Regions of interest include the thoracic spine, lumbar spine, and sacroiliac joints.

MRI and CT: For early diagnose of sacroiliitis • DD of spondylodiskitis • In difficult cases • With complications such as fracture, spondylolysis, or neurologic symptoms.

▸ **General**

Destructive and proliferative • Ankylosis.

▸ **Radiographic findings**

Squaring of the vertebral bodies: Anterior contour of vertebral body is straight • *Biconvex vertebrae:* Convex anterior contour of vertebral body • Disk calcifications • *Syndesmophytes:* Ossification of the peripheral fibers of the annulus fibrosus and between the intervertebral disk and anterior longitudinal ligament • *Anterior spondylitis:* Spondylitis of the anterior superior and inferior margins of the vertebra, occasionally posterior as well. Sclerosis with or without erosion.

Aseptic spondylodiskitis:

- Inflammatory type: Destructive granulomatous process in the region of the endplate.
- Noninflammatory type: Stress or insufficiency fracture.

Erosion on the spinous processes • Arthritis of the facet joints • Ligament calcifications • *Full radiologic picture of sacroiliitis:* Destruction, subchondral sclerosis, and bony ankylosis, generally bilaterally.

▸ **CT findings**

High sensitivity for identifying sacroiliitis • Involvement of the costovertebral joints • Evaluation of fractures.

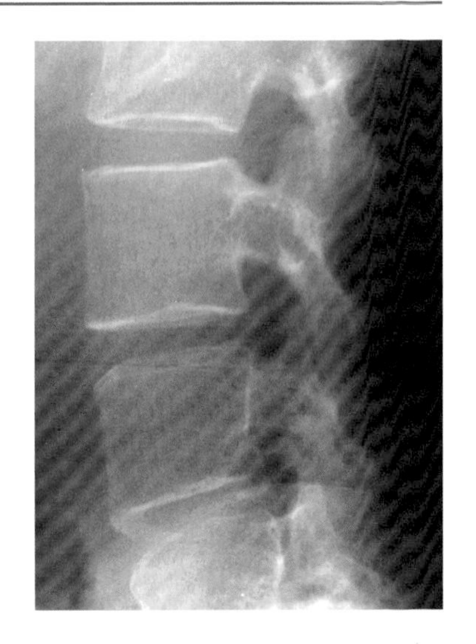

Fig. 4.18 Conventional lateral radiograph of the lumbar spine. Anterior vertebral body squaring from periosteal remodeling secondary to anterior osteitis.

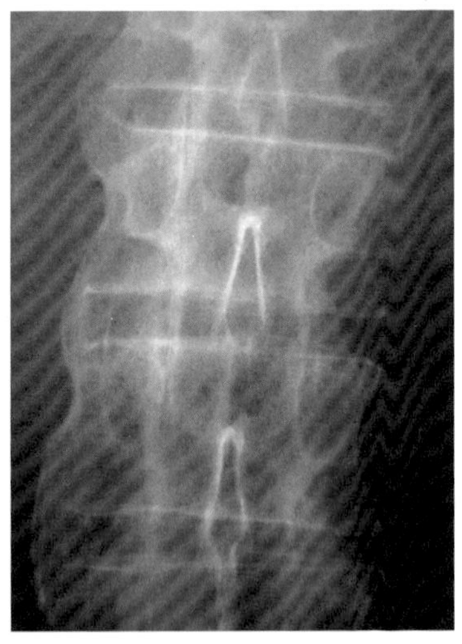

Fig. 4.19 Conventional A-P radiograph of the upper lumbar spine (detail). Syndesmophytes.

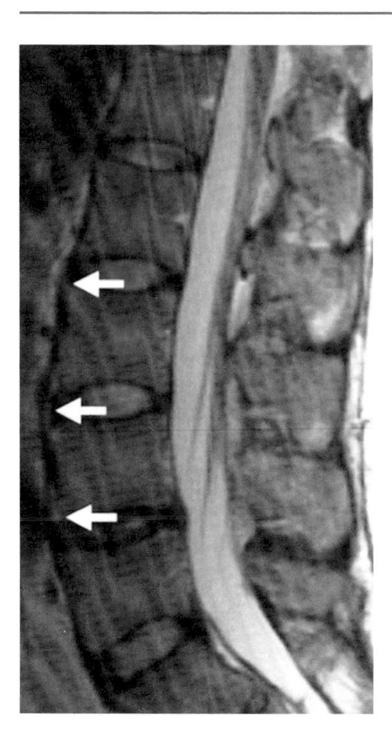

Fig. 4.20 MR image of the lumbar spine (sagittal, T2). Syndesmophytes (arrows).

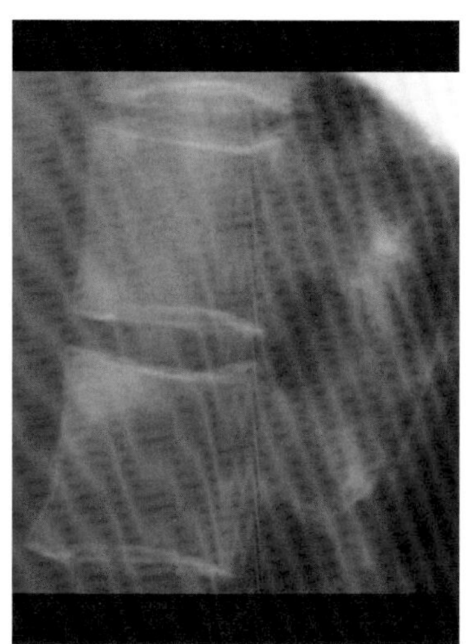

Fig. 4.21 Conventional lateral radiograph of the thoracic spine (detail). Anterior spondylitis with a predominantly sclerotic component.

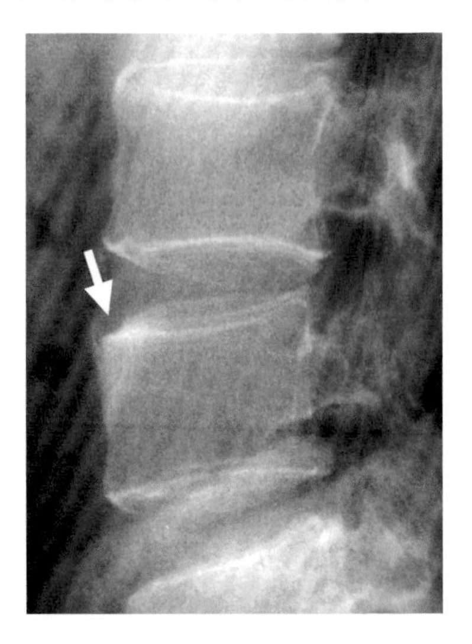

Fig. 4.22 Conventional lateral radiograph of the lumbar spine (detail). Anterior spondylitis with sclerosis and active erosion (arrow).

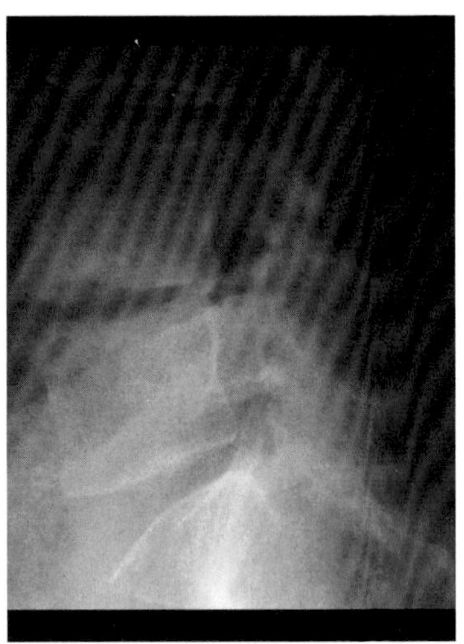

Fig. 4.23 Conventional lateral radiograph of the lumbar spine. Spondylodiskitis at L4–L5.

▸ **MRI findings**
Bone marrow edema: Hypointense on T1-weighted, hyperintense on T2-weighted and STIR images, enhances with contrast • Spinal stenosis and neural foramina stenosis • Arachnoiditis with cauda equina syndrome.

Clinical Aspects

▸ **Typical presentation**
Begins with unspecific symptoms in lower thoracic spine, lumbar spine, and sacrum • Low back pain at night • Buttock pain • Stiffness • Peripheral arthritis • Inflammation and pain in musculotendinous insertions.

▸ **Therapeutic options**
Physical therapy • *Medical therapy:* NSAIDs, sulfasalazine, methotrexate, anti-TNF.

Differential Diagnosis

Reiter syndrome	– Arthritis of peripheral joints in the lower extremity – Mucocutaneous changes, uveitis, conjunctivitis – Previous infection
Psoriasis	– Skin changes – Appearance of peripheral arthritis – Asymmetric sacroiliitis
DISH, Forestier disease	– No sacroiliitis – Widespread ossification of the paraspinal ligaments – Facet joints

Selected References

Dihlmann W. Spondylitis ankylosans. In: Dihlmann W. Gelenke – Wirbelverbindungen. Stuttgart: Thieme 1987: 591–605

Elyan M, Khan MA. Diagnosing ankylosing spondylitis. J Rheumatol Suppl 2006; 78: 12–23

Leeb BF et al. Diagnosis and therapy of chronic polyarthritis. Radiologe 1996; 36: 657–662

Levine DS, Forbat SM, Saifuddin A. MRI of the axial skeletal manifestations of ankylosing spondylitis. Clin Radiol 2004; 59: 400–413

Vinson EN, Major NM. MR imaging of ankylosing spondylitis. Semin Musculoskelet Radiol 2003; 7: 103–113

Definition

Up to 20% of all patients with ankylosing spondylitis eventually develop severe disabilities due to progressive ankylosis and ligament ossification.

Imaging Signs

- **Modality of choice**
  Conventional radiographs in two planes.
  MRI and CT where there are complications such as fracture, spondylolysis, or neurologic symptoms.
- **Radiographic findings**
  Ankylosis of the affected joints • Extensive ligament ossification • "Double railroad track" sign: Ankylosis of the facet joints and calcification of the interspinous and supraspinous ligaments • *"Bamboo spine":* Undulating contour from syndesmophytes • Fixed deformity • Atlantoaxial subluxation.
- **CT findings**
  Visualization of fractures and pseudarthroses.
- **MRI findings**
  Stenosis of spinal canal and neural foramina • Cauda equina syndrome resulting from arachnoiditis with formation of diverticula and erosion of the vertebral arches.

Clinical Aspects

- **Typical presentation**
  Postural deformity • Restricted mobility • Increased risk of fracture and spondylolysis.
- **Therapeutic options**
  Physical therapy • Treatment is symptomatic and depends on disease activity.

Selected References

Dihlmann W. Spondylitis ankylosans. In: Dihlmann W. Gelenke – Wirbelverbindungen. Stuttgart: Thieme 1987: 591–605

Hanson JA, Mirza S. Predisposition for spinal fracture in ankylosing spondylitis. AJR 2000; 174: 150

Resnick D. Ankylosing Spondylitis. In: Resnick D, ed. Bone and Joint Imaging. 2nd ed. Philadelphia: Saunders 1996: 246–264

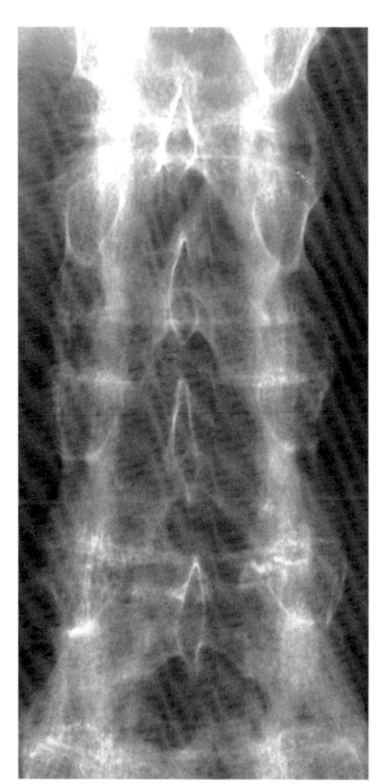

Fig. 4.24 Conventional A-P radiograph of the lumbar spine (detail). Ankylosis of the facet joints and bridging syndesmophytes ("bamboo" sign).

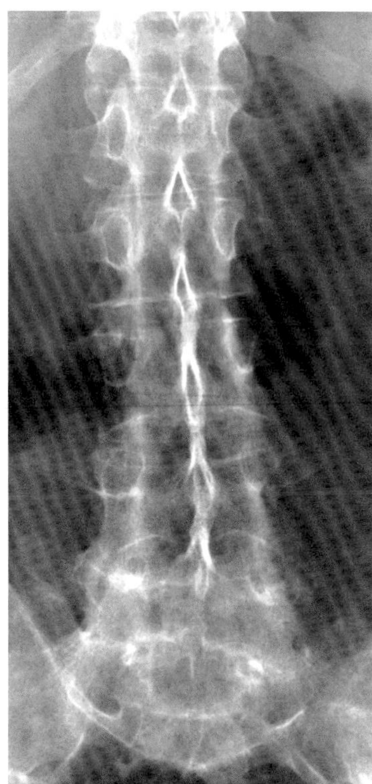

Fig. 4.25 Conventional A-P radiograph of the lumbar spine (detail). Ankylosis of the facet joints and ossification of the interspinous and supraspinous ligaments.

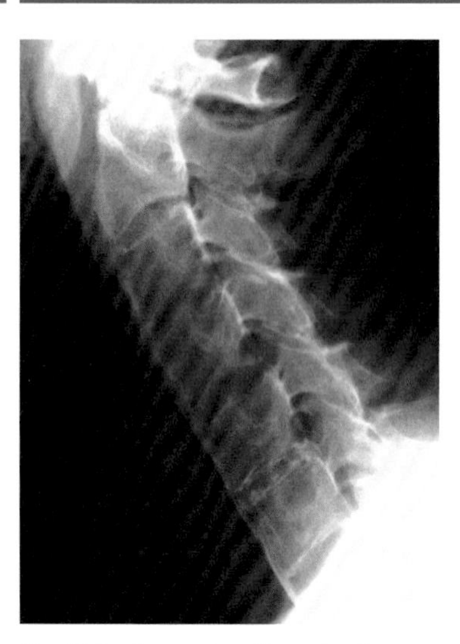

Fig. 4.26 Conventional lateral radiograph of the cervical spine. Ossification of the anterior longitudinal ligament with squaring of the vertebral body anteriorly.

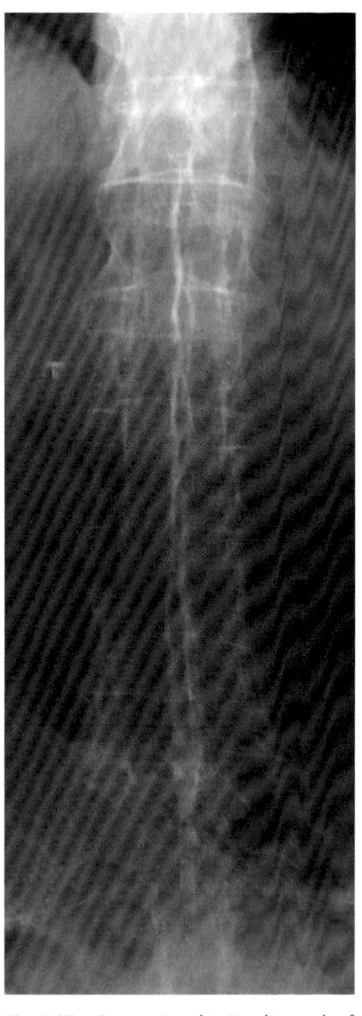

Fig. 4.27 Conventional A-P radiograph of the lumbar spine. Ankylosis of the facet joints, "bamboo spine," ossification of the interspinous and supraspinous ligaments.

Definition

- **Epidemiology**
  Prevalence of fractures is up to four times higher (up to 17%) in patients with ankylosing spondylitis than in the normal population • Patients with ankylosing spondylitis account for 1.2–1.5% of all patients with spinal cord injuries • Increased risk (up to 8%) of paralytic spinal injury • 75% of all fractures involve the cervical spine • Second most common fracture site is the thoracolumbar junction.
- **Etiology, pathophysiology, pathogenesis**
  Transverse fracture through the vertebral body or disk and the posterior elements (traumatic spondylolysis) and/or dislocation of the facet joints • Rupture of the ligament complex • Often associated with listhesis • Typical injury with minimal trauma • Flexion–distraction injury (B2) • Advanced ankylosing spondylitis increases the risk of fracture, mainly due to the altered biomechanics and also due to osteoporosis.

Imaging Signs

- **Modality of choice**
  Conventional radiography is acceptable as the primary imaging modality.
  CT and MRI (the latter especially where neurologic symptoms are present) are indicated because of their greater sensitivity compared with conventional radiographs.
- **General**
  Prompt radiologic examination is indicated in patients with ankylosing spondylitis presenting with minimal trauma and/or onset or aggravation of pain • In cervical fractures, it is important to exclude injury to the vertebral arteries.
- **Radiographic findings**
  Focal kyphosis • Abnormal vertical distance between the facet joints and spinous process • Discontinuity in calcified ligaments • Subluxation • Osteopenia and changes due to the underlying disorder can mask fractures.
- **CT findings**
  With multiplanar reconstruction, multislice CT in particular is significantly better than conventional radiographs for evaluating fractures.
- **MRI findings**
  Evaluation of spinal cord and spinal nerves.

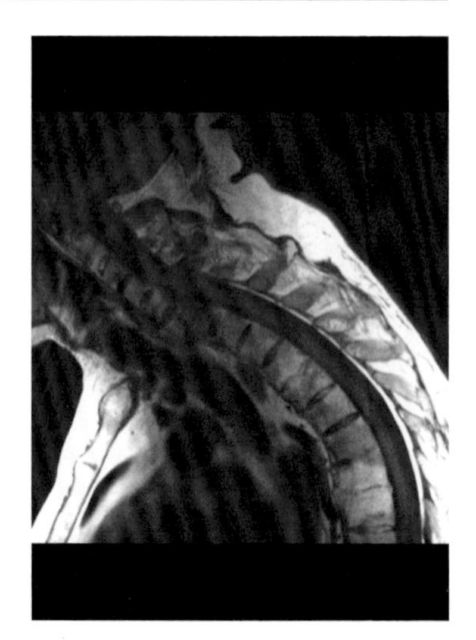

Fig. 4.28 MR image of the cervical spine (sagittal, T1). Transverse shear fracture at C6–C7 with anterior subluxation. Rupture of the ligament complex, associated vertebral fracture, facet joint dislocation, and compression of the spinal cord. Osteoporosis. Complication in ankylosing spondylitis (syndesmophytes, Andersson lesion at T3–T4 and T7–T8, ligament ossification).

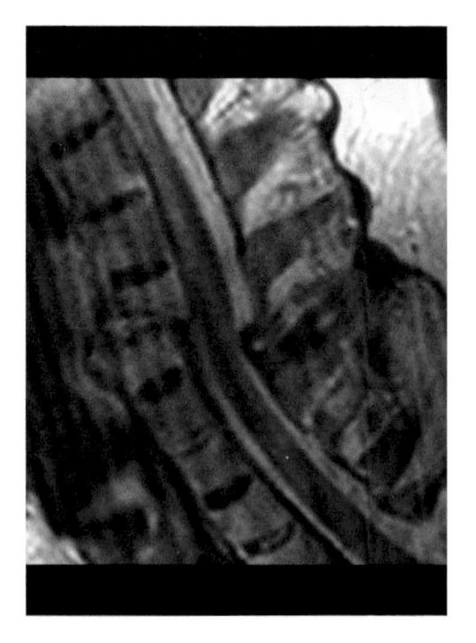

Fig. 4.29 MR image of the cervical spine (sagittal, T2). Transverse shear fracture at C4–C5 with anterior subluxation. Rupture of the ligament complex, associated vertebral fracture, facet joint dislocation, and compression of the spinal cord. Osteoporosis. Complication in ankylosing spondylitis (syndesmophytes, ligament ossification).

Clinical Aspects

- **Typical presentation**
  Ankylosing spondylitis • Minimal trauma produces symptoms • Sudden onset or aggravation of pain • Minor trauma can cause severe neurologic problems.
- **Therapeutic options**
  Conservative therapy (cervical collar, halo brace) is not generally indicated • Surgical management aims to achieve:
  - Reduction of the fracture.
  - Stabilization.
  - Decompression of the spinal canal where indicated.

Selected References

Hunter T, Durbo HI. Spinal fractures complicating ankylosing spondylitis. Long-term follow-up study. Arthritis Rheum 1983; 26: 751–759

May PJ, Raunest J, Herdmann J, Jonas M. Behandlung der Wirbelsäulenfraktur bei ankylosierender Spondylitis. Unfallchirurg 2002; 105: 165–169.

Weinstein PR, Karpmann RR, Gall EP, et al. Spinal cord injury, spinal fracture, and spinal stenosis in ankylosing spondylitis. J Neurosurg 1982; 57: 609–616

Definition

- **Epidemiology**
  Peak ages are 10–30 and 50–70 • The lower lumbar spine is the focus of the disorder.
- **Etiology, pathophysiology, pathogenesis**
  Bacterial spondylitis, spondylodiskitis • Usually caused by *Staphylococcus aureus* • Primarily hematogenous (venous, arterial), occasionally by extension (as from a retropharyngeal abscess) or postoperatively • Usually begins in the subchondral region.

Imaging Signs

- **Modality of choice**
  Early diagnosis:
  - MRI (T1, T2, STIR, T1 with contrast).
  - Scintigraphy.

  Diagnosis during clinical course:
  - Conventional A-P and lateral radiographs.
  - Scintigraphy.

  With complications:
  - MRI (T1, T2, T1 with contrast).
- **Radiographic findings**
  Narrowed disk interspace with irregular osteochondral border and increased subchondral sclerosis • Retrolisthesis.
- **MRI findings**
  Disk appears narrowed, hyperintense on T1-weighted and STIR sequences, with an irregular osteochondral border and surrounded by a bone marrow edema • Significant enhancement after contrast administration, occasionally in the epidural region • Soft tissue edema, rarely abscess.
  First signs of healing:
  - Sclerosis.
  - Reduced focal uptake on scintigraphy.
  - Conversion of fatty marrow and reduced enhancement on MRI.

Clinical Aspects

- **Typical presentation**
  Usually there is marked pain and tenderness to palpation in the affected area • Fever • Erythrocyte sedimentation rate is elevated.
- **Therapeutic options**
  Long-term antibiotics • Stabilization of the spine (corset, surgery) • Surgical removal of abscess where indicated.

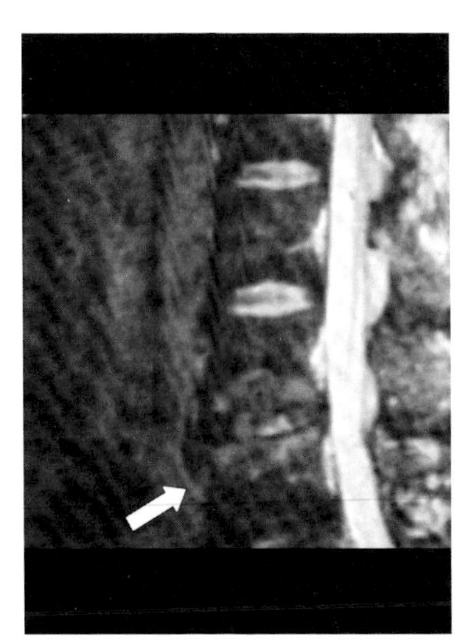

Fig. 4.30 MR image of the lumbar spine (sagittal, T2). Subchondral hyperintensity (edema) at L2–L3 with a fine halo (sclerosis, fibrosis). There is partial destruction of the cortex (superior and inferior endplates). Disk height is reduced and there are abnormal changes in the nucleus pulposus (hypointense longitudinal ligament cannot be differentiated; 1–2 weeks before onset of clinical symptoms).

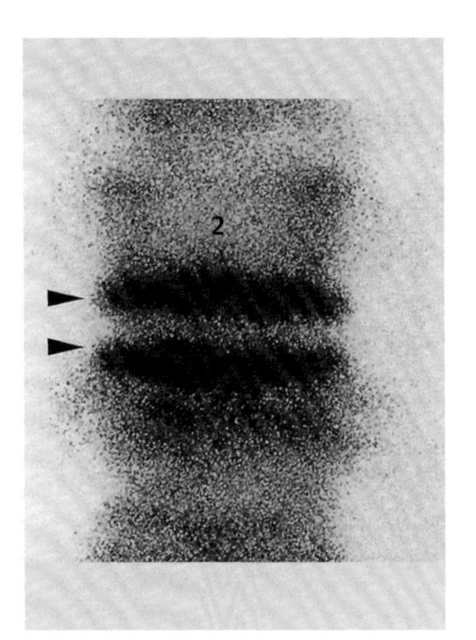

Fig. 4.31 Bone scan of L2–L3 (detail). Abnormal focal uptake in the subchondral region at L2–L3, disk narrowing with increased focal uptake. Typical picture of spondylodiskitis (1–2 weeks after onset of clinical symptoms).

▸ **Course and prognosis**

With early treatment, the prognosis is very good • 25% of cases become chronic • *Complications:* Abscess, sequestration • *Late complications* ("healing"): Scoliosis, kyphosis, fused vertebrae.

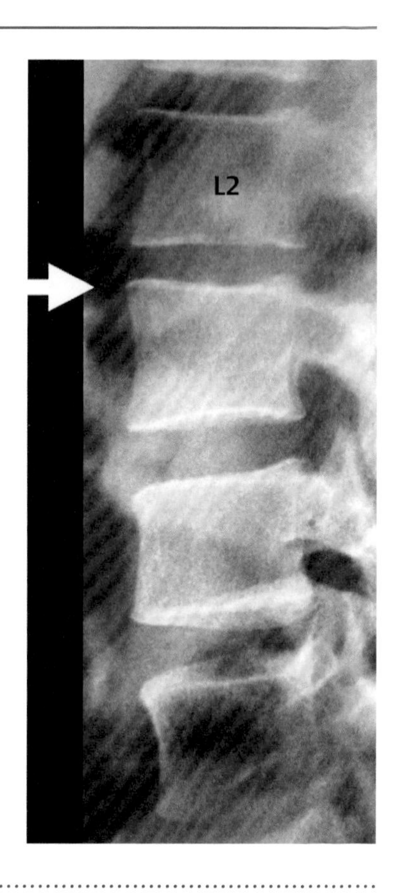

Fig. 4.32 Conventional lateral radiograph of the lumbar spine. Discrete disk narrowing at L2–L3 (6–8 weeks after onset of clinical symptoms).

Differential Diagnosis

Specific spondylitis	– History – Clinical symptoms are usually less severe, less disk involvement, extensive abscesses, soft tissue swelling, calcification
Vertebral fracture	– Osteoporosis, trauma – Contrast images: no inflammation or abscesses
Metastasis	– Changes in vertebral body; disk is not usually involved – History of underlying malignant disorder – Diffusion sequence (reduced diffusion)
Epidural abscess	– History – Distributed over several segments – Vertebral body and disk are not the focus of the disorder

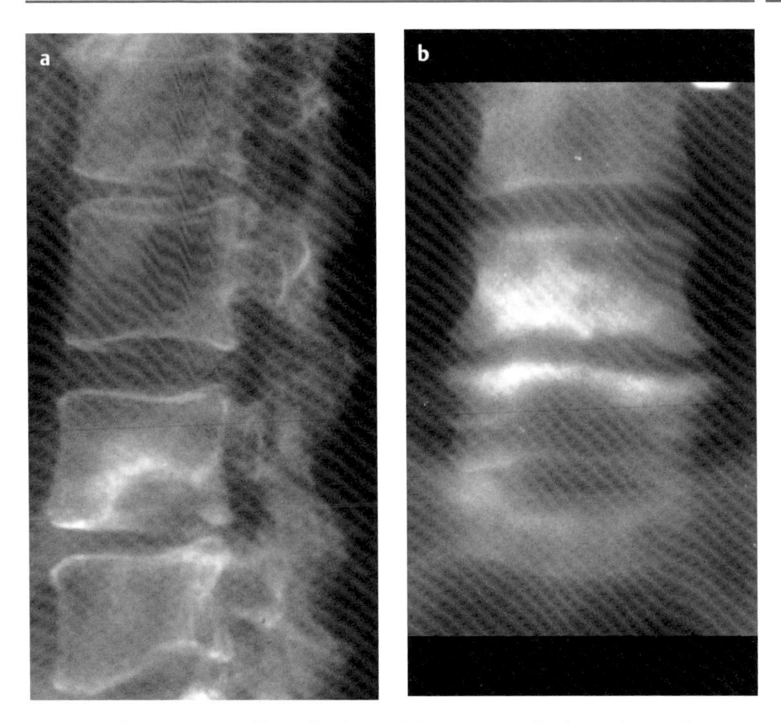

Fig. 4.33 a, b Conventional lateral radiograph (**a**). Circumscribed osteolysis with posteroinferior marginal sclerosis of vertebra L3 with narrowing of the L3–L4 disk. Conventional A-P tomography (**b**). Narrowing of the L4–L5 disk with significant subchondral sclerosis and irregular osteolysis. Typical findings in chronic spondylodiskitis. The sclerosis is an initial sign of healing.

Selected References

Dagirmanjian A, et al. MR of vertebral osteomyelitis revisited. AJR1996; 167: 1539–1543

Imhof H, Kramer J, Rand T, Trattnig S. Knochenentzündungen (einschließlich Spondylitis). Orthopäde 1994; 23: 323

Tali ET. Spinal infections. European Journal of Radiology 2004; 50: 120–133

Vahlensieck M, Reiser M. MRT des Bewegungsapparates, 3rd ed. Stuttgart: Thieme 2006

Vorbeck F, Morscher M, Ba-Ssalamah A, Imhof H. Infektiöse Spondylitis beim Erwachsenen. Radiologe 1996; 36: 795

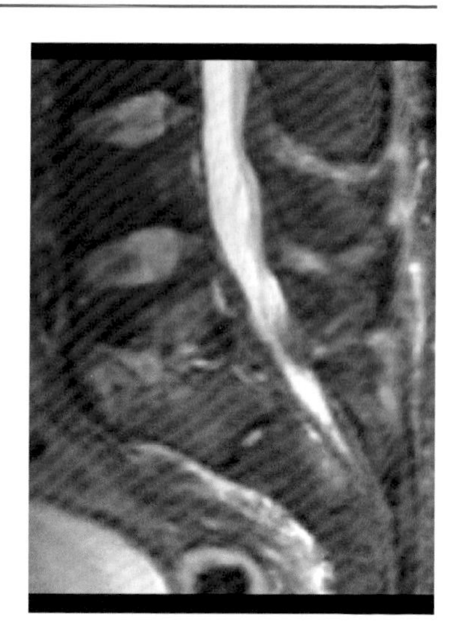

Fig. 4.34 MR image of the lumbar spine (sagittal, STIR). The image shows destruction of the L5–S1 disk. The subchondral regions of the adjacent vertebral bodies are also affected.

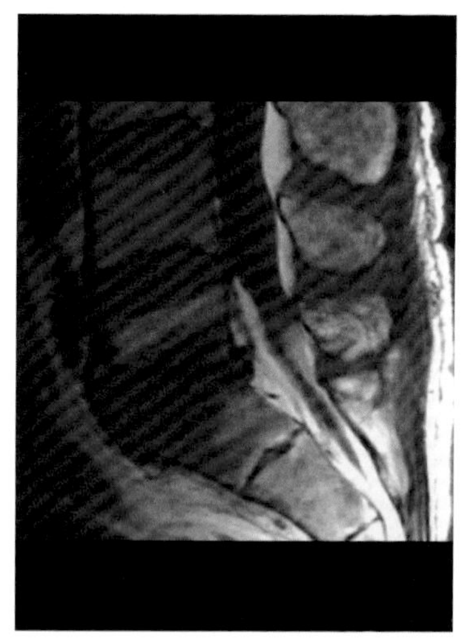

Fig. 4.35 MR image of the lumbar spine (sagittal, T1). Vertebral and disk destruction (hypointensity).

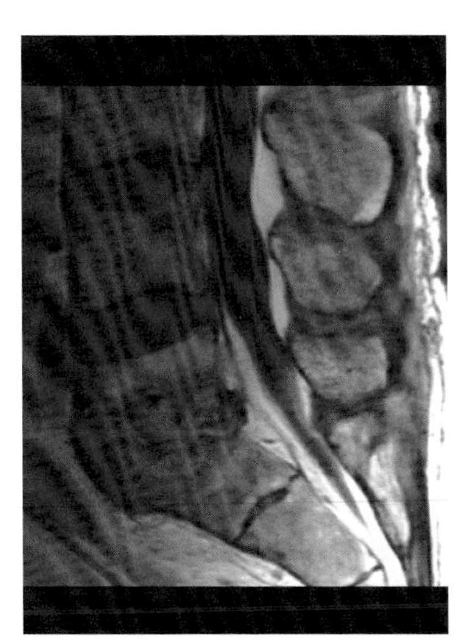

Fig. 4.36 MR image of the lumbar spine (sagittal, T1 with contrast). Enhancement of the inflammatory tissue. This is not an abscess.

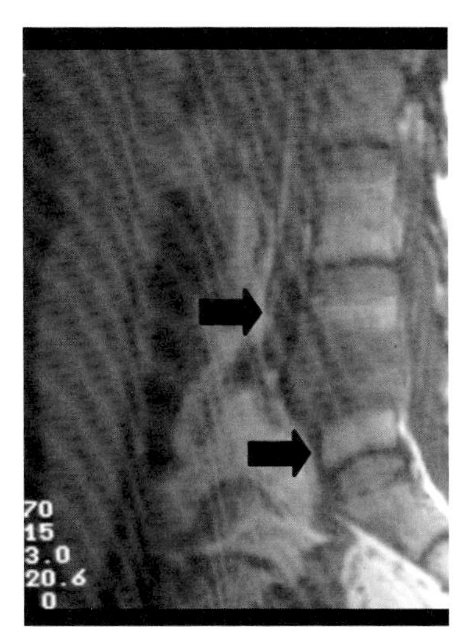

Fig. 4.37 MR image of the lumbar spine (sagittal, T1 with contrast). The image shows complete destruction of the L4–L5 disk. An area of subchondral inflammation is present. Anterior paravertebral soft tissue swelling (inflammation).

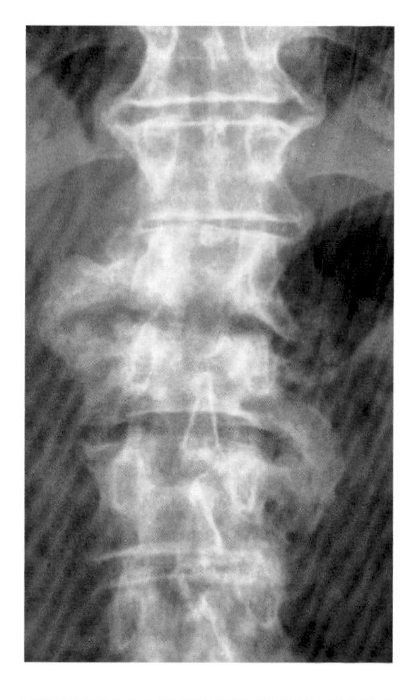

Fig. 4.38 Conventional A-P radiograph. The T11–T12 and T12–L1 disk interspaces are narrowed with irregular margins, indicating sclerosis with pronounced bridging osteophytes. Chronic (healed) spondylitis.

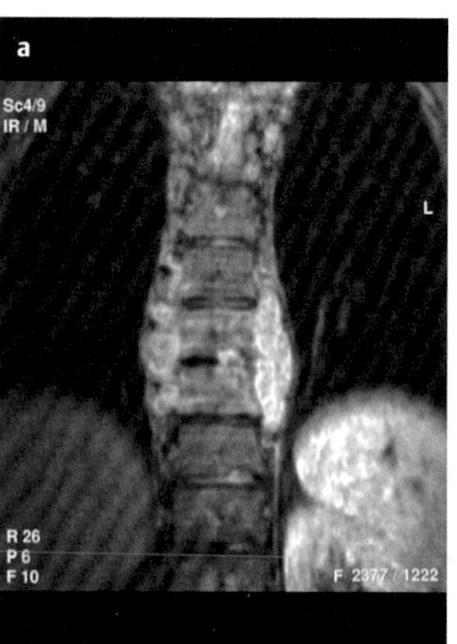

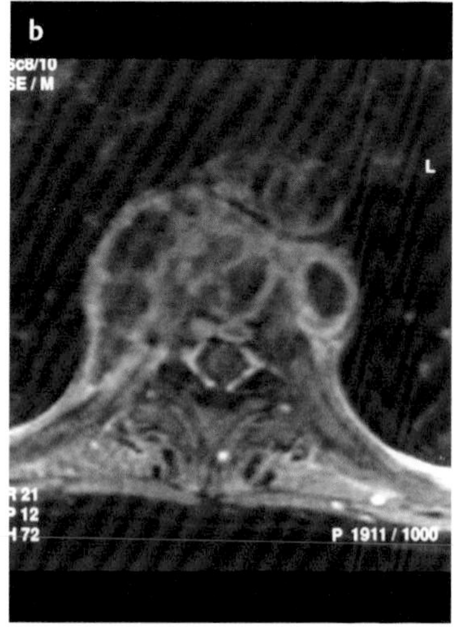

Fig. 4.39 a, b MR image of the lower thoracic spine (coronal, axial, STIR, T1 with contrast). Paravertebral soft tissue swelling at T9–T10 with formation of a paravertebral abscess. Intervertebral disks T9 and T10 are hyperintense (= edema).

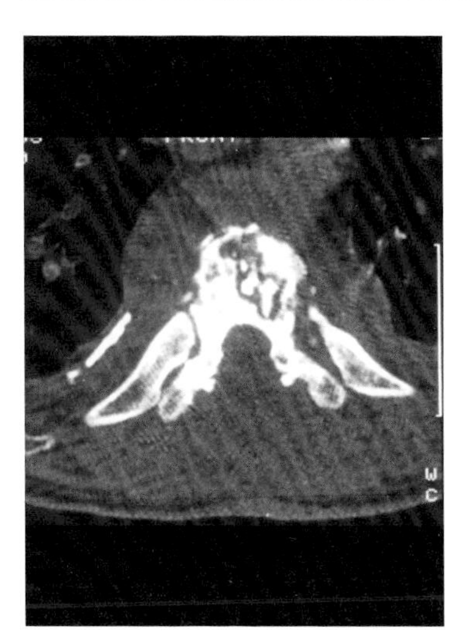

Fig. 4.40 CT of vertebra T12 (axial). Sequestrum in the vertebral body. The vertebral body and parts of the vertebral arch are abnormally dense. Marked soft tissue swelling.

Definition

- **Epidemiology**
  Peak incidence is at 20–40 years • Spinal involvement is present in only 1% of patients with tuberculosis, usually at the thoracolumbar junction • 10% of the patients with spinal tuberculosis also have lung involvement.
- **Etiology, pathophysiology, pathogenesis**
  Tuberculous infestation of the spine • Tuberculous spondylitis or Pott disease; kyphosis in this disease is known as Pott's curvature • Fungi (*Aspergillus*) • Pseudotuberculous spondylitis • Immunosuppressed patients are at risk.
  Typical findings:
  - Multisegmental involvement.
  - Soft tissue tumor.
  - Calcification in 30% of cases.

Imaging Signs

- **Modality of choice**
  Early diagnosis:
  - MRI.
  - Scintigraphy.

  Diagnosis during clinical course (late diagnosis):
  - Conventional radiographs.
  - MRI (with complications).
- **Radiographic findings**
  Inflammatory destruction of bone, diffuse sclerosis (visible on radiographs later than on cross-sectional images) • Disk space may be narrowed with an irregular margin • Secondary spinal deformities (gibbus) and fused vertebrae are well visualized on plain films.
- **CT findings**
  CT also shows typical signs of osteomyelitis with bony destruction; these may occur first in the anterior portion of the vertebral body • Sequestra are well visualized as are typical calcifications of the paravertebral abscesses.
- **MRI findings**
  Always obtain contrast images • Typical inflammatory signal in the vertebral body (osteomyelitis)—hyperintense on STIR images, hypointense on T1-weighted images, significantly enhancing, often at the periphery with a sequestrum or necrosis in the center • There may be anterior involvement (anterior spondylitis) • Several vertebral bodies may be affected with dissemination along the posterior longitudinal ligament, possibly sparing the disks • Disk involvement appears as an inhomogeneously enhancing disk, hyperintense on STIR and T2-weighted images, with irregular margins • Soft tissue abscesses typically occur in the psoas or epidural regions, appearing hyperintense on STIR and T2-weighted images and hypointense on T1-weighted images, with significant marginal enhancement.

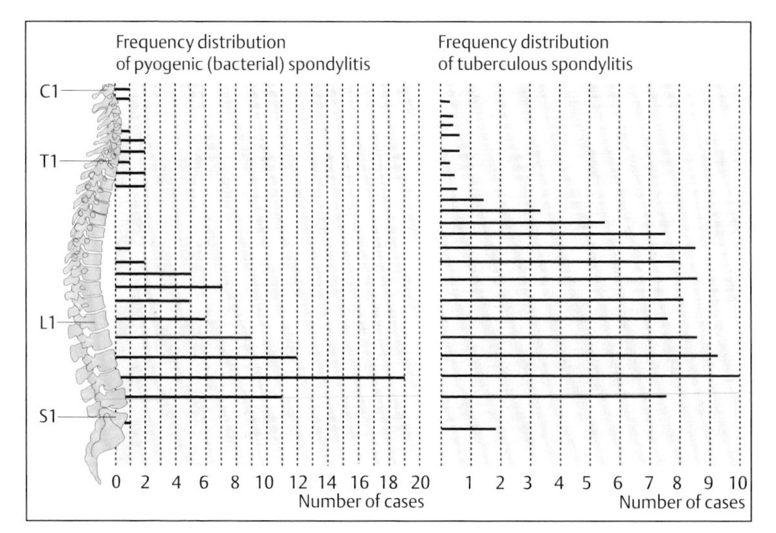

Fig. 4.41 a, b Frequency distribution of pyogenic (bacterial) spondylitis (**a**) and tuberculous spondylitis (**b**).

Clinical Aspects

- **Typical presentation**
  Chronic lumbago, occasionally with kyphosis • Neurologic deficits may be present • Subfebrile • There may be a history of residence in an endemic area.
- **Therapeutic options**
  Abscess drainage • Long-term antibiotics • Stabilization of the spine (corset, surgery).
- **Course and prognosis**
  With prompt treatment, the prognosis is good • Neurologic deficits may persist.

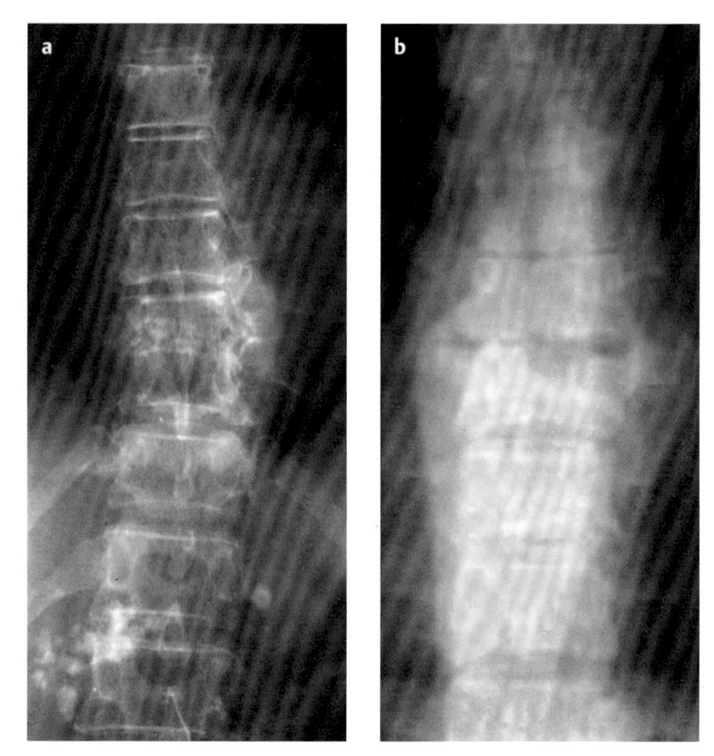

Fig. 4.42 a, b Conventional A-P radiograph (**a**) and conventional tomogram (**b**) of the thoracic spine. Narrowing of the disk, right lateral subchondral osteolysis, fine marginal sclerosis, significant soft tissue swelling spreading to T7 and T10. Reactive osteophytes.

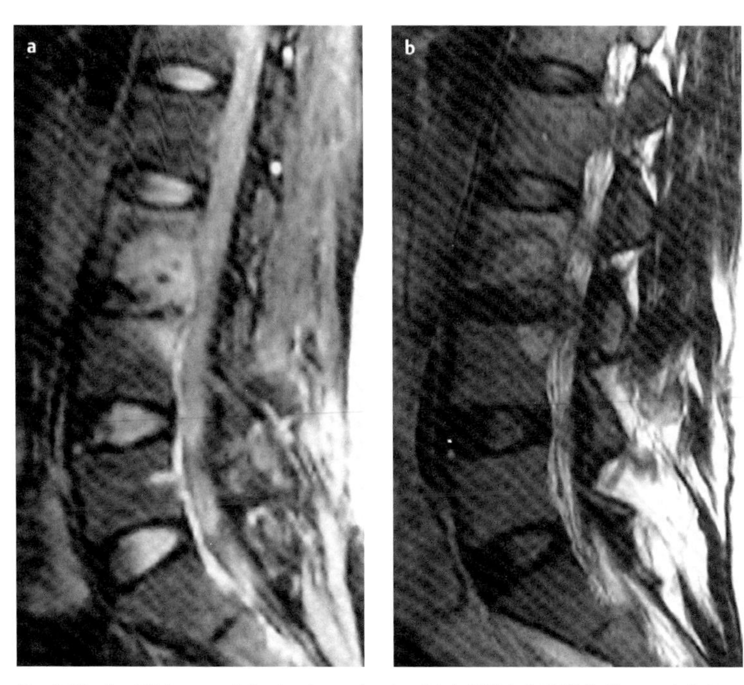

Fig. 4.43 a, b MR image of the lumbar spine (sagittal, STIR [**a**], T2 [**b**]). Posteroinferior hyperintensity in L3 and posterior hyperintensity in L4. Disk is partially hyperintense with reduced height.

Differential Diagnosis

Bacterial spondylitis	– History – Peak ages 10–30 and 50–70 years – Predilection for the lower lumbar spine – Spondylodiskitis
Vertebral fracture	– Osteoporosis, trauma – Contrast images: no inflammation or abscesses
Metastasis	– Changes in vertebral body; disk is not usually involved – No paravertebral abscesses – History of underlying malignant disorder – Diffusion sequence (reduced diffusion)
Epidural abscess	– History – Distributed over several segments – Vertebral body and disk are not the focus of the disorder
Fungal infection	– History – Indistinguishable on imaging studies

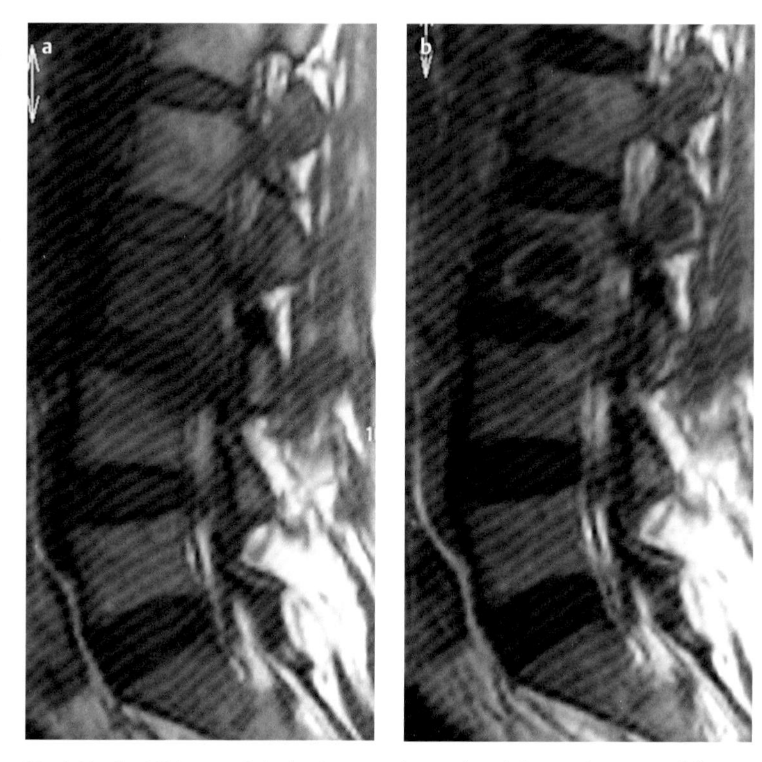

Fig. 4.44 a, b MR image of the lumbar spine (sagittal, T1 [**a**], T1 with contrast [**b**]). L3 appears hypointense with an enhancing halo after IV contrast administration (edema with abscess and granulation tissue). Posterior soft tissue swelling spreading to L4.

Selected References

Bohndorf K, Imhof H. Radiologische Diagnostik der Knochen und Gelenke, 2nd ed. Stuttgart: Thieme 2006

Tali ET. Spinal infections. European Journal of Radiology 2004; 50: 120–133

Vahlensieck M, Reiser M. MRT des Bewegungsapparates, 3rd ed. Stuttgart: Thieme 2006

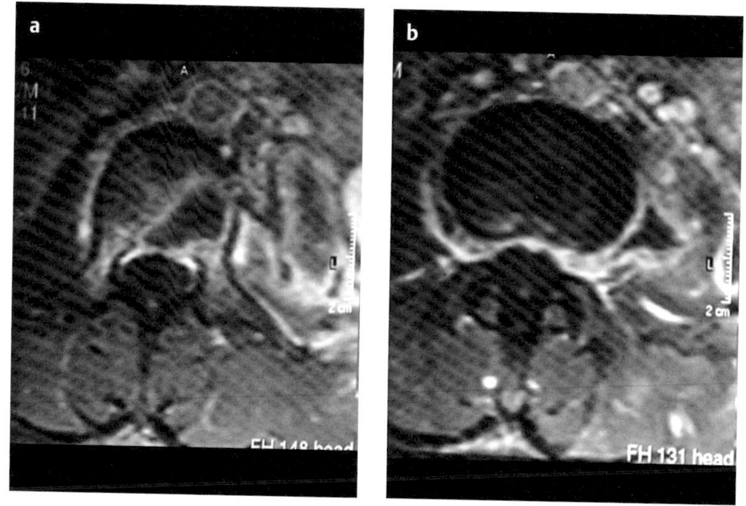

Fig. 4.45 a, b MR image of L3 (axial, T1 with fat saturation and contrast). The area of liquefaction has broken through the cortex posteriorly (with spread along the posterior longitudinal ligament) and in the left lateral region. Large psoas abscesses are present.

Definition

▸ **Epidemiology**
More common in men than in women • Highest incidence is at age 50–60 years • Most common pathogens: *Staphylococcus aureus*, streptococci, *Escherichia coli, Pseudomonas*; less often anaerobes, mycobacteria, and fungi.

▸ **Etiology, pathophysiology, pathogenesis**
Accumulation of pus between the dura mater of the spinal cord and the vertebral periosteum • *Hematogenous dissemination* (occurring in 60% of cases): Skin and soft tissue infection, infectious endocarditis, pneumonia, urogenital tract infection • *By extension:* vertebral osteomyelitis, psoas abscess, paraspinal abscess, trauma • *Iatrogenic:* lumbar puncture, epidural anesthesia, postoperatively.

Imaging Signs

▸ **Modality of choice**
MRI:
- Sagittal: T1, T2, STIR (bone), T1 with contrast and fat saturation.
- Axial: T1 with contrast and fat saturation.
- Coronal (one sequence): Visualization of the paraspinal extension (psoas major).

Conventional radiographs:
- To demonstrate associated osteomyelitis.

▸ **CT findings**
Used where MRI is contraindicated • Fluid accumulation in the epidural space • CT myelography is sensitive but invasive • CT-guided biopsy to identify the pathogen.

▸ **MRI findings**
Epidural mass compressing the spinal cord and displacing the dura mater, more often anterior than posterior • May spread through the neural foramina to cause abscess in the psoas major • Signal alteration in the adjacent vertebral bodies and disks with simultaneous spondylodiskitis.
T1:
- Hypointense mass, contrast improves demarcation of the abscess membrane.

T2:
- Homogeneously hyperintense to spinal cord and isointense to CSF.

DWI:
- Hyperintense signal with corresponding hypointensity on the apparent diffusion coefficient (ADC) evaluation image.

Clinical Aspects

▸ **Typical presentation**
Back pain, radicular pain • Weakness in the legs • Sphincter dysfunction • Fever.

▸ **Therapeutic options**
Surgical decompression via laminectomy and drainage • Systemic antibiotic therapy.

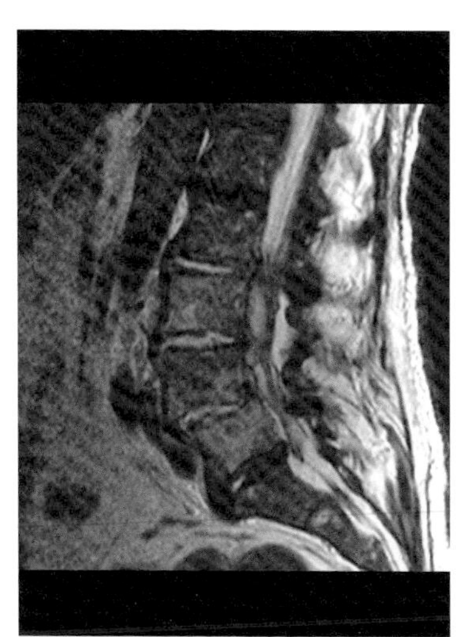

Fig. 4.46 Recurrence of pain with elevated inflammatory markers (generalized sepsis) after spondylodiskitis. MR image of the lumbar spine (sagittal, T2). Biconvex epidural mass at the level of vertebra L3. The mass is homogeneously hyperintense and demarcated from the spinal cord by a hypointense membrane. Hyperintense intervertebral disks at levels L2–L3 through L4–L5.

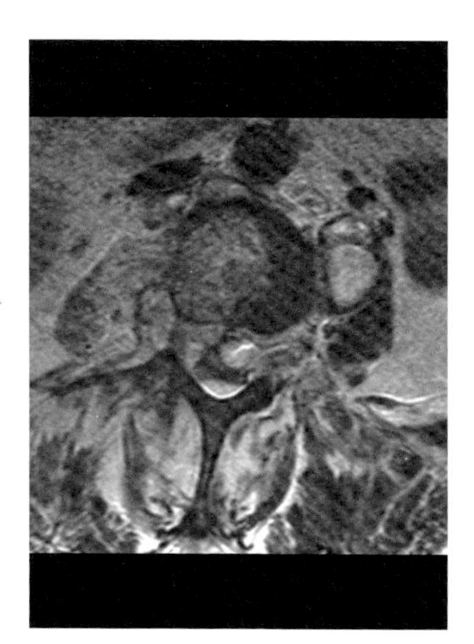

Fig. 4.47 MR image of L3 (axial, T2). The lesion has spread through the left neural foramen, with abscess formation in the left psoas major.

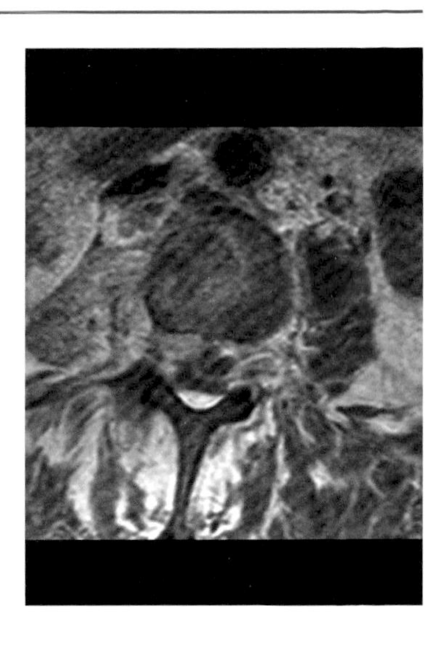

Fig. 4.48 MR image of L3 (axial, T1 with contrast and fat saturation). Psoas major abscess and epidural abscess.

▸ **Course and prognosis**
Mortality 5–10% • Neurologic status at the time of the diagnosis is an important prognostic factor.

Differential Diagnosis

Epidural hematoma	– History (trauma, anticoagulation) – Acute onset of clinical symptoms – Inflammatory markers
Vertebral body osteomyelitis	– Limited to the bone
Spondylodiskitis	– Intervertebral disk is involved
Disk herniation	– Signal differs on T1- and T2-weighted images – Pathology limited to one segment – No enhancement (except sequestra)
Guillain–Barré syndrome (postinfectious polyneuropathy)	– No mass effect

Selected References

Joshi SM et al. Spinal epidural abscess: a diagnostic challenge. Br J Neurosurg 2003; 17: 160–163

Nussbaum ES et al. Spinal epidural abscess: a report of 40 cases and review. Surg Neurol 1992; 38: 225–231

Ruiz A et al. MR imaging of infections of the cervical spine. Magn Reson Imaging Clin N Am. 2000; 8: 561–80

Definition

Inflammatory disorders of the spinal cord and spinal canal of different etiologies, characterized by granuloma formation.

▸ **Selected clinical conditions**

Sarcoidosis: Neurologic symptoms occur in 5% of cases • Spinal manifestation is rare, most often between 30 and 40 years • Most often in the cervical spine (> 50%) and thoracic spine (< 40%).

Wegener granulomatosis: Neurologic involvement is present in 30–50% of cases.

Tuberculosis: Neurologic involvement is usually cerebral, rarely spinal • More common in immunocompromised persons (elderly people, children, and patients with HIV or diabetes).

Imaging Signs

▸ **Modality of choice**

MRI:
- Sagittal: T1, T2, T1 with contrast.
- Axial: T1 with contrast, T2.
- Study should include the cerebrum.

CSF examination:
- CNS sarcoidosis: Pleocytosis, elevated protein content, elevated IgG, and elevated ACE (nonspecific).
- Wegener granulomatosis: Pleocytosis, elevated protein content, elevated IgG ("sterile meningitis," nonspecific).
- Tuberculosis: Pleocytosis, elevated protein content, depressed glucose content; PCR identifies the pathogen.

Biopsy:
- Granulomas are seen.
- Wegener granulomatosis: c-ANCA is detected.
- Tuberculosis: PCR identifies the pathogen.

▸ **Conventional radiographs and CT findings**

Associated bony changes are seen • *Tuberculous spondylodiskitis:* Destruction of the vertebral body, often multisegmental • *Sarcoidosis:* Nodular pattern of bony sclerosis in the axial skeleton (nonspecific), lytic and cystic changes in the phalanges and metacarpals (arthritis).

▸ **MRI findings**

Leptomeningitis:
- Linear enhancement after contrast administration, along the spinal cord, nerve roots, and cauda equina.
- Epidural granulomas and tuberculomas.
- Enhancing nodular or plaquelike dural deposits.

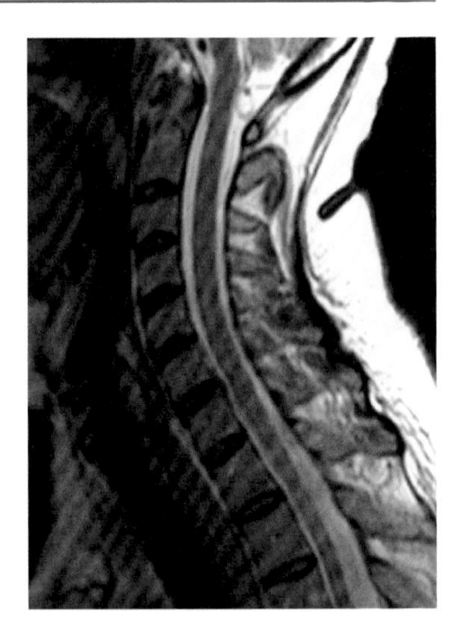

Fig. 4.49 This patient with known Wegener granulomatosis since several years developed gait disturbances and sensory deficits at various levels in the past few weeks. MR image of the cervical spine (sagittal, T2). Numerous indistinct hyperintense signal alterations in the spinal cord.

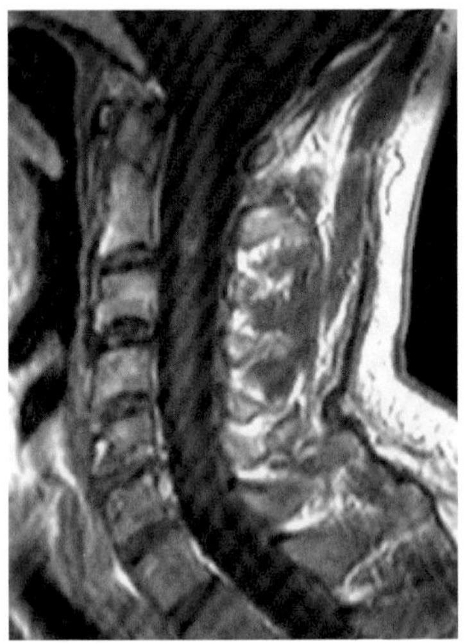

Fig. 4.50 Patient with known sarcoidosis, on cortisone therapy, complaining of headache in the past few weeks. Neurologic examination suggests involvement of long pathways. MR image of the cervical spine (sagittal, T1 with contrast). An enhancing spinal cord lesion is seen at C1–C2, as are two lesions in the caudal portion of the pons (cerebral involvement was present in the underlying disorder). *Caution:* With cortisone therapy there is usually no meningeal enhancement.

Intramedullary granulomas and tuberculomas:
- T1: Isointense or hypointense.
- T2: Isointense, hypointense, or hyperintense.
- Nodular or ring enhancement.
- Perifocal edema (hyperintense on T2-weighted images).

Tuberculous spondylodiskitis (p. 166)

Clinical Aspects

- **Typical presentation**
  Back pain • Fever • Cauda equina syndrome • Weakness in the legs • Paraparesis and tetraparesis.
- **Therapeutic options**
  Wegener granulomatosis:
  - High dose cyclophosphamide therapy (alternatively: azathioprine, methotrexate).
  - Usually remits but often recurs.

  Tuberculosis:
  - Tuberculostatic agents.
  - Microsurgical resection of intramedullary tuberculomas.

  Sarcoidosis:
  - Corticosteroids, usually over several months.
  - Recurrence is possible.

Differential Diagnosis

Leptomeningeal metastases	- History - In metastatic leptomeningeal malignancies, the leptomeningeal thickening is more often nodular and irregular.
Arachnoiditis	- History: postoperative condition, trauma, infection - No intramedullary involvement
Intramedullary tumors	
Multiple sclerosis	
Acute transverse myelitis	

Selected References

Lexa FJ et al. MR of sarcoidosis in the head and spine: spectrum of manifestations and radiographic response to steroid therapy. AJNR Am J Neuroradiol 1994; 15: 973–982

Moorthy S et al. Spectrum of MR imaging findings in spinal tuberculosis. AJR Am J Roentgenol 2002; 179: 979–983

Nishino H et al. Neurological involvement in Wegener's granulomatosis: an analysis of 324 consecutive patients at the Mayo Clinic. Ann Neurol 1993; 33: 4–9

Definition

- **Epidemiology**
  Incidence is increasing due to the increasing number of immunocompromised patients.
- **Etiology, pathophysiology, pathogenesis**
  Inflammatory disorder of meninges and subarachnoid space • Inflammation with fibrinous exudate.
  Pathogenesis:
  - Postoperative and posttraumatic.
  - Infectious (bacteria, viruses, fungi, parasites).
  - Intrathecal application of oil-containing contrast agents (no longer permitted), anesthetics, antibiotics, and steroids.
  - Intraspinal hemorrhage.

  Complications: Syringomyelia, spinal arachnoid cysts, arachnoiditis ossificans.

Imaging Signs

- **Modality of choice**
  MRI:
  - Sagittal (T1, T2, STIR).
  - Axial (T2).
  - Sagittal and axial (T1-weighted) contrast sequences with fat suppression.
- **CT findings**
  CT myelography (where MRI is contraindicated):
  - Irregular accumulation of contrast agent around thickened nerve roots.
  - Contrast filling defects from granulation tissue.
- **MRI findings**
  Types:
  - Type I: Adhesions form conglomerates around nerve roots.
  - Type II: *"Empty thecal sac":* The fibers of the cauda equina adhere to the dural sac, creating the impression of an "empty" dural sac on axial images.
  - Type III: Soft tissue mass in the dural sac is seen in the final stage of the inflammation process.

  T1:
  - CSF signal is increased so that the outer contour of the spinal cord is no longer clearly demarcated.
  - Usually the meninges and fibers of the cauda equina show homogeneous linear enhancement, rarely nodular enhancement.
  - Diffuse intradural enhancement is seen where the dural sac is filled with inflammatory soft tissue.

  T2:
  - Thickened nerve roots with adhesions.
  - Subarachnoid space obliterated by granulation tissue.
  - Leptomeningeal adhesions.

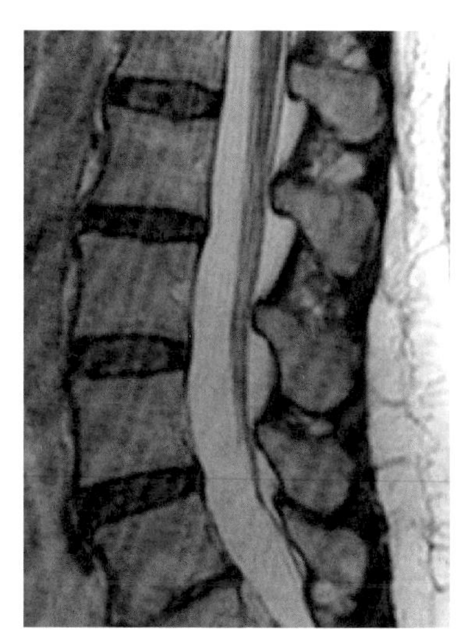

Fig. 4.51 Several months after surgery for a herniated disk at L4–L5 the patient complained of increasing pain in both legs and then urine retention. Clinical examination revealed "saddle" anesthesia and residual urine. Elevated inflammatory markers. MR image of the lumbar spine (sagittal, T2). Cauda equina fibers cannot be distinguished; some edema is present in vertebrae L5–S1.

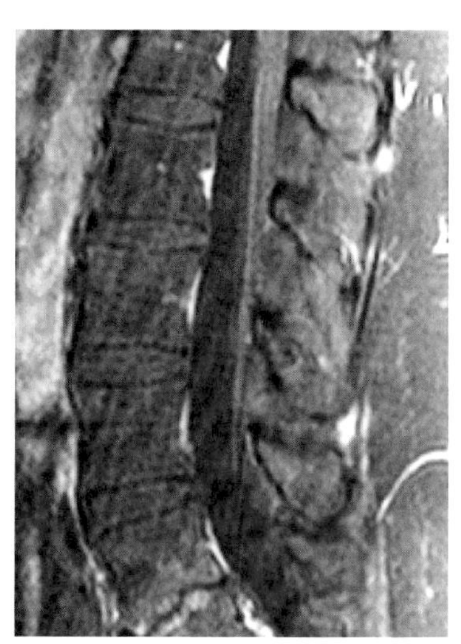

Fig. 4.52 MR image of the lumbar spine (sagittal, T1 with contrast). The thickened cauda equina fibers and L4–L5 disk are enhanced, early spondylodiskitis at L5–S1.

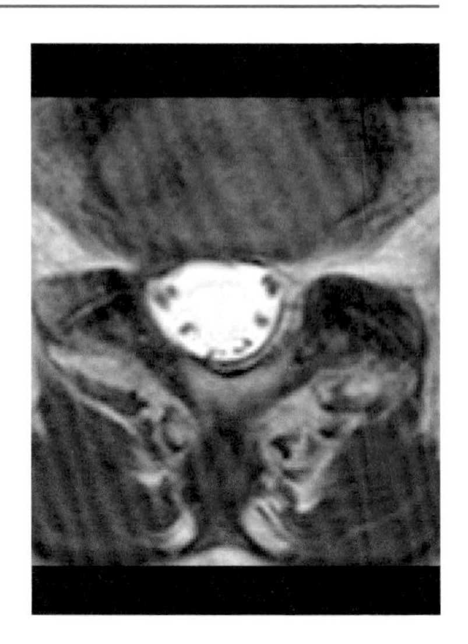

Fig. 4.53 MR image of L4 (axial, T2). The cauda equina fibers are adherent to the dural sac, creating the impression of an "empty" dural sac (type II).

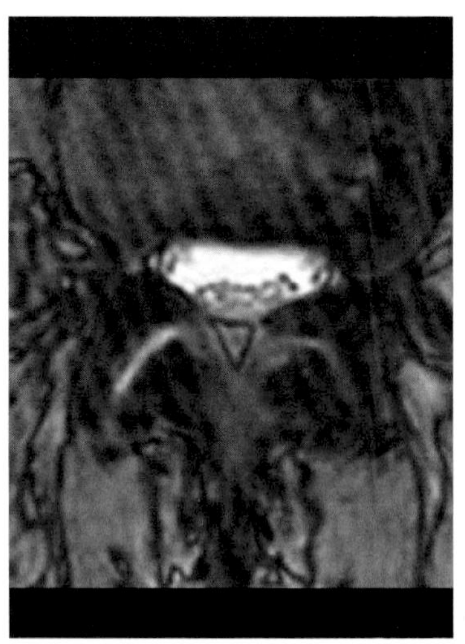

Fig. 4.54 MR image of L4 (axial, T2). Normal pattern of cauda equina fibers.

Clinical Aspects

- **Typical presentation**
  Chronic low back pain • Paresis from tethering and/or compression of the spinal cord • Leg weakness • Neurogenic bladder and bowel dysfunction.
- **Therapeutic options**
  Symptomatic medical treatment • Surgical lysis of adhesions.

Differential Diagnosis

Leptomeningeal metastases	– Enhancement is usually more intense in metastatic leptomeningeal malignancies – Leptomeningeal thickening is more often nodular, irregular, and asymmetric – Not always clearly distinguishable from benign arachnoiditis on MRI – History is crucial to diagnosis
Intradural tumor	– History – Tumor usually shows more pronounced enhancement
Sarcoidosis	– Enhancing leptomeningeal lesion usually accompanied by enhancing intramedullary focal lesions – Bony changes in the vertebral bodies

Selected References

Fitt GJ et al. Postoperative arachnoiditis diagnosed by high resolution fast spin-echo MRI of the lumbar spine. Neuroradiology 1995; 37: 139–145

Ross JS et al. MR imaging of lumbar arachnoiditis. AJR Am J Roentgenol 1987; 149: 1025–1032

Struffert T et al. Lumbar arachnoiditis as differential chronic spinal symptoms diagnosis. Radiologe 2001; 41: 987–992

Definition

- **Epidemiology**
  Bimodal age distribution with peaks at 10–20 and 30–40 years • Predilection for the cervical and thoracic spine.
- **Etiology, pathophysiology, pathogenesis**
  Clinical syndrome characterized by dysfunction of motor, sensory, and autonomous nerve pathways due to an acute focal spinal cord inflammation • *Diagnostic criteria:* MRI demonstrates an enhancing lesion and CSF examination reveals pleocytosis or elevated IgG.
  Causes:
  - ADEM: Acute inflammation of the brain and spinal cord; postinfectious, postvaccinal, or sporadic.
  - Parainfectious: Viral (herpes simplex, herpes zoster, cytomegalovirus, enteroviruses, Epstein–Barr virus, HIV, influenza, rabies), bacterial (mycoplasmas, syphilis, borreliosis, tuberculosis).
  - Systemic disorders: Systemic lupus erythematosus, Sjögren syndrome, sarcoidosis.
  - Multiple sclerosis.
  - Paraneoplastic syndrome.
  - Vascular causes (arteriovenous malformation, vasculitis, spinal thrombosis).
  - Radiation myelopathy.
  - Idiopathic.
  - Atopic.

Imaging Signs

- **Modality of choice**
  Acute indication for MRI:
  - Sagittal: STIR, T2, T1 (with and without contrast).
  - Axial: T2, T1 with contrast.

  CSF examination:
  - Oligoclonal bands, PCR, IgG index, antibodies (mycoplasmas, *Borrelia*).
  - Serologic tests according to clinical findings.

  CT myelography:
  - Where MRI is not feasible or available. (Caution: Spinal puncture can cause spinal cord swelling.)
- **MRI findings**
  General:
  - Slight to significant expansion of the spinal cord. For this reason, imaging studies must be done prior to spinal puncture.
  - Lesion extends over more than two-thirds of the cross-sectional area of the spinal cord.
  - Can extend across several spinal segments (prognosis is poor where more than 10 segments are involved).

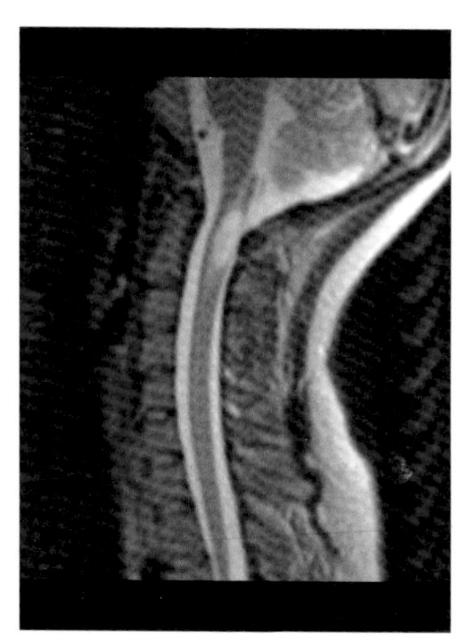

Fig. 4.55 This patient reported weakness in the arm and leg, increasing over the course of a single day and more pronounced on the right side. Neurologic status included loss of right corneal reflex and crescentic sensory deficit in the face. MR image of the cervical spine (sagittal, T2). Intramedullary hyperintense signal alteration at the level of C1–C2, where the spinal cord is distended. On the axial T2-weighted sequence, the signal alterations appear more pronounced on the right side.

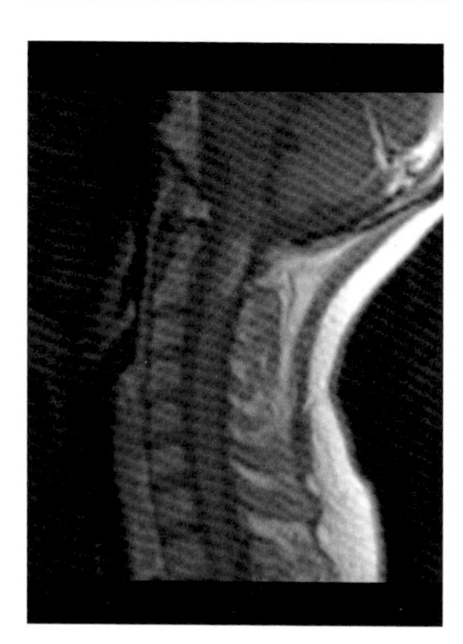

Fig. 4.56 MR image of the cervical spine (sagittal, T1 with contrast). Lesion shows partial enhancement.

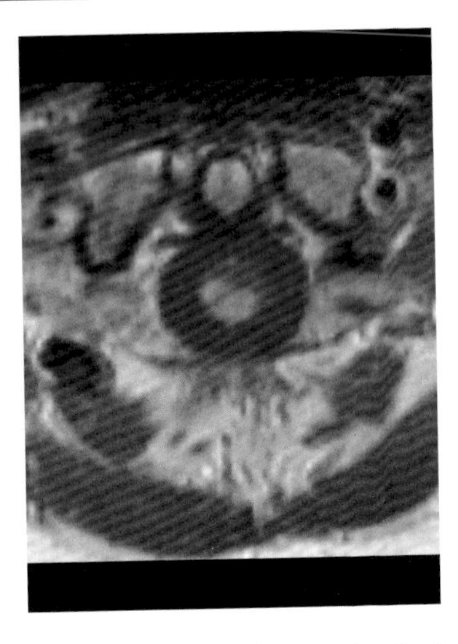

Fig. 4.57 MR image of C1 (axial, T1 with contrast). Delayed enhancement of the lesion.

- Skip lesions are observed, normal areas in the spinal cord between involved segments.

T1:
- Inhomogeneous.
- Marginal enhancement (inconstant, transient, and often only briefly detectable).
- Enhancement is often delayed, so late sequences should be obtained (several T1-weighted sequences after contrast administration).

T2:
- Hyperintense central lesion
- Isointense area in the center ("central dot sign")
- Sharply demarcated.

Clinical Aspects

▸ **Typical presentation**

The full clinical picture develops within 24 hours in 45% of patients • Almost all patients have weakness in the legs • Bladder dysfunction • Paresthesia • Back pain, radicular pain.

▸ **Therapeutic options**

Acute management:
- High-dose intravenous corticosteroid therapy.
- Plasmapheresis.
- Antibiotics in infectious cases.

- Anticoagulation in patients with systemic lupus erythematosus and antiphospholipid antibodies.
- Neurosurgical intervention where indicated.

Long-term management:
- Rehabilitation.
- Pain medication.
- Muscle relaxants.

▸ **Course and prognosis**

Partial or complete regression of clinical symptoms occurs after 1–3 months • Usually a monophasic disorder, although recurrent manifestation is possible where there is a predisposing underlying disorder.

Differential Diagnosis

Disseminated encephalomyelitis	– Asymmetric clinical symptoms with predominantly sensory dysfunction – Oligoclonal bands in CSF (also in ADEM) – Eccentric signal increase in the white matter – Lesion involves fewer than two segments; there are multiple lesions – Enhancement within the lesion in acute episodes
Spinal infarction	– Predilection for gray matter – Usually anterior, in the area supplied by the anterior spinal artery
Intramedullary tumors (such as astrocytoma)	– Inhomogeneously hyperintense (T2) – Entire cross- section affected – Blood breakdown products (hyperintense on T1-weighted images) – No skip lesions – There may be intense heterogeneous enhancement

Selected References

Kerr DA et al. Proposed diagnostic criteria and nosology of acute transverse myelitis. Neurology 2002; 59: 499–505

Kerr DA et al. Immunopathogenesis of transverse myelitis. Current Opinion In Neurology 2002; 15: 339–347

Uhlenbrock D. Akute Querschnittsmyelitis. In: Uhlenbrock (Hrsg.) MRT der Wirbelsäule und des Spinalkanals. Stuttgart: Thieme 2000

Definition

- **Epidemiology**
  Spinal lesions occur in 55–75% of patients with multiple sclerosis • Isolated spinal lesions occur in 20% of cases; 67% of these develop in the cervical spine • Age at which lesions occur is variable • Twice as common in men than in women.
- **Etiology, pathophysiology, pathogenesis**
  Focal demyelination in the spinal cord • MRI findings do not always correlate with clinical symptoms • Histologic findings include lymphoplasmacytic infiltrates (usually perivenous) and selective demyelination, later gliosis and scarring.

Imaging Signs

- **Modality of choice**
  - Indication for MRI: T1, T2, STIR (sagittal), T2 (axial) for proved lesions • Contrast administration (double dose, longer delay) is required to evaluate activity of the lesions.
  - Supplementary cerebral MRI is indicated with any newly detected spinal multiple sclerosis.
  - CSF examination is indicated to confirm the diagnosis (findings include oligoclonal bands).
- **CT findings**
  CT is not indicated.
- **MRI findings**
  General:
  - Plaquelike lesions with nodular, ring-shaped, or arched configuration.
  - Spinal cord involvement is eccentric, especially affecting the posterior and lateral aspects.
  - Less than 50% of the cross-sectional area of the spinal cord is affected.
  - Spinal cord is expanded in the acute phase.
  - Focal or extensive spinal cord atrophy occurs in chronic cases.

  T1:
  - Acute: Isointense to slightly hypointense lesions • Lesions shows marked ring to solid enhancement (detectable for 2–8 weeks).
  - Chronic: Lack of enhancement • Associated spinal cord atrophy.

  T2:
  - Hyperintense lesions.
  - In an acute episode, there may be a diffuse perifocal signal increase and expansion of the spinal cord due to associated edema.

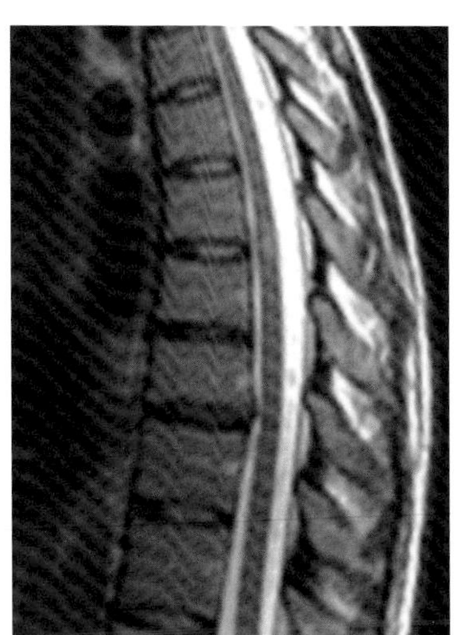

Fig. 4.58 A 33-year-old woman with a 5-week history of paresthesias and progressive motor weakness in both extremities. MR image of the middle thoracic spine (sagittal, T2). A hyperintense intramedullary lesion is seen at the level of T4.

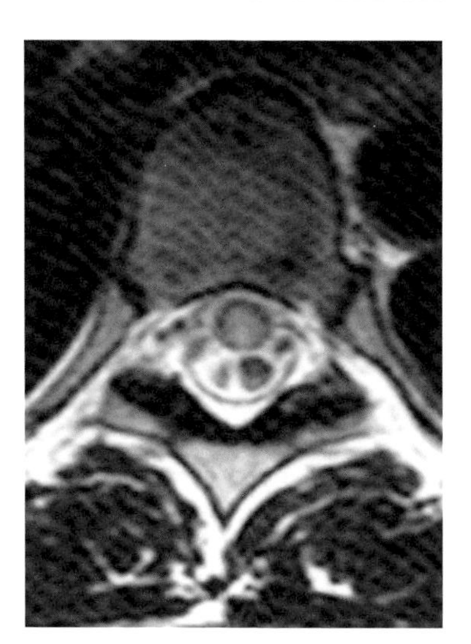

Fig. 4.59 MR image of T2 (axial, T2). The intramedullary lesion is located in the right posterolateral region.

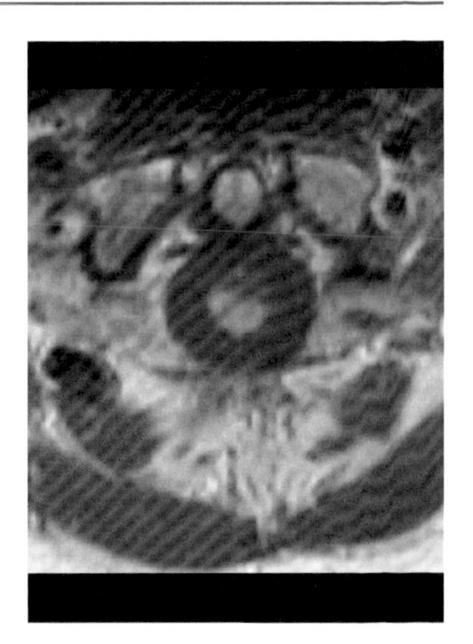

Fig. 4.60 MR image of the thoracic spine (sagittal, diffusion-weighted). Here, too, the lesion appears hyperintense.

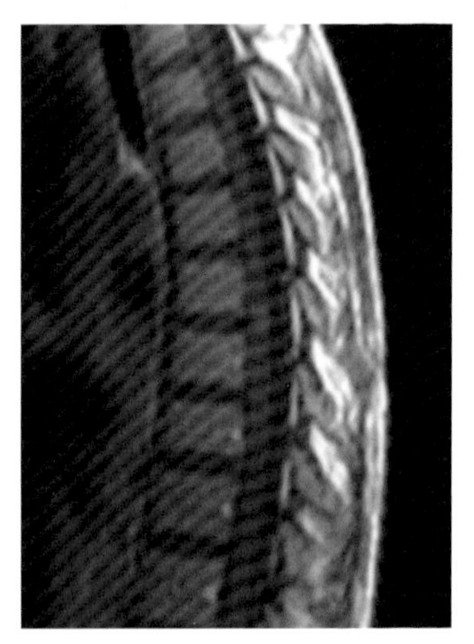

Fig. 4.61 MR image of the thoracic spine (sagittal, T1 with contrast). Enhancing lesion.

Clinical Aspects

- **Typical presentation**
  Sensory deficits • Spastic paresis • Neurogenic bladder and bowel dysfunction • *Devic disease* (neuromyelitis optica): Bilateral optic neuritis and high paraplegia • Clinical course is episodic with complete or incomplete remission between episodes.
- **Therapeutic options**
  Glucocorticoids during the episode • Prophylaxis with interferon, copolymer 1, azathioprine, mitoxantrone (patients with severe clinical course), low-dose methotrexate • Symptomatic medical therapy.

Differential Diagnosis

Astrocytoma	– Usually extends over a longer distance (more than two vertebrae) – Rarely multifocal
Ependymoma	– Central intramedullary location – Extends over a long distance – Associated cysts
Acute transverse myelitis	– Extends over a longer longitudinal distance than multiple sclerosis, often involves more than 50% of the cross-sectional area of the spinal cord – History (infectious, toxic, autoimmune)
Acute spinal infarction	– Paramedian involvement of posterior spinal cord, less often anterior spinal cord
Sarcoidosis	– Enhancing parenchymal lesions and possibly linear leptomeningeal enhancement are also present – When in doubt, biopsy can confirm the diagnosis
Systemic lupus erythematosus	– Picture of transverse myelitis

Selected References

Hickman SJ, Miller DH. Imaging of the spine in multiple sclerosis. Neuroimaging Clin N Am. 2000 Nov; 10: 689–704

Losseff NA et al. T1 hypointensity of the spinal cord in multiple sclerosis. J Neurol 2001; 248: 517–521

Tartaglino LM et al. Multiple sclerosis in the spinal cord: MR appearance and correlation with clinical parameters. Radiology 1995; 195: 725–732

Definition

- **Epidemiology**
  Common (prevalence is 10% of the population) • Primarily affects the thoracic spine.
- **Etiology, pathophysiology, pathogenesis**
  Benign vascular tumor (cavernous, capillary, venous) • Usually an incidental finding (possibly malformation) • Usually limited to the vertebral body • In rare cases, the posterior elements are also involved • Cystic angiomatosis (diffuse skeletal form) • Vertebral collapse can occur as complication • Aggressive (symptomatic) form is rare and characterized by growth, vertebral collapse, lack of fat storage, and an extraosseous component.

Imaging Signs

- **Modality of choice**
  Conventional radiographs.
  Where clinical symptoms are present: MRI (enhancement, size), CT.
- **General**
  Typical configuration of trabeculae • Typical radiologic picture (conventional radiographs, CT, MRI).
- **Radiographic findings**
  Circumscribed osteolysis (defect) • Thickened, “stranded” trabeculae aligned axially.
- **CT findings**
  Circumscribed osteolysis (defect) • Thickened, “stranded” trabeculae aligned axially (multiplanar reconstruction) • Fat deposits.
- **MRI findings**
  T1 hyperintensity • Pronounced T2 hyperintensity (fat deposit) • Complications (spinal cord or nerve root compression) • Moderate to pronounced enhancement • Aggressive hemangioma is hypointense on T1-weighted images, hyperintense on T2-weighted images • Epidural spread and fracture often present.

Clinical Aspects

- **Typical presentation**
  Clinically occult • *Aggressive form:* Localized pain due to vertebral collapse, radiculopathy, myelopathy.
- **Therapeutic options**
  Only the aggressive form requires treatment (vertebroplasty, embolization; radiation therapy) • *With suspected compression:* Surgical stabilization.

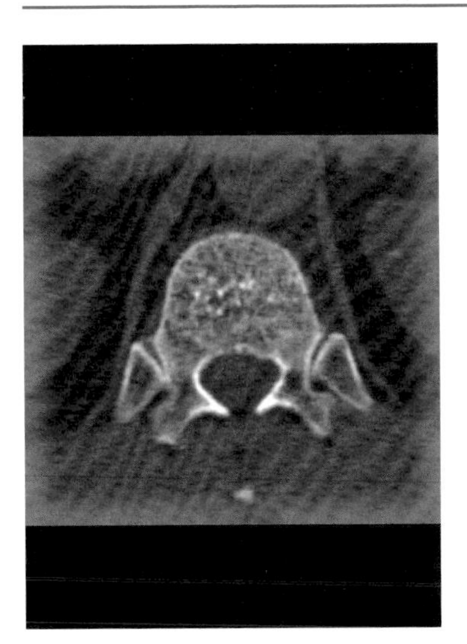

Fig. 5.1 Normal clinical findings. CT (axial). Typically thickened trabeculae showing craniocaudal alignment (salt and pepper pattern).

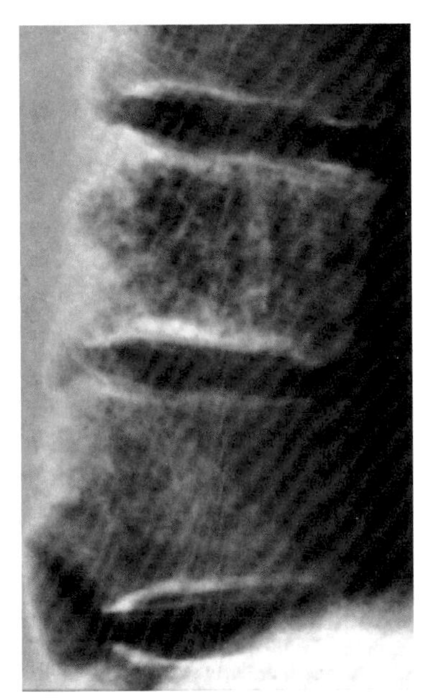

Fig. 5.2 Conventional lateral radiograph of the middle thoracic spine (detail). Coarse, stranded cancellous bone structure. Normal-sized vertebrae.

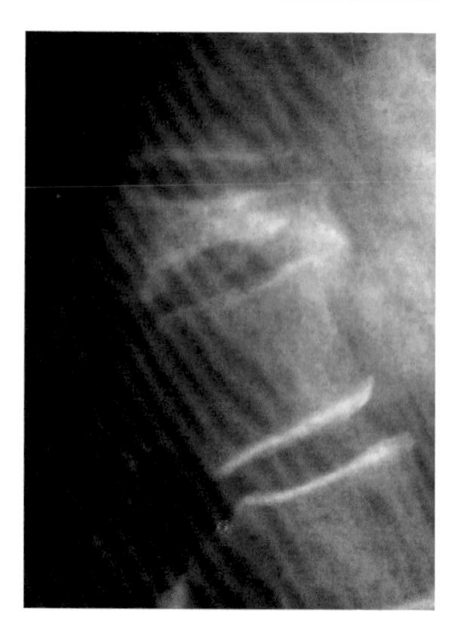

Fig. 5.3 Conventional lateral radiograph of the middle thoracic spine (detail). Compressed vertebra in hemangioma with anterior and posterior displacement (spinal stenosis).

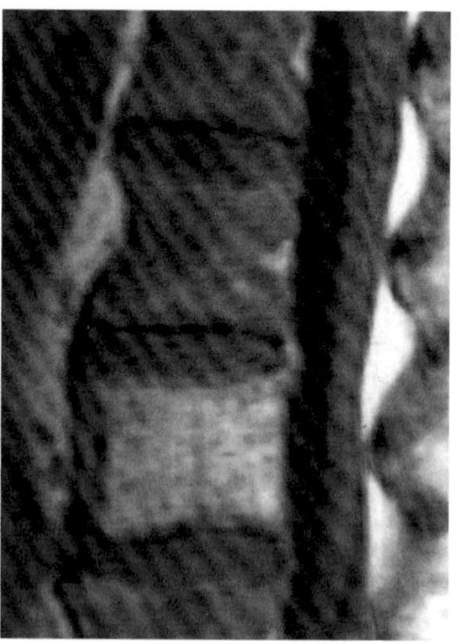

Fig. 5.4 MR image of the middle thoracic spine (sagittal, T1, detail). Vertebral hemangioma with fatty marrow (markedly hyperintense).

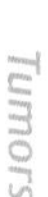

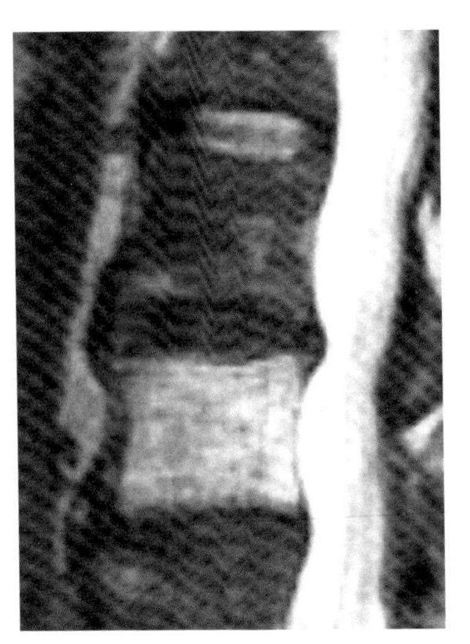

Fig. 5.5 MR image of the middle thoracic spine (sagittal, T2, detail). Vertebral hemangioma with fatty deposits (markedly hyperintense).

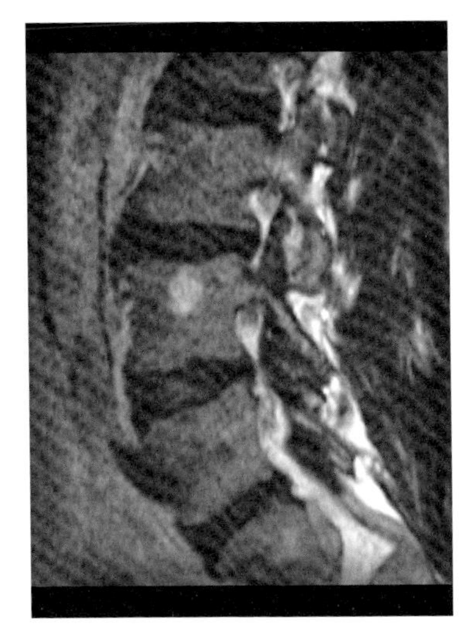

Fig. 5.6 MR image of the lumbar spine (sagittal, T2). Circumscribed subchondral hemangioma.

Differential Diagnosis

Metastasis	– T1 hypointensity – Soft tissue component – Pedicles are often involved – Bony destruction
Remnant of the notochord	– Eccentric

Selected References

Baudrez V. Benign vertebral hemangioma: MR-histological correlation. Skeletal Radiol 2001; 30: 442–426

Heyd R. Radiotherapy in vertebral hemangioma. Rontgenpraxis 2001; 53: 208–220

Manning HJ. Symptomatic hemangioma of the spine. Radiology 1951; 56: 58–65

Sar C. Double thoracic vertebral hemangioma causing complete paraplegia. Am J Orthop 2004; 33: 81–84, 57

Definition

- **Epidemiology**
  Age 0–30 years • More common in males than females • Occurs in the spine (posterior elements) in 10% of cases • In order of decreasing frequency: femur (50% of cases), tibia, hand and foot, intraarticular sites.
- **Etiology, pathophysiology, pathogenesis**
  Benign, osteoblastic tumor • Highly vascularized central nidus and significant marginal sclerosis • Classic clinical symptoms include nighttime pain. Responds to salicylates in 50% of cases. Responds to NSAIDs.

Imaging Signs

- **Modality of choice**
  Conventional radiographs.
  CT.
- **General**
  Central noncalcified nidus (lysis) with reactive marginal sclerosis • Smaller than 1.5 cm (> 1.5 cm = osteoblastoma) • *Typical location:* Vertebral arch, base of the pedicles (posterior half of the vertebra).
- **Radiographic findings**
  Bone sclerosis with a central radiolucency (nidus).
- **CT findings**
  Central hypodense nidus, halo of bone sclerosis • Periosteal thickening • Soft tissue tumor may be present • Very rapidly enhancing.
- **MRI findings**
  Nidus is hypointense on T1, hyperintense on T2 • Sclerosis is hypointense on T1 and T2.
- **Nuclear medicine (SPECT)**
  Uptake is greatly increased in nidus and increased in sclerotic halo • FDG-PET (highest specificity).

Clinical Aspects

- **Typical presentation**
  Nighttime pain that responds to salicylates in 50% of cases • Painful scoliosis • Muscle atrophy • Focal radicular pain.
- **Therapeutic options**
  Surgical resection of the nidus • CT-guided percutaneous procedure to sclerose the nidus.

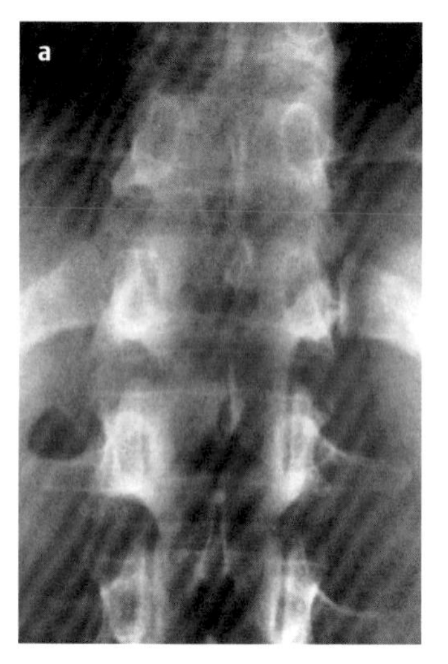

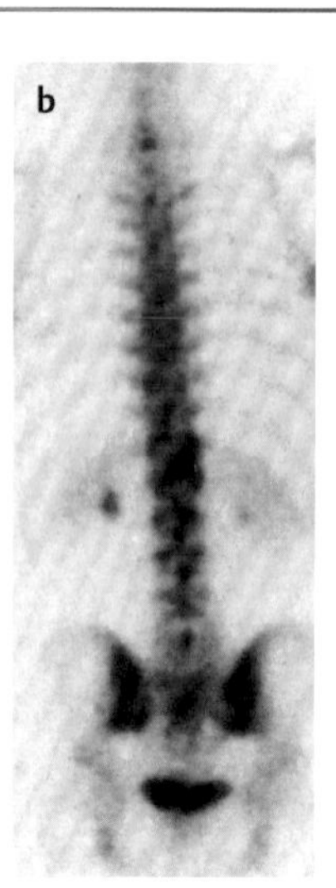

Fig. 5.7 a, b Nighttime back pain. Slight scoliosis. Pain eliminated with salicylates. A-P radiograph of the thoracolumbar junction (detail; **a**). Fine sclerosis in the right pedicle of vertebra T12. P-A bone scan (**b**). Increased uptake on the right in vertebra T12.

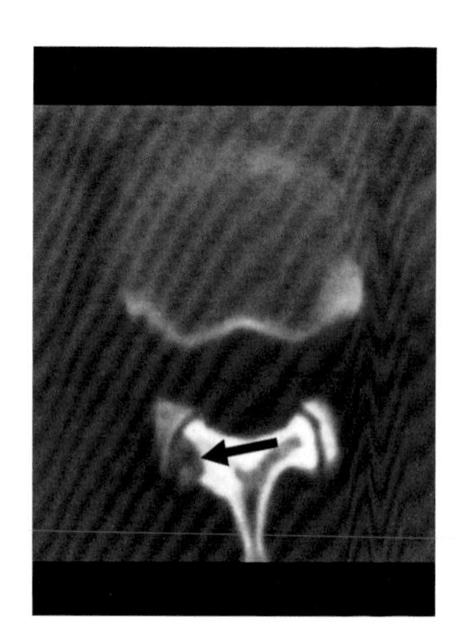

Fig. 5.8 CT (axial). Subarticular nidus with slight sclerosis.

Differential Diagnosis

Osteoblastoma (> 1.5 cm)	
Stress fracture of the pedicle	
Osteoblastic metastasis breast carcinoma lymphoma, prostate carcinoma	– Older patients – Pedicles and/or anterior vertebral bodies often involved
Aneurysmal bone cyst	– Multicystic, expansile, fluid sign
Sclerotic bone islands	– No nidus – No clinical symptoms – Normal scintigraphy findings
Inflammation (Brodie's abscess, sequestrum)	– Slowly enhancing

Tips and Pitfalls

Often misdiagnosed as the MRI resolution chosen is insufficient for examining details.

Selected References

Cioni R. CT-guided radiofrequency ablation of osteoid osteoma: long-term results. Eur Radiol 2004; 14: 1203–1208

Lindner NJ. Percutaneous radiofrequency ablation in osteoid osteoma. J Bone Joint Surg Br 2001; 83: 391–396

Ozaki T. Osteoid osteoma and osteoblastoma of the spine: experiences with 22 patients. Clin Orthop 2002; 397: 394–402

Definition

- **Epidemiology**
  Age 0–30 years (70% of cases aged 10–30 years) • Occurs in order of decreasing frequency in the cervical spine (40%), lumbar spine (20%), thoracic spine, and sacral region • Sites in order of decreasing frequency include the spine, flat bones (skull, mandible, pelvis), long bones (primarily in the diaphysis) • More common in males than females.
- **Etiology, pathophysiology, pathogenesis**
  Highly vascularized osteoid-forming tumor larger than 1.5 cm • Benign, expansile, usually osteolytic • Typically occurs in the posterior half of the vertebra.
  Benign type: Primarily sclerotic. *Aggressive type:* Osteolytic with a soft tissue component. Fifty percent of all lesions recur; no metastases!

Imaging Signs

- **Modality of choice**
  Conventional radiographs.
  CT.
- **General**
  Sharply demarcated oval lytic tumor (50% of cases) with marginal sclerosis • *Caution:* Soft tissue component, periosteal reaction, and cortical thinning can occur.
- **Conventional radiography and CT findings**
  Expansile, usually sclerosing tumor of the vertebral arch and pedicle • Newly formed bone has a ground-glass structure.
- **MRI findings**
  Sclerosis hypodense on T1 and T2 • Osteolysis and soft tissue component appear as T1 hypointensities and T2 hyperintensities • *Caution:* Edema can mimic a malignant tumor and/or inflammation • Marked peritumoral edema.

Clinical Aspects

- **Typical presentation**
  Pain that can only be partially alleviated with salicylates or NSAIDs • Painful scoliosis • Focal radicular pain • Muscle atrophy.
- **Therapeutic options**
  Surgical resection • Embolization.

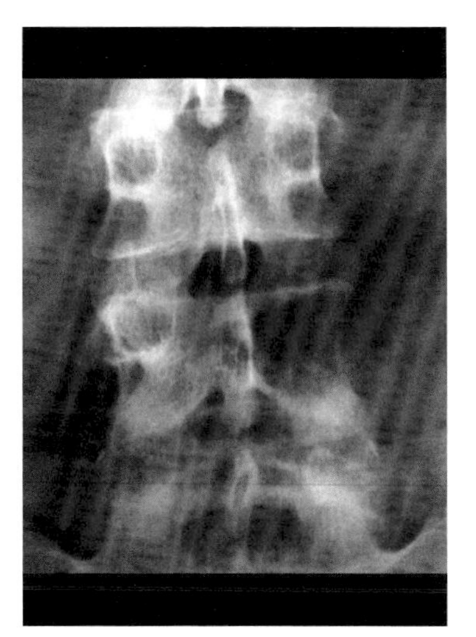

Fig. 5.9 Nighttime pain and increasing scoliosis. Conventional A-P radiograph of the lower lumbar spine. Destruction of the right pedicle and transverse process in vertebra L4.

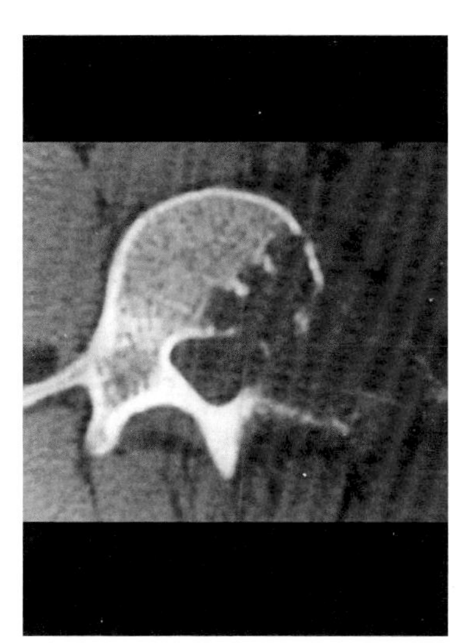

Fig. 5.10 CT of vertebra L4 (axial). Expansile osteolytic lesion (osteoblastoma) surrounded by a fine sclerotic halo.

Differential Diagnosis

Osteoid osteoma (< 1.5 cm)	
Osteoblastic metastasis breast carcinoma lymphoma, prostate carcinoma	– Older patients – Pedicles and/or anterior vertebral body often involved – Destruction instead of expansion
Aneurysmal bone cyst	– Multicystic, fluid sign; yet they also occur with osteoblastomas – Secondary aneurysmal bone cyst in osteoblastoma
Sclerotic bone islands	– No nidus – No clinical symptoms – Normal scintigraphy findings
Primary bone tumors	– Fibrous dysplasia – Histiocytosis X (primarily vertebral body) – Giant cell tumor (10–40 years; primarily vertebral body) – Enchondroma, osteochondroma (popcorn-like matrix calcification) – Osteosarcoma (extremely rare in the spine)

Selected References

Chew FS. Cervical spine osteoblastoma. AJR Am J Roentgenol. 1998; 171: 1244

Schneider M. Destructive osteoblastoma of the cervical spine with complete neurologic recovery. Spinal Cord 2002; 40: 248–252

Sonel B. Osteoblastoma of the lumbar spine as a cause of chronic low back pain. Rheumatol Int 2002; 21: 253–255

Definition

- **Epidemiology**
  Primarily 10–30 years of age • More common in females than males • Frequency of osteochondroma in the spine is less than 7% • Predilection for the cervical spine, most often C2 (50% of cases).
- **Etiology, pathophysiology, pathogenesis**
  Exostosis (solitary or multiple, sessile or peduncular) • Painless and slow-growing • *Caution:* Irritation of spinal cord, nerve roots, or vascular structures may occur • Rapid growth and a cartilage cap thicker than 1.5 cm are signs of malignant transformation (chondrosarcoma) • Osteochondromas can increase in size during skeletal growth but remain the same size in adults • In growing children, the cartilage cap can be thicker (up to 3 cm) • *Caution:* This is not a sign of malignancy • Osteochondromas are occasionally associated with systemic disorders:
  - Pseudohypoparathyroidism.
  - Pseudopseudohypoparathyroidism.
  - Myositis ossificans.
  - Hereditary multiple exostoses (spinal involvement in approximately 10% of cases).

  Osteochondromas occasionally occur after radiation therapy (at the margins after a latent period of about 2 years).

Imaging Signs

- **Modality of choice**
  Conventional radiographs • MRI (cartilage cap on cartilage sequence) • CT (continuity with vertebral bone).
- **General**
  Bony outgrowth arising from vertebra (cortex and cancellous bony are continuous) • Cartilage cap.
- **Conventional radiography and CT findings**
  Exostosis with a cartilage cap arising from the vertebra, occasionally pedunculated • Scintigraphy and PET are helpful in evaluating malignant transformation (increased uptake).
- **MRI findings**
  Central (mature fatty marrow): T1 and T2 hyperintensity • *Cortex:* T1 and T2 hypointensity • *Cartilage cap* (hyaline cartilage): T1 hyperintensity or hypointensity, T2 hyperintensity.

Clinical Aspects

- **Typical presentation**
  Incidental finding, clinically silent • Palpable tumor • Hoarseness • Dysphagia • Restricted mobility • Painless growth • Complications can occur due to secondary irritation of spinal cord, nerve root, or vascular structures.

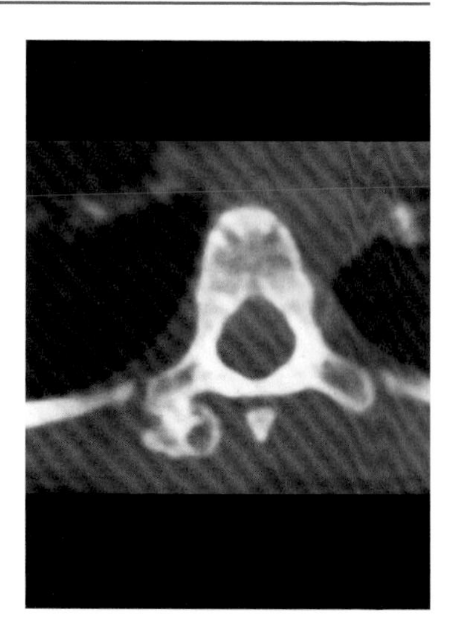

Fig. 5.11 CT of vertebra T12 (axial). Cartilaginous exostosis (osteochondroma) in the right transverse process.

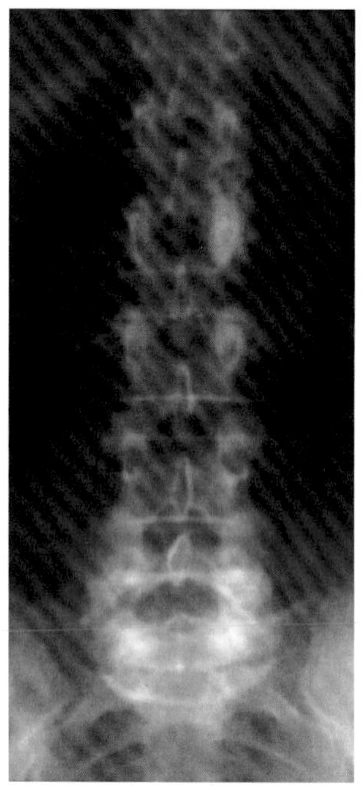

Fig. 5.12 Conventional A-P radiograph. Circumscribed osteolytic expansion of the L2 vertebral arch with left marginal sclerosis.

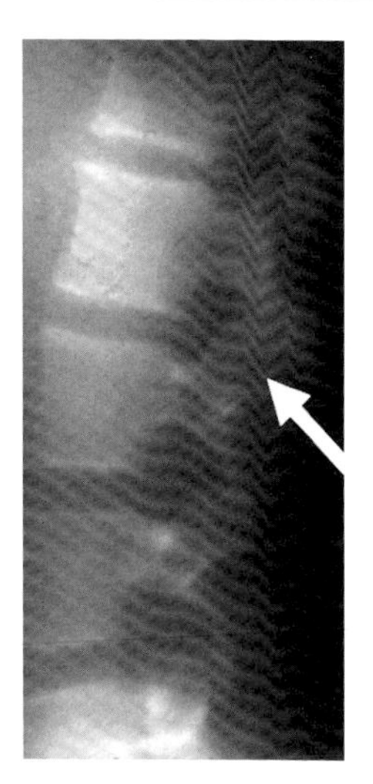

Fig. 5.13 Conventional lateral tomography. Circumscribed thickened osteolytic expansion of the L2 pedicle, a typical chondroma, not an osteochondroma!

▶ **Therapeutic options**

Resection (spontaneous remissions are rare) • Recurrences are extremely rare • Multiple exostoses are hereditary; malignant degeneration occurs in 3–5% of cases.

Differential Diagnosis

Chondrosarcoma	– Rapid growth – Cartilage cap thicker than 1.5 cm – Aggressive – Pain – 1% of all osteochondromas
Parosteal osteosarcoma	– Extremely rare in the spine – Aggressive bone remodeling

Selected References

Aoki J. FDG PET of primary benign and malignant bone tumors: standardized uptake value in 52 lesions. Radiology 2001; 219: 774–777

Gorospe L. Radiation-induced osteochondroma of the T4 vertebra causing spinal cord compression. Eur Radiol 2002; 12: 844–888

Jose Alcaraz Mexia M. Osteochondroma of the thoracic spine and scoliosis. Spine 2001; 26: 1082–1085

Definition

- **Epidemiology**
  Peak age 10–30 years • Lesions occur in order of increasing frequency in the thoracic spine, lumbar spine, cervical spine, and sacrum • Typically they involve the posterior elements and spread into the vertebral body • 55–60% of aneurysmal bone cysts are primary lesions • Approximately 45% of all aneurysmal bone cysts are secondary lesions occurring with a giant cell tumor, osteoblastoma, chondroblastoma, fibrous dysplasia, chondromyxofibroma, etc. • *Solid aneurysmal bone cysts:* Rare form (< 5%).
- **Etiology, pathophysiology, pathogenesis**
  Expansive, thin-walled, multilobulated, blood-filled bone cysts (“egg shells”) • Blood or fluid signs, septa, solid components • Cortical thinning • Occasionally associated with preexisting bone pathology (trauma, tumor) • *Caution:* Underlying malignant process; malignant degeneration may occur.

Imaging Signs

- **Modality of choice**
  CT • MRI (in spinal cord compression).
- **General**
  Expansile, multicystic lesion of the vertebral arch extending into the vertebral body • Blood or fluid sign.
- **Radiographic findings**
  Expansile, multicystic osteolysis (“egg shells”).
- **CT findings**
  Expansile, multilobulated cysts with a thin sclerotic halo (“egg shell” appearance) • Blood or fluid sign • Compression of the dural sac and nerve roots • Septa and solid components enhance after contrast administration.
- **MRI findings**
  Hypointensity on T1, hyperintensity on T2 and STIR sequences. (*Caution:* Signal behavior of the blood components varies depending on the breakdown stage) • Blood or fluid sign • Compression of the dural sac and nerve roots. *Secondary aneurysmatic bone cyst:* intravenous contrast adminstration; enhancement of the primary tumor.
- **Nuclear medicine**
  Marginal uptake with ring sign.

Clinical Aspects

- **Typical presentation**
  Pain and scoliosis • Myelopathy, radiculopathy (compression) • Compression fracture • Rapid growth.
- **Therapeutic options**
  Surgical resection • Embolization • Radiation therapy where resection is not feasible.

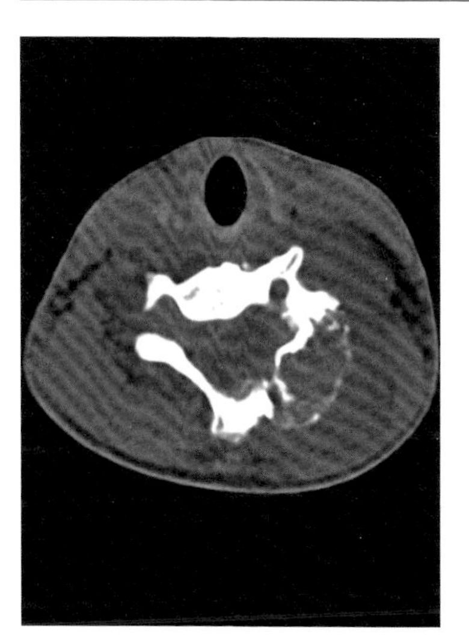

Fig. 5.14 Back pain with scoliosis. CT of C6 (axial). Extensive expansile osteolysis and intraspinal soft tissue component.

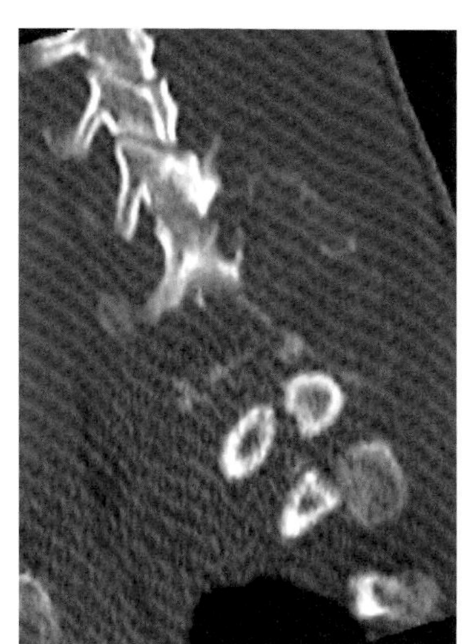

Fig. 5.15 CT sagittal reconstruction of the cervical spine. Expansile osteolysis extending across several segments. Partial destruction of vertebra C6.

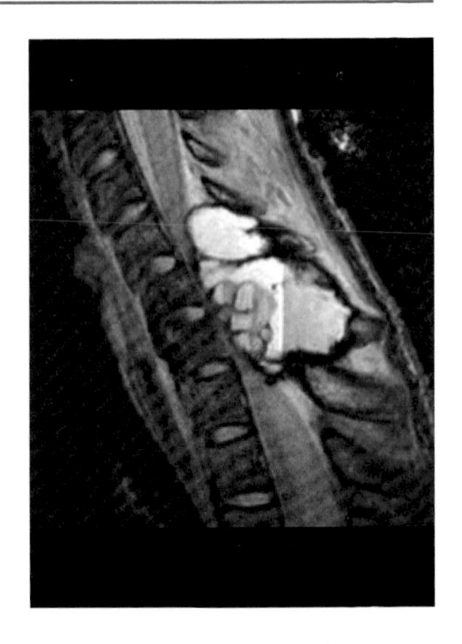

Fig. 5.16 MR image of the cervical spine (sagittal, T2). Expansile, cystic mass with blood or fluid sign (characteristic but not pathognomonic).

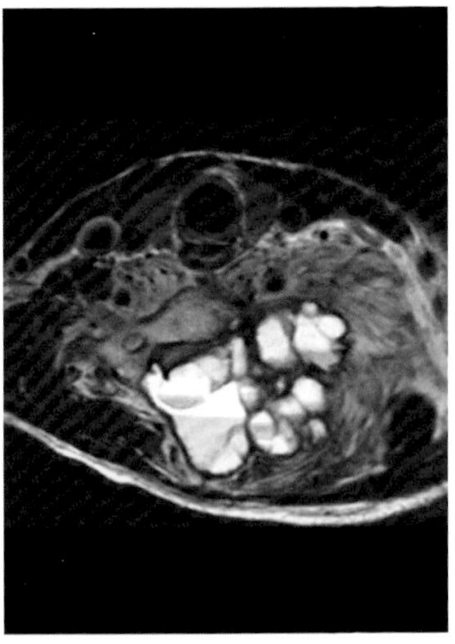

Fig. 5.17 MR image of C6 (axial, T2). Multicystic mass with blood or fluid sign. Extensive marginal edema.

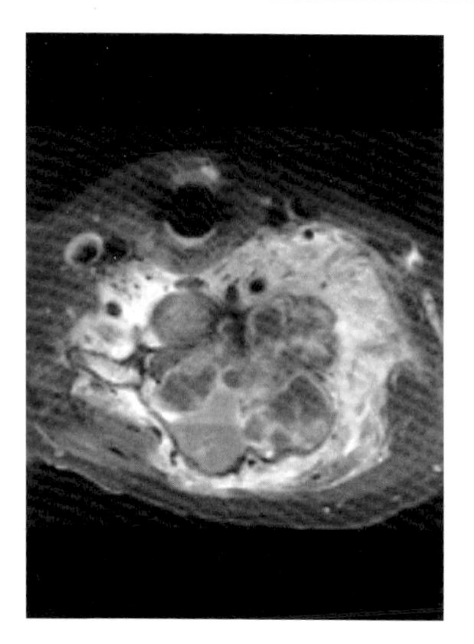

Fig. 5.18 MR image (axial, T1 with contrast). Aneurysmal bone cyst showing marked marginal enhancement and marked enhancement of the surrounding soft tissue.

▸ **Course and prognosis**
Rate of recurrence is about 10–30%.

Differential Diagnosis

Osteoblastoma, giant cell tumor, fibrous dysplasia	– Blood or fluid sign
Metastases with bleeding	– Higher peak age, different location – Caution: Aneurysmal bone cysts skip the disk interspaces and can mimic metastases – Manifestation in several bones – Soft tissue component – Compression fracture of the vertebral body
Giant cell tumor	– Older peak age, over 30 years

Selected References

de Kleuver M. Aneurysmal bone cyst of the spine: 31 cases and the importance of the surgical approach. J Pediatr Orthop B 1998; 7: 286–292

Murphey MD. From the archives of the AFIP. Primary tumors of the spine: radiologic pathologic correlation. Radiographics 1996; 16: 1131–1158

Erlemann R. Imaging and differential diagnosis of primary bone tumors and tumor-like lesions of the spine. Eur J Radiol 2006; 58: 48–67

Definition

- **Epidemiology**
  Peak age 20–40 years • Account for approximately 20% of all benign bone tumors and 10% of all primary spinal tumors • Initially malignant giant cell tumors are rare (1–2% of cases) • High recurrence rate (approximately 60%) • *Typical location:* Sacrum, vertebral bodies.
- **Etiology, pathophysiology, pathogenesis**
  Osteolytic locally aggressive tumor with osteoclast-like giant cells ("semi-malignant" tumor with lymph node metastases in 1–2% of cases) • Multicentric manifestation (lung metastases) • Osteolysis of the anterior vertebral body; the posterior elements may be involved • Tumor consists of multinucleated giant cells, connective tissue, and a fatty component • Angiogenesis and hemorrhages are common.

Imaging Signs

- **Modality of choice**
  CT • MRI (spread into spinal canal).
- **General**
  Expansive osteolysis • No matrix calcification • Slight or absent marginal sclerosis • Soft tissue component.
- **Radiographic findings**
  Expansive osteolysis.
- **CT findings**
  Expansive osteolysis • Evaluation of articular and neurovascular involvement.
- **MRI findings**
  Inhomogeneous signal behavior (T1 hypointensity, T2 hyperintensity) • Inhomogeneous, usually marginal enhancement (less often homogeneous) • Evaluation of the soft tissue component and involvement of the spinal canal and neurovascular structures • Occasionally blood or fluid sign (less often than with aneurysmal bone cyst).

Clinical Aspects

- **Typical presentation**
  Pathologic fracture • Radicular symptoms • Upper back pain.
- **Therapeutic options**
  Resection and cryotherapy or thermocoagulation • Eventual sequential embolization.
- **Course and prognosis**
  Malignant degeneration can occur secondary to radiation therapy.

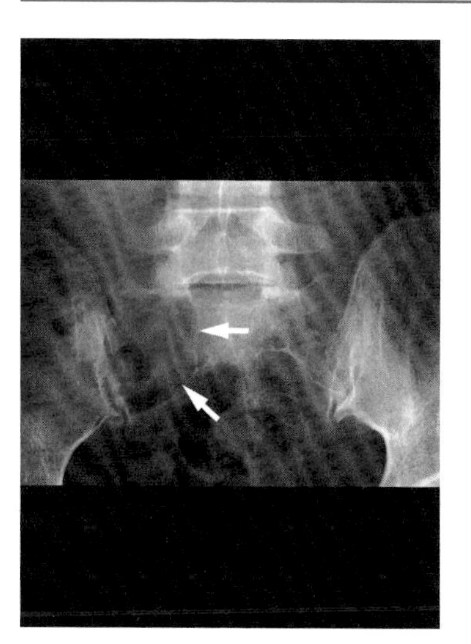

Fig. 5.19 Conventional radiograph of the sacrum. Large osteolytic defect in the right sacrum (S2–S5). Histologic diagnosis: Giant cell tumor.

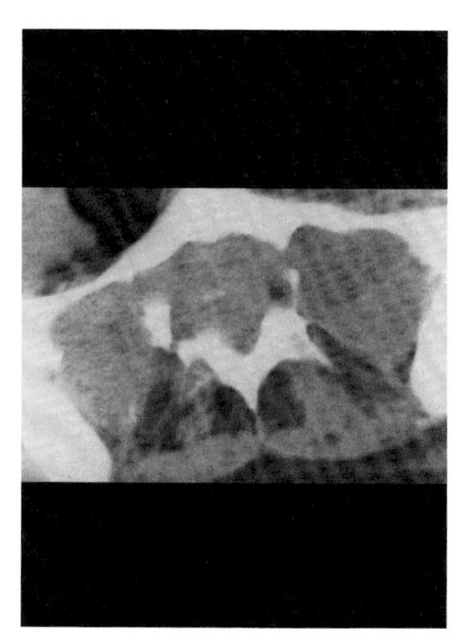

Fig. 5.20 CT (axial). Sharply demarcated solid osteolytic defect in the lateral masses and body of the sacrum. Histologic diagnosis: Giant cell tumor (DD: chordoma, metastasis).

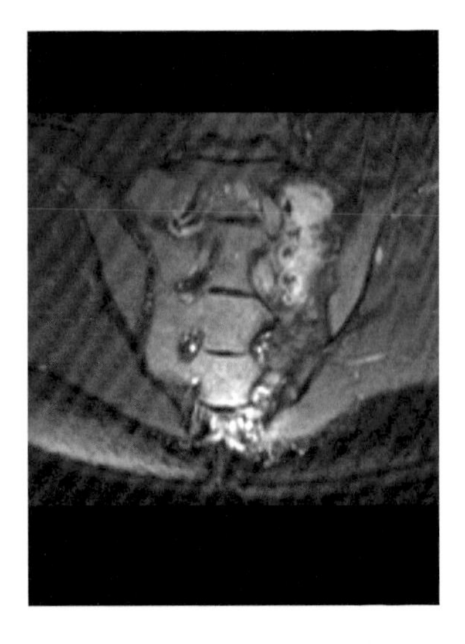

Fig. 5.21 MR image of the sacrum (coronal, T2, STIR). Hyperintense, partially lobulated lesion in the left lateral mass (S1–S3). The tumor extends as far as the sacroiliac joint and has spread to the foramina.

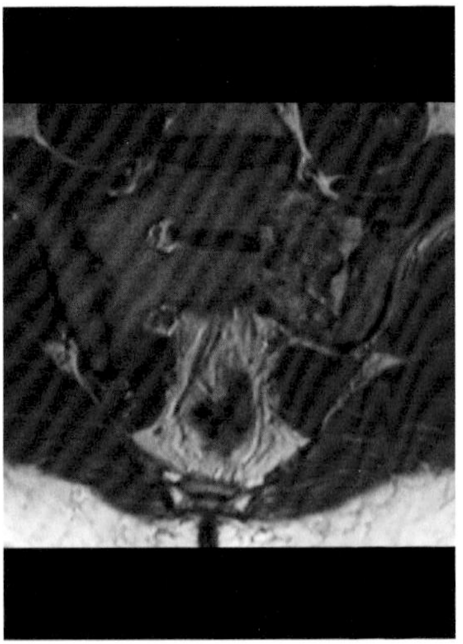

Fig. 5.22 MR image of the sacrum (coronal, T1). Hypointense mass in the left lateral mass.

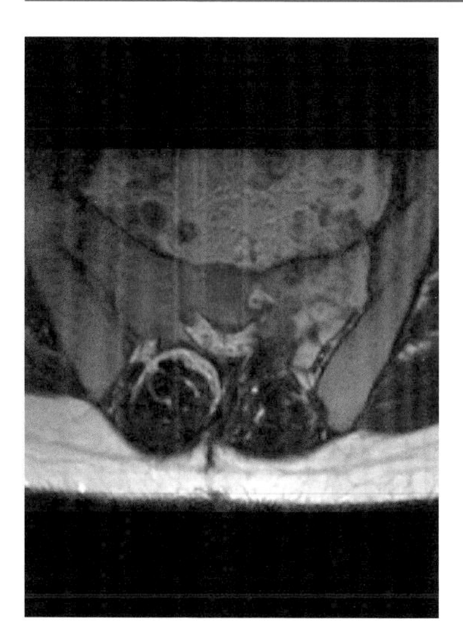

Fig. 5.23 MR image of the sacrum (axial, T1 with contrast). Tumor shows significant enhancement. Slightly inhomogeneous.

Differential Diagnosis

Metastasis	– Usually multiple, in older patients
Aneurysmal bone cyst	– Usually proceeds from the posterior elements (Caution: Blood or fluid signs occur in both entities) – Aneurysmal bone cysts and giant cell tumors can occur together

Selected References

Bloem JL, Kroon HM, Mulder JD, Ooosterhuis JW, Schütte HE, Taconis WK, Taminian AHM. Radiologic Atlas of Bone Tumors. Elsevier 1993

Freyschmidt J, Ostertag H, Hundh G. Knochentumoren. Berlin: Springer 1998

Definition

- **Epidemiology**
  Age 5–15 years • 10–20% of cases are polyostotic • Occurs in order of decreasing frequency in the thoracic (50% of cases), lumbar, and cervical spine.
- **Etiology, pathophysiology, pathogenesis**
  Synonyms: Histiocytosis X, eosinophilic granuloma (bony manifestation) • Rapidly growing, permeative osteolysis primarily occurring in children • Course is invariably benign.

Imaging Signs

- **Modality of choice**
  Conventional radiographs • MRI (multiplanar) • CT (spread in bone).
- **General**
  Osteolytic destruction of the vertebral body; the intervertebral disk is spared • Vertebra plana or wedge-shaped vertebral bodies in children.
- **Radiographic findings**
  Permeative osteolysis without a sclerotic halo • Central bone fragment (DD: Sequestrum) • Vertebra plana.
- **CT findings**
  Osteolysis without a sclerotic halo • Soft tissue component • Homogeneous enhancement.
- **MRI findings**
  T1 hypointensity, T2 hyperintensity • Moderate, homogeneous enhancement after contrast administration • Soft tissue component (*Caution:* spinal stenosis).
- **Nuclear medicine**
  Unspecific • Up to 30% false negative scans.

Clinical Aspects

- **Typical presentation**
  Pain • Fever.
  Chronic disseminated form: Before age 5 years (Hand–Schüller–Christian disease): Skeletal, visceral, and reticuloendothelial manifestation, 10% mortality.
  Fulminant form: Before age 3 years (Letterer–Siwe disease): Skin, liver, spleen, lymph nodes, skeleton; high mortality.
  New classification:
  - Circumscribed Langerhans cell histiocytosis.
  - Extensive Langerhans cell histiocytosis.
- **Therapeutic options**
  Spontaneous remission (3 months to 2 years) • Orthopedic support is required • Intralesional steroid injections • Surgical excision is indicated where conservative therapy fails.

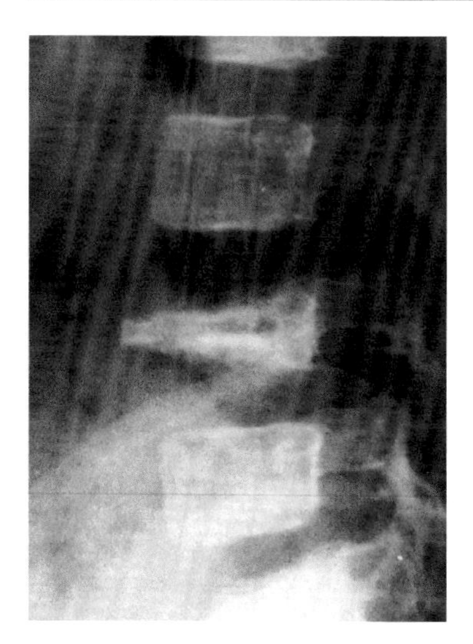

Fig. 5.24 Conventional lateral radiograph of the lumbar spine in an 8-year-old child. Vertebra plana. Disk height is normal.

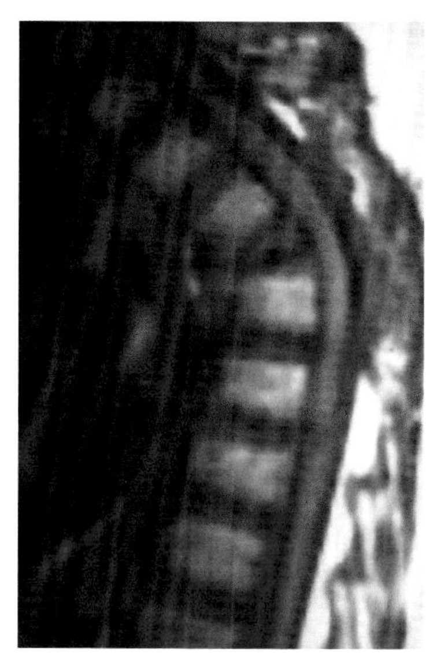

Fig. 5.25 MR image of the thoracic spine (sagittal, T1). Vertebra plana with hypointensity in vertebra T8.

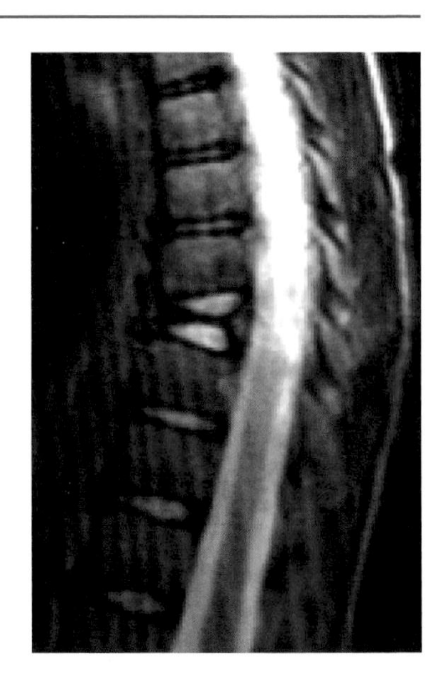

Fig. 5.26 MR image of the thoracic spine (sagittal, T2). Vertebra plana at T8. The disks show reactive hyperintensity and thickening ("tram tracking" of the spine). Small anterior soft tissue tumor mass.

Differential Diagnosis

Ewing sarcoma	– Large soft tissue tumor
Lymphoma	
Metastasis	– Later age
Infection	– Spondylodiskitis – Intervertebral disk is also involved
Giant cell tumor	– Over 30 years of age

Selected References

Azouz EM. Langerhans' cell histiocytosis: pathology, imaging and treatment of skeletal involvement. Pediatr Radiol 2004; 28

Raab P. Minimal invasive therapy of localized Langerhans-cell histiocytosis of bone. Z Orthop Ihre Grenzgeb 2000; 138: 140–145

Malignancy criteria

- **Growth**
  - Matrix.
  - Permeative or moth-eaten: Narrow transitional zone or none at all (rapid growth).
  - Geographic: Broad transitional zone (slow growth).
  - Smoothly demarcated, sclerotic (minimal or absent growth).
- **Periosteal reaction (decreasing aggressiveness)**
  - Sunburst.
  - Hair on end.
  - “Onion peel” appearance.
  - Codman triangle.
  - Double layer cortex.
- **Morphology (highly aggressive lesion)**
  - Widespread bone marrow edema.
  - Marked enhancement.
  - Large soft tissue component.
- **Tissue type (benign and malignant)**
  - Bone matrix (osteoid osteoma, osteoblastoma, osteosarcoma).
  - Cartilage matrix (chondroma, chondroblastoma, chondrosarcoma).
  - Myxoid matrix (chondromyxofibroma).
  - Dedifferentiation.
  - Bone marrow (multiple myeloma and lymphoma).
  - Unclear (aneurysmal bone cyst, giant cell tumor).
- **Ages (benign and malignant)**
  - 0–20: Ewing sarcoma.
  - 10–30: Osteosarcoma, osteoid osteoma, osteoblastoma, aneurysmal bone cyst.
  - > 30: Lymphoma, giant cell tumor.
  - > 40: Metastases (above age 40 the most common bony pathology); multiple myeloma.

Definition

- **Epidemiology**
  Primarily affects people over 40 years • Most common spinal neoplasm • Approximately 40% of bone metastases • Often occurs in the thoracic spine, less often in the lumbar spine.
- **Etiology, pathophysiology, pathogenesis**
  Primarily hematogenous metastases (medulla): venous (Batson vertebral plexus), arterial, rarely by extension (neck, bronchus) • Primarily in pedicle and anterior vertebral body (blood supply) • Localization depends on levels of local osteoprotegerin.
  Osteolytic: Bronchial carcinoma, thyroid carcinoma, renal carcinoma, etc.).
  Osteoblastic: Prostate carcinoma, breast carcinoma, carcinoid, nasopharyngeal and bladder malignancies, medulloblastoma.
  Mixed (osteolytic and osteoblastic): Breast carcinoma, bronchial carcinoma, cervical carcinoma, ovarian carcinoma.
  Occult primary tumor in approximately 20% of cases.

Imaging Signs

- **Modality of choice**
  MRI (T1, STIR, T1 with contrast) • Scintigraphy (whole body examination with possible lesions primarily in the skull, ribs, and pelvis).
- **General**
  - *Osteoblastic:* Circumscribed sclerosis (irregular).
  - *Osteolytic:* Circumscribed void with a sharply demarcated or ill-defined border, cortical destruction, localized widening of paravertebral soft tissue structures.
  - Pathologic compression fracture (DD: osteoporosis, trauma, steroid therapy).
- **Radiographic findings**
  Osteolytic metastases are only visible where there is 50% loss of substance in a lesion with a minimum size of 1 cm • Large expansive osteolytic lesion: Renal carcinoma, thyroid carcinoma • Predilection for pedicle and vertebral body.
- **CT findings**
  Bone destruction and/or irregularly demarcated bony sclerosis • Soft tissue component • Variable enhancement after contrast administration.
- **MRI findings**
  Main imaging plane: Sagittal • Bone marrow reaction • Soft tissue component • Intervertebral disks are usually not affected • T1 hypointensity (natural contrast to mature bone marrow) • STIR hyperintensity (may be absent with calcification) • *T1 with contrast:* Significant enhancement • Whole-body MRI is useful for staging and searching for the primary tumor.
- **Nuclear medicine**
  Staging • *PET:* high specificity.

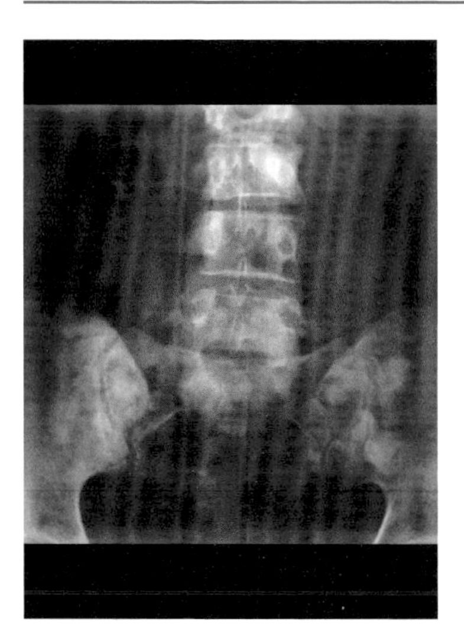

Fig. 5.27 Conventional A-P radiograph of the lumbar spine. Multiple osteoblastic metastases of a breast carcinoma.

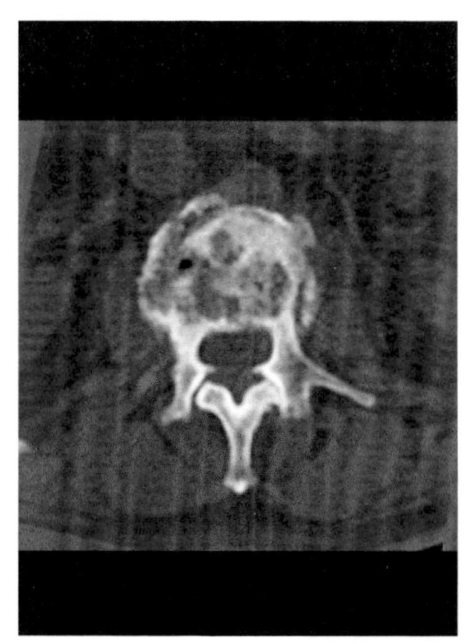

Fig. 5.28 CT of vertebra L1 (axial). Mixed metastasis of a prostate carcinoma.

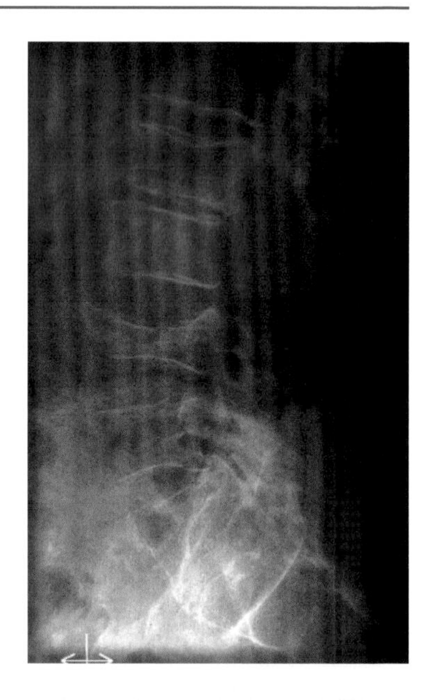

Fig. 5.29 Conventional lateral radiograph of the lumbar spine. Osteolytic metastasis of a hypernephroma in the posterior vertebra.

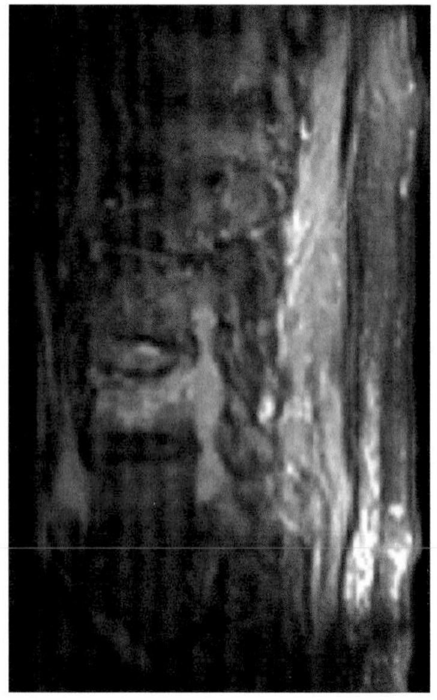

Fig. 5.30 MR image of the lumbar spine (sagittal, STIR). Metastasis with a significant soft tissue component in vertebra L3, spreading into the adjacent vertebral body. Colon carcinoma.

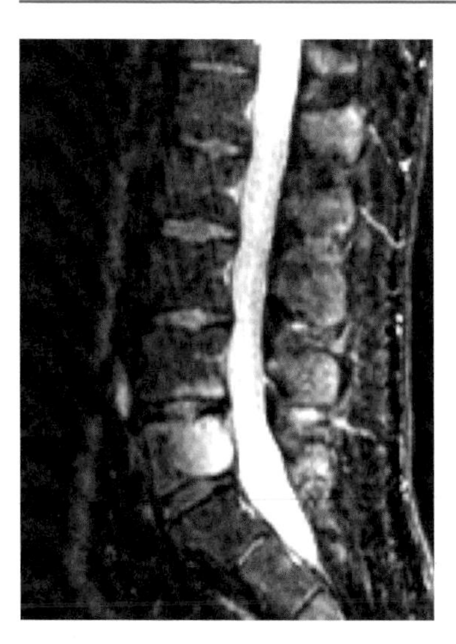

Fig. 5.31 MR image of the lumbar spine (sagittal, T2). Metastasis of a bronchial carcinoma in the posterior vertebral body of L5.

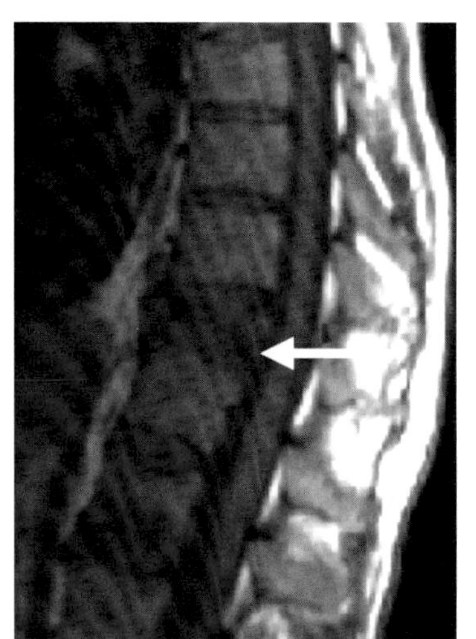

Fig. 5.32 MR image of the thoracolumbar junction (sagittal, T1) in the same patient as in Fig. 5.**3**.

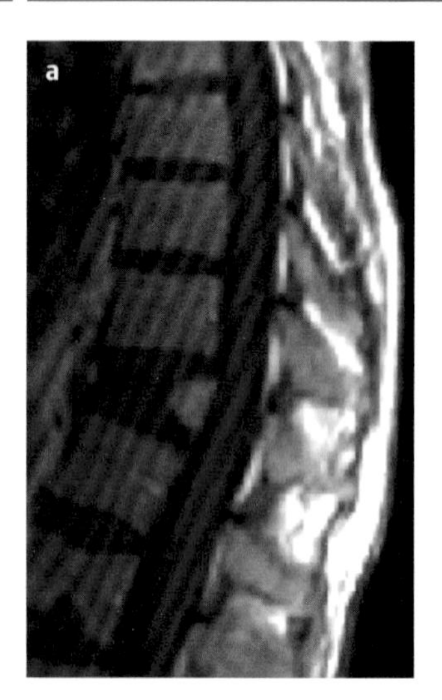

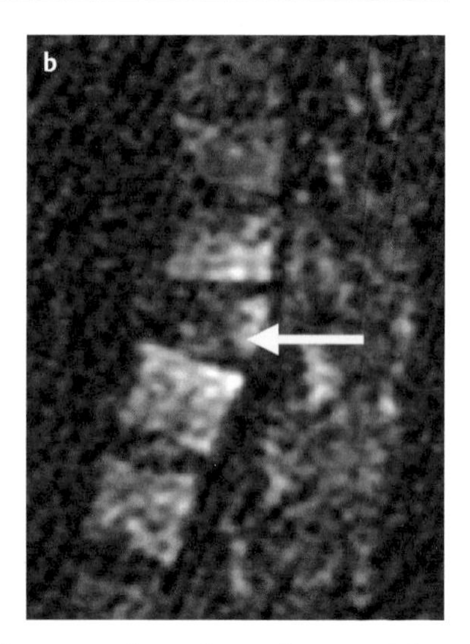

Fig. 5.33 a, b MR image of the thoracolumbar junction (sagittal, T1 with contrast [**a**], diffusion-weighted [**b**]), showing posterior enhancement in vertebra T12. Anterior necrosis is present. Diffusion is not restricted (**b**), so this is an osteoporotic vertebral collapse.

Clinical Aspects

- **Typical presentation**
  Pain (especially with exercise and improving significantly with rest, invariably increasing pain consistent with an incipient insufficiency fracture) • Angular deformity • Pathologic vertebral collapse • Radiculopathy, myelopathy (extradural spinal cord compression) • Occurs in order of decreasing frequency in the thoracic (70%), lumbar (20%), and cervical spine.
- **Therapeutic options**
  These depend on the primary tumor • Radiation therapy • Chemotherapy • Surgical management (with neurologic symptoms) • Vertebroplasty • Immunotherapy (experimental).

Differential Diagnosis

Acute vertebral collapse in osteoporosis	– Cannot be clearly distinguished from pathologic vertebral collapse (bone marrow edema) – Follow-up examination: Edema will remain unchanged in a pathologic fracture but will regress in an osteoporotic fracture – DWI: Reduced diffusion indicates benign lesion; increased diffusion indicates malignancy – Fluid sign
Primary bone tumors (rare, monostotic)	
Hematopoietic tumors (lymphoma, plasmacytoma)	
Circumscribed bone marrow inhomogeneity	– Fat fibrosis in older patients, red bone marrow indicates increased hematopoiesis – Signs of a benign lesion include: Intact posterior wall and/or sparing of the posterior vertebral elements, no soft tissue component

Selected References

Dominkus M. Surgical therapy of spinal metastases. Orthopäde. 1998; 27: 282–286

Herneth AM et al. Diffusion weighted imaging for bone marrow pathologies. Eur J Radiol 2005; 55: 74–83

Link TM: Spinal metastases. Value of diagnostic procedures in the initial diagnosis and follow-up. Radiologe 1995; 35: 21–27

Lodwick GS. Determining growth rates of focal lesions of bone from radiographs. Radiology 1980; 134: 577–583

Moulopoulos LA. MR prediction of benign and malignant vertebral compression fractures. J Magn Reson Imaging 1996; 6: 667–674

Yoshida S. The generation of anti-tumoral cells using dentritic cells from the peripheral bloood of patients with malignant brain tumors. Cancer Immunol Immunother 2001; 50: 321–327

Definition

- **Epidemiology**
  Most common primary malignant bone tumor • Occurs in people over 60 years.
- **Etiology, pathophysiology, pathogenesis**
  Solitary myeloma (plasmacytoma): A single lesion as opposed to multiple myeloma • The vertebral body and posterior elements are the most common sites of plasmacytoma • Plasma cell infiltration of the medulla.

Imaging Signs

- **Modality of choice**
  Conventional radiographs • MRI (T1 and STIR).
- **General**
  One or more sharply demarcated osteolytic subcortical lesions.
- **Radiographic findings**
  Findings are normal in early stages or diffuse osteopenia • Solitary (plasmacytoma) or multiple (multiple myeloma) round, smoothly demarcated osteolytic lesions • Endosteal bony destruction • Vertebral body compression • Secondary sclerosis (after vertebral fracture, radiation therapy, chemotherapy).
- **CT findings**
  Osteolysis arising in the medulla • Soft tissue tumor • Sclerotic in 3% of cases • Can infiltrate the intervertebral disk (see also Chordoma) • Minimal enhancement.
- **MRI findings**
  T1 hypointensity (isointense to muscle) • Moderate enhancement after contrast administration • Soft tissue tumor • T2 hyperintensity (possibly inhomogeneous) • STIR hyperintensity (diffuse or local).
- **Nuclear medicine**
  Bone scan is typically normal (only sclerotic lesions are positive) • *FDG-PET:* Active multiple myeloma can be precisely identified.

Clinical Aspects

- **Typical presentation**
  Asymptomatic (in 20% of cases) • Anemia (multiple myeloma) • Bence Jones proteinuria • Amyloidosis • Local pain • Vertebral collapse • Electrophoresis (monoclonal gammopathy).
- **Therapeutic options**
  Radiation therapy (plasmacytoma) • Chemotherapy (multiple myeloma) • Bisphosphonate therapy • Bone marrow transplantation (multiple myeloma).
- **Course and prognosis**
  Plasmacytoma: Average survival is 10 years • *Multiple myeloma:* Average survival is 3–4 years.

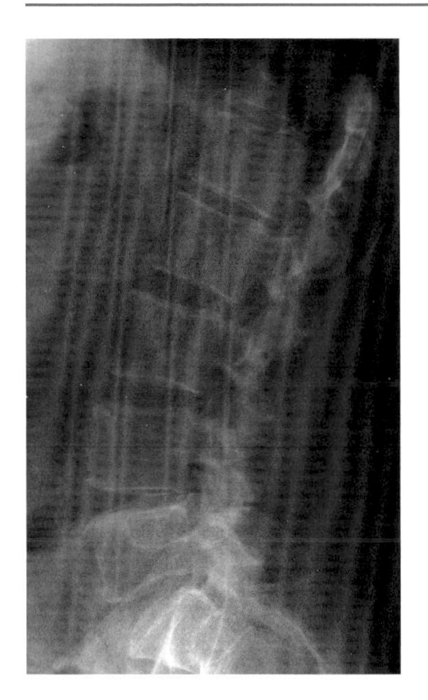

Fig. 5.34 General fatigue and exhaustion, with markedly raised erythrocyte sedimentation rate. Conventional lateral radiograph. Multiple osteolytic lesions in vertebrae L1–L3 and L5.

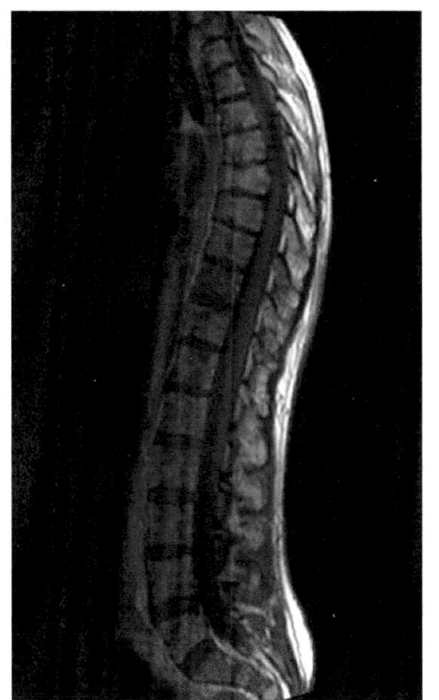

Fig. 5.35 MR image of the thoracic spine (sagittal, T1 with contrast). The bone marrow is diffusely permeated with hyperintense enhancing lesions. Vertebral collapse at several sites in the middle thoracic spine.

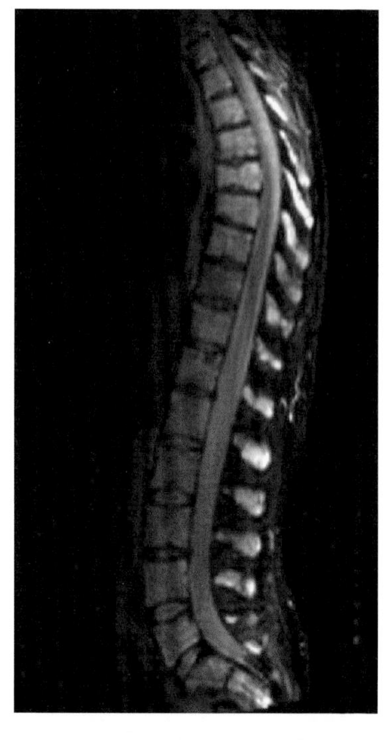

Fig. 5.36 MR image of the thoracic and lumbar spine (sagittal, T2 with fat suppression). Nodular lesions are present throughout the bone marrow. Normal bone has largely been replaced in the middle thoracic spine.

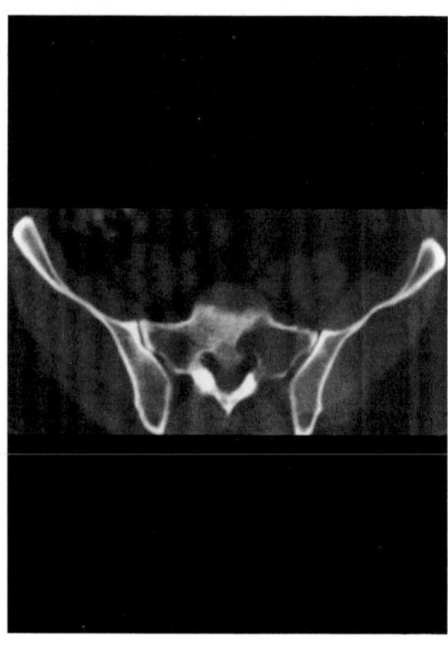

Fig. 5.37 Pelvic CT (axial). A circumscribed lytic tumor is present in the left lateral mass. There is no soft tissue tumor.

Differential Diagnosis

Metastasis	– Disk not infiltrated (usually)
Aggressive hemangioma	
Vertebral collapse in osteoporosis	– Follow-up examination – DWI

Selected References

Baur A. The diagnosis of plasmocytoma with MRT. Radiologe 2000; 40: 716–722
Rand T. Percutaneous radiologically-guided vertebroplasty in the treatment of osteoporotic and tumorous spinal body lesions. Radiologe 2003; 43: 723–728
Sirohi B. Multiple myeloma. Lancet 2004; 363: 875–887

Definition

- **Epidemiology**
  Rare malignant tumor derived from the notochord • Peak age 40–60 years • Twice as common in men than in women • Occurs in order of decreasing frequency in the sacral region (50%), sphenooccipital region (30%), and cervical spine.
- **Etiology, pathophysiology, pathogenesis**
  Chordomas arise from remnants of the notochord (third to seventh week of embryonal development) which arises anterior to the neural tube (sella to coccyx) • The tumor destroys the vertebral body (causing vertebral collapse and secondary sclerosis) • Locally aggressive and metastasizes early • Metastases occur in about 50% of cases (lung, liver, bone, lymph nodes) • Can spread into the intervertebral disk • Calcifications (approximately 40–60% of cases) along the midline, mucoid material. *Three histologic types:* Conventional, chondroid, dedifferentiated.

Imaging Signs

- **Modality of choice**
  Conventional radiographs • CT (spread in bone) • MRI (spread in soft tissue, involvement of neurovascular structures).
- **General**
  Bony destruction • Infiltration of the nerve roots and adjacent soft tissue structures • Calcification, fibrosis, cystic necrosis.
- **Radiographic findings**
  Circumscribed bony destruction (aggressive) • Calcification • *Typical site:* Midline, from sacrum to sphenooccipital region.
- **CT findings**
  Hypodense, osteolytic tumor with matrix calcifications (40–60% of all cases) • Slight to moderate enhancement after contrast administration • Soft tissue compartment • Sclerosis at tumor edges.
- **MRI findings**
  Inhomogeneously structured multilobulated osteolytic tumor • T1 hypointensity or hyperintensity; T2 hyperintensity (hyperintense to disk) • Calcifications (T1 and T2 hypointensity) • Slight to moderate enhancement.

Clinical Aspects

- **Typical presentation**
  Pain • Paresthesias (nerve root infiltration) • Vertebral collapse (pain, angular deformity) • Chromosome abnormalities.
- **Therapeutic options**
  Resection.
- **Course and prognosis**
  High rate of recurrence (90%) • 5-year survival rate is 80% • 10-year survival rate is 40%.

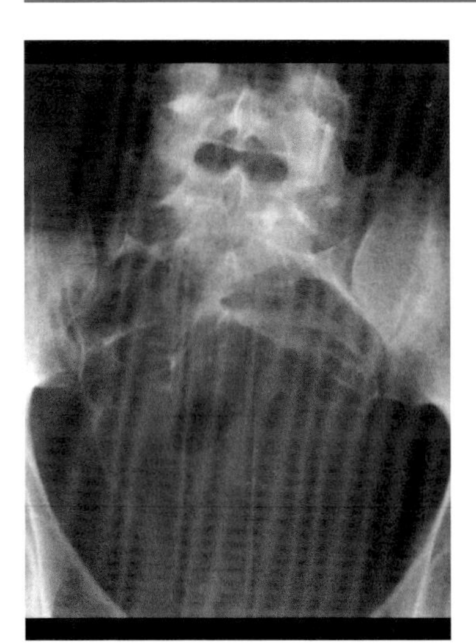

Fig. 5.38 Patient with six-month history of increasing pain in the sacral region. Conventional A-P radiograph of the sacrum. Geographic lytic lesion.

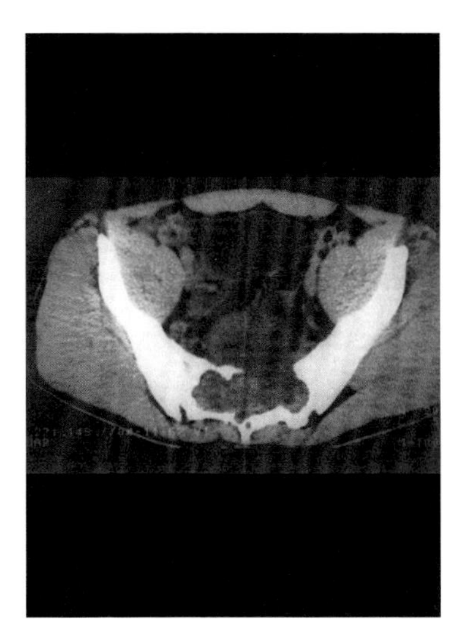

Fig. 5.39 Pelvic CT (axial). Sharply demarcated lobulated sacral lesion with large anterior extraosseous soft tissue tumor.

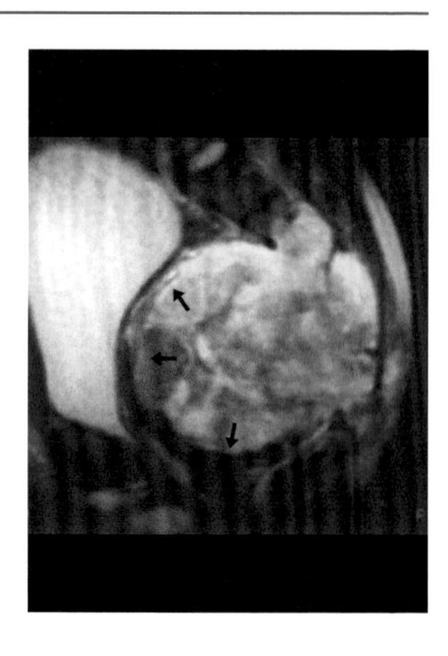

Fig. 5.40 Pelvic MR image (sagittal, T2). Large inhomogeneously structured solid tumor arising from the sacrum and spreading anteriorly. Impression of the bladder. Lesion has a pseudocapsule.

Differential Diagnosis

Metastases	– Later age – Multifocal
Giant cell tumor	– T2 hypointensity – Hemorrhages may be present
Chondrosarcoma	– Primarily in the posterior spine, cartilage matrix. Chondroid chordoma can be differentiated only on histological examination.
Plasmacytoma, lymphoma, neurogenic tumors	
Malignant fibrous histiocytoma	– Dedifferentiated chordoma can be differentiated only on histological examination

Selected References

Diel J. The sacrum: pathologic spectrum, multimodality imaging, and subspecialty approach. Radiographics 2001; 21: 83–104

Flemming DJ. Primary tumors of the spine. Semin Musculoskelet Radiol 2000; 4: 299–320

Pease AP. Radiographic, computed tomographic and histopathologic appearance of a presumed spinal chordoma in a dog. Vet Radiol Ultrasound 2002; 43: 338–342

Wacker A. Chordomas-diagnostic steps and therapeutic consequences. Dtsch Med Wochenschr 2002; 127: 1389–1391

Definition

- **Epidemiology**
  Rare highly malignant tumor (round-cell sarcoma) occurring in childhood and adolescence • Age 5–20 years.
- **Etiology, pathophysiology, pathogenesis**
  Closely related to PNET • Permeative osteolytic tumor arising from the medulla, usually with a large soft tissue component • The intervertebral disk is spared • Arises from the vertebral body (occasionally from two) • Only 5% of lesions are sclerotic • Extraosseous soft tissue component in over 50% of cases • Metastases (lung, bone, lymph nodes) arise in over 20% of cases.

Imaging Signs

- **Modality of choice**
  Conventional radiographs, CT (diagnosis) • MRI (extent of tumor).
- **General**
  Aggressive permeative (moth-eaten) osteolysis • Periosteal reaction • Soft tissue component (50% of lesions).
- **Radiographic findings**
  Permeative bony destruction with a broad transitional zone • Periosteal reaction ("onion peel" appearance, "hair on end," Codman triangle) on the vertebral bodies is often not distinct • Compression fracture.
- **CT findings**
  Bony destruction • Infiltration of paravertebral structures • Soft tissue component.
- **MRI findings**
  T1 hypointensity, significant enhancement after contrast administration • T2 and STIR hyperintensity • Evaluation of soft tissue component • Infiltration of paravertebral and intraspinal structures • *Caution:* Hemorrhage and necrosis can alter the appearance of the lesion.
- **Nuclear medicine**
  Pronounced radionuclide uptake (searching for metastases).

Clinical Aspects

- **Typical presentation**
  Pain • Fever and leukocytosis (mimics osteomyelitis) • Swelling • Developmental anomaly • Pathologic fractures present in over 10% of cases.
- **Therapeutic options**
  Preoperative chemotherapy (goal: 90% reduction in tumor size); combination modality therapy • Resection followed by chemotherapy.
- **Course and prognosis**
  In 50% of cases with localized disease, survival is good • Rate of tumor recurrence is over 15%.

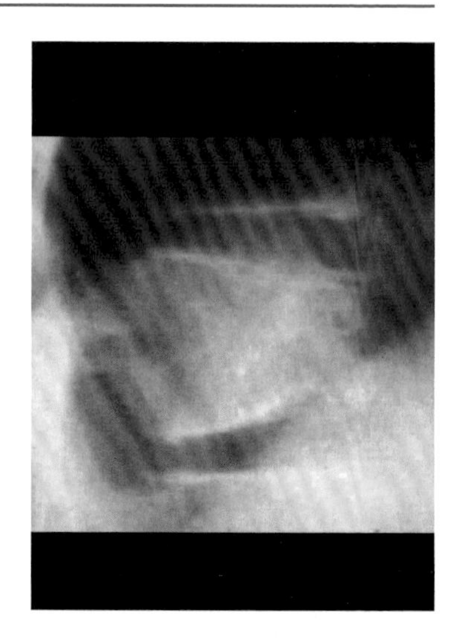

Fig. 5.41 Fatigue, slightly elevated temperature, leukocytosis. Conventional lateral radiograph of the thoracic spine (detail). Moderately sclerotic anteriorly compressed vertebral body. Tumor has penetrated the posterior cortex. The matrix is highly inhomogeneous, a sign of osteoblastic and osteolytic posterior bone remodeling.

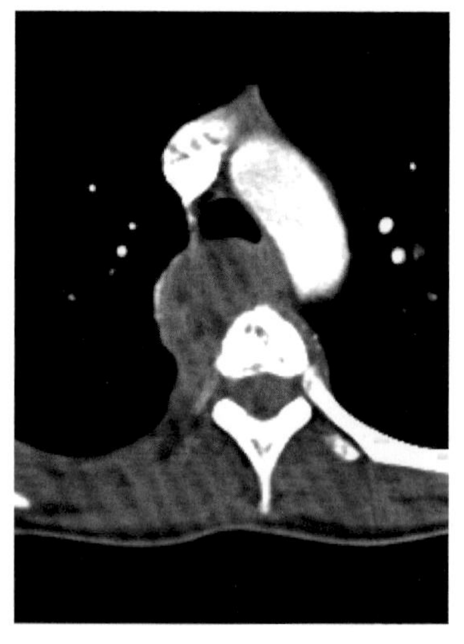

Fig. 5.42 CT of the thoracic spine (axial). Large right anterolateral soft tissue tumor with impression of the trachea. Lesion extends to the aortic arch.

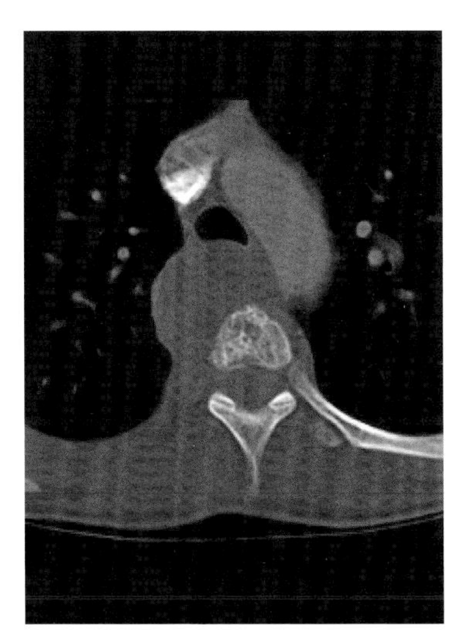

Fig. 5.43 CT of vertebra T8 (axial, bone window). Extensive osteolysis of the vertebral body with paravertebral tumor masses isodense to soft tissue.

Differential Diagnosis

Neuroblastoma	– PNET can only be distinguished by histologic examination
Langerhans cell histiocytosis	– More geographic lesions
Osteosarcoma	– 80% involve matrix calcification
Eosinophilic granuloma	– Histiocytosis X
Osteomyelitis	– Fever, leukocytosis, elevated erythrocyte sedimentation rate – Intervertebral disk also affected

Selected References

Donaldson SS. Ewing sarcoma: radiation dose and target volume. Pediatr Blood Cancer 2004; 42: 471–476

Flemming DJ. Primary tumors of the spine. Semin Musculoskelet Radiol 2000; 4: 299–320

Greenspan A, Remagen W. Differential Diagnosis of Tumors and Tumor-like Lesions of Bones and Joints. Lippincott-Raven 1998

Hoffer FA. Primary skeletal neoplasms: osteosarcoma and ewing sarcoma. Top Magn Reson Imaging 2002; 13: 231–239

Definition

- **Epidemiology**
  Peak age 30–70 years • 85% are non-Hodgkin lymphomas (< 80% are B cell lymphomas) • Initial manifestation is in bone (accounting for 4% of primary bone tumors) • Secondary manifestation (30% of systemic lymphomas metastasize to bone).
- **Etiology, pathophysiology, pathogenesis**
  Lymphoreticular neoplasm • Secondary involvement (bone to leptomeninges) • Lesions are encountered in order of increasing frequency in bone, at extradural sites, at intradural sites, and in bone marrow • Lesions are highly variable in appearance, rendering differential diagnosis difficult.

Imaging Signs

- **Modality of choice**
  Conventional radiographs and CT (bony structures) • MRI with contrast (leptomeningeal and intramedullary lesions).
- **General**
  Caution: Because of their highly variable appearance, lymphomas can mimic many other disorders.
- **Radiographic findings with bony lesions**
  Osteolysis • Rarely sclerosis ("ivory" vertebral body).
- **CT findings with bony lesions**
  Permeative bony destruction (osteolytic and, less often, sclerotic) • Usually multisegmental with infiltration of the disk interspaces • Soft tissue component.
- **MRI findings with bony lesions**
  T1 hypointensity, T2 hyperintensity • Dynamic contrast MRI shows rapid enhancement • Soft tissue tumor • Homogeneous enhancement after contrast administration.
- **Nuclear medicine with bony lesions**
  Bone scan is abnormal, showing increased uptake • FDG-PET is used for staging and follow-up of treatment.
- **CT findings with leptomeningeal and/or intramedullary lesions**
  Solid tumor mass that may exhibit bony infiltration • Homogeneous enhancement after contrast administration.
- **MRI findings with leptomeningeal and/or intramedullary lesions**
  Tumor mass:
  - On T1: hypointense to isointense.
  - On T2: isointense to hyperintense (tumor and edema).
  - On T1 with contrast: pronounced enhancement.

  Thickened nerve roots.

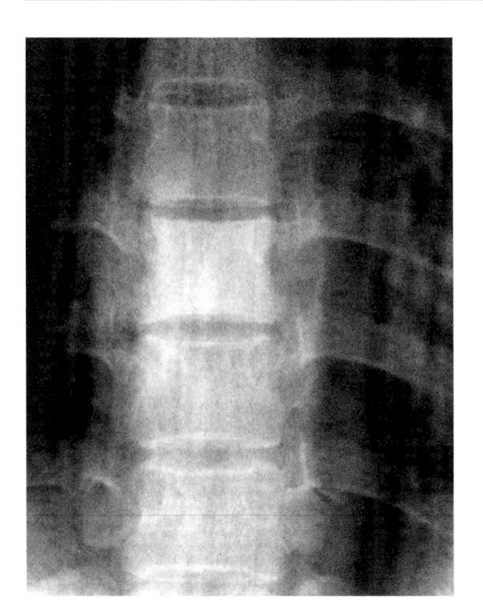

Fig. 5.44 Conventional A-P radiograph of the thoracic spine. Sclerosis in lymphomatous vertebra T5 ("ivory" vertebral body). Paravertebral soft tissue appears broadened.

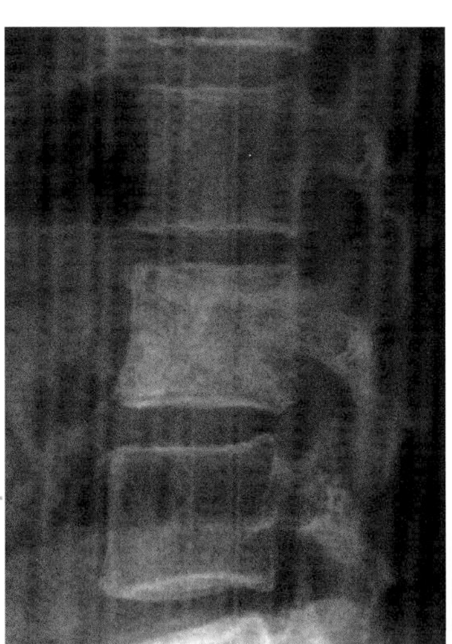

Fig. 5.45 Conventional lateral radiograph of the lumbar spine. Sclerosis in lymphomatous vertebra L1 ("ivory" vertebral body). The sclerosis is highly inhomogeneous. Isolated lytic areas are present.

Clinical Aspects

- **Typical presentation**
  Uncharacteristic back pain.
- **Therapeutic options**
  Lymphomas typically respond well to chemotherapy and/or radiation therapy • Surgical decompression is indicated for acute neurologic symptoms.

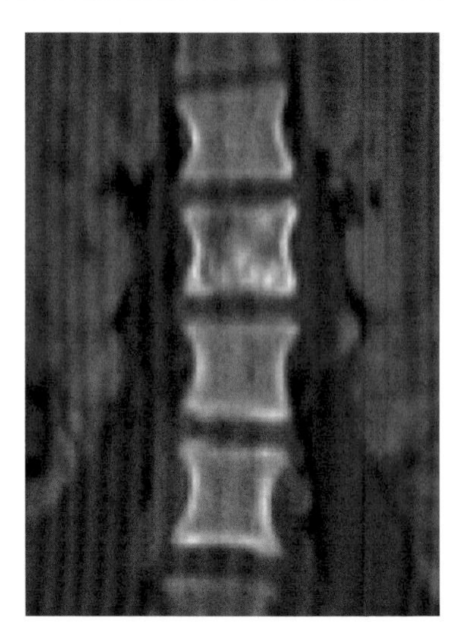

Fig. 5.46 CT of the thoracolumbar junction (A-P). Mixed lymphoma.

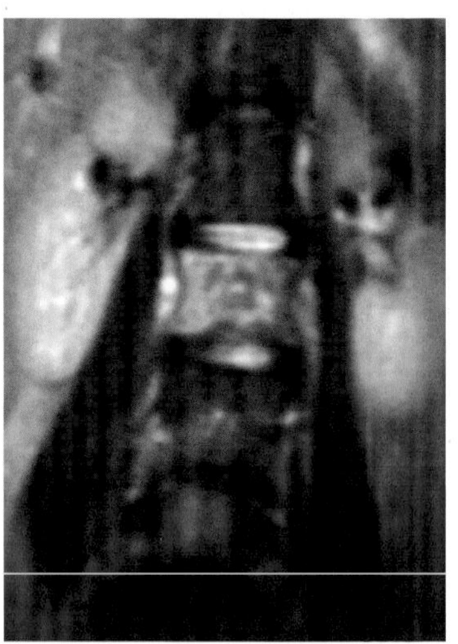

Fig. 5.47 MR image of thoracolumbar junction (coronal STIR). Hyperintense lymphoma in vertebra L3.

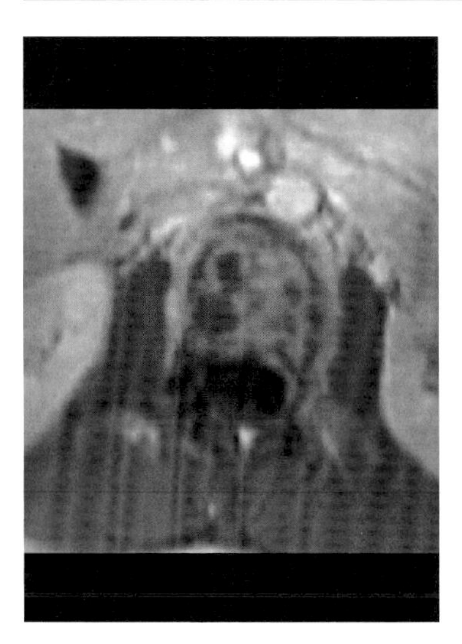

Fig. 5.48 MR image of T12 (axial, T1 with contrast). The solid areas of the lymphoma show significant enhancement. Osteolytic necrotic areas are also present. A fine mantle of soft tissue tumor surrounds the vertebral body. On the left side, the tumor extends into the vertebral arch.

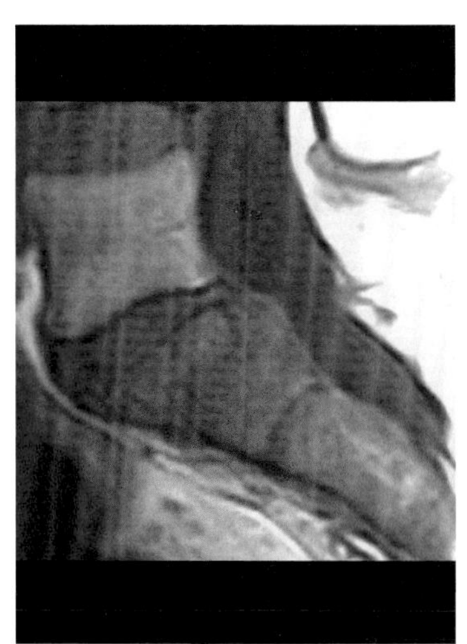

Fig. 5.49 MR image of the sacrum (sagittal, T1). Epidural soft tissue mass with cortical destruction.

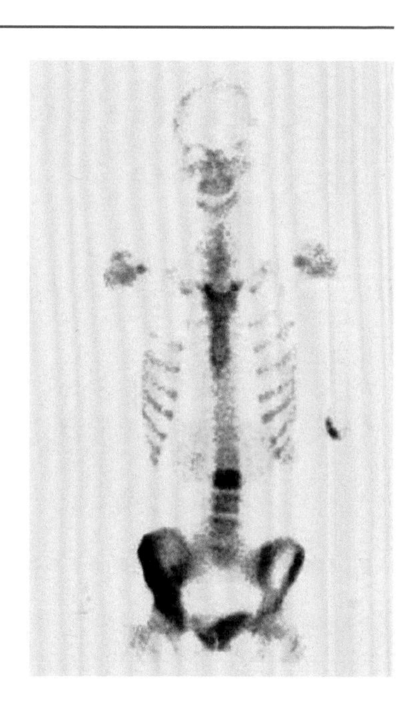

Fig. 5.50 Bone scan. Lymphoma appears as a "hot spot" in vertebra L3. Lymphoma is also visualized in the right anterior iliac crest.

Differential Diagnosis

Bony	– Metastases – Paget disease ("ivory" vertebral body) – Langerhans cell histiocytosis
Leptomeningeal and/or intramedullary	– Hematoma – Metastasis – Meningitis – Astrocytoma – Ependymoma

Selected References

Drevelegas A. Imaging of primary bone tumors of the spine. Eur Radiol 2003; 13: 1859–1871

Murphey MD. From the archives of the AFIP. Primary tumors of the spine: radiologic pathologic correlation. Radiographics 1996; 16: 1131–1158

Definition

- **Epidemiology**
  Peak frequency is at 30–40 years • These account for 25% of spinal tumors • Most common intradural and extramedullary tumors • Predilection for the thoracic spine.
- **Etiology, pathophysiology, pathogenesis**
  Occurrence in neurofibromatosis type II:
  - Tumors arising from the Schwann cells of the nerve sheaths.
  - Tumors have a capsule.
  - Usually benign; malignant degeneration is rare.
  - Usually small encapsulated tumors, rarely giant Schwannomas (> 2.5 cm) with extraspinal components (especially in the lumbosacral and intrasacral regions).

  Occurrence in neurofibromatosis type I:
  - Neurofibroma.
  - Arising directly from the nerve fibers (surrounded by nerve fibers).
  - No capsule.
  - Malignant (sarcomatous) degeneration may occur.

  Histology:
  - Type A schwannoma (Antoni): Densely packed spindle cells.
  - Type B schwannoma (Antoni): Sparse, myxomatous tissue structure, hypocellular.
  - Neurofibroma: Increased connective tissue content, inclusion of nerve roots.

Imaging Signs

- **Modality of choice**
  MRI:
  - Sagittal: T1 with and without contrast, T2.
  - Axial: T1 with contrast, T2.
  - Coronal: Course along the nerve roots.
  - Examination should include cerebrum (cranial nerve schwannomas occur in neurofibromatosis type II).

  Conventional radiographs and CT:
  - Preoperative evaluation of bony destruction in giant schwannoma.
  - Evaluation of spinal stability.
- **Radiographic findings**
  Benign erosion of the posterior margins of the vertebral body (“scalloping”) • Widening of the neural foramina • Erosion of the pedicles.
- **CT findings**
  Hypodense enhancing paraspinal and/or intraspinal mass • Fusiform expansion of the nerve roots • CT myelography • CSF flow is obstructed.

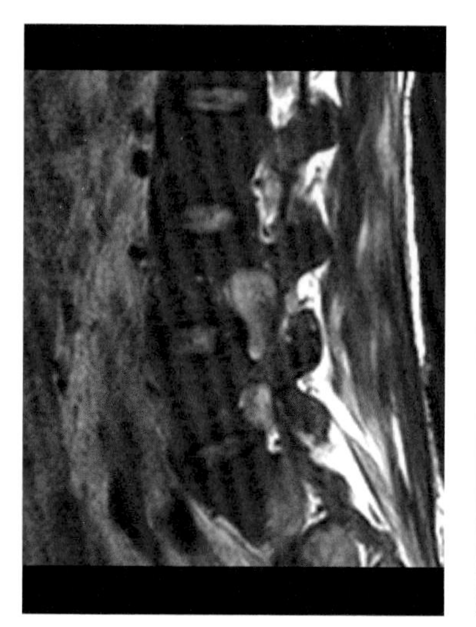

Fig. 5.51 Patient with history of increasing radicular deficits for several months with lateral hypesthesia in the thigh, weakness while extending the leg, and early signs of quadriceps atrophy. MR image of the lumbar spine (sagittal, T2). The bony nerve root canal of L5 is widened, but not eroded. It is filled by a structure isointense to the nerve roots lying cranial and caudal to it.

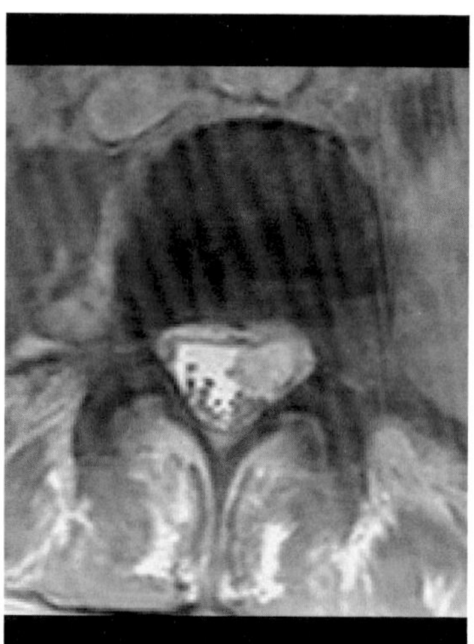

Fig. 5.52 MR image of L5 (axial, T2). Image shows left lateral intraspinal extension of the mass.

▸ **MRI findings**

General:
- Intradural extramedullary mass (rarely intramedullary).
- Dumbbell-shaped extension of large tumors across the neural foramina into the extraspinal region.
- Extraspinal components are cystic.
- Schwannoma: Sharply demarcated, encapsulated, eccentric.
- Neurofibroma: Encasement and/or fusiform expansion of the posterior nerve root.

T1:
- Signal is isointense to slightly hyperintense to the spinal cord and slightly hyperintense to CSF.
- Usually significant enhancement after contrast administration, occasionally homogeneous, occasionally heterogeneous ring enhancement.

T2:
- Schwannoma: Usually a hyperintense mass.
- Neurofibroma: Heterogeneous signal behavior due to cysts, hemorrhage, or collagen deposits.
- Signs of malignant (sarcomatous) degeneration (very rare): Increase in tumor size • Tumor size exceeding 5 cm • Ill-defined margin with infiltrative growth • Heterogeneous signal behavior.

Clinical Aspects

▸ **Typical presentation**
Radicular pain • Motor weakness • Unsteady gait • Sensory deficits • Bladder and bowel dysfunction.

▸ **Therapeutic options**
Surgical tumor resection (not indicated in asymptomatic patients with neurofibromatosis type I) • Small nerve sheath tumors are easily resected • Neurofibromas lack a capsule and extend into the extraspinal region, often rendering total resection unfeasible. Resection can result in an iatrogenic neurologic deficit as functioning nerve fibers are usually resected along with the tumor • Subtotal resection carries a risk of recurrence.

Differential Diagnosis

Disk prolapse, sequestration	– No widening of the neural foramina – Associated with degenerative changes in the vertebral bodies – Does not enhance
Meningioma	– Broad base in contact with the dura with "dural tail" sign (adjacent dura mater enhances after contrast administration) – Usually isointense to the spinal cord on T2-weighted sequences – Different peak age (40–60 years)
Filum terminale ependymoma	– Both may occur in neurofibromatosis type II; morphologically they are practically indistinguishable

Selected References

Conti P et al. Spinal neurinoma: retrospective analysis and long-term outcome of 179 consecutively operated cases and review of the literature. Surg Neurol 2004; 61: 34–43

Khong P et al. MR imaging of spinal tumors in children with neurofibromatosis I. AJR Am J Neurorad 2003; 180: 413–.417

Sridhar K et al. Giant invasive spinal schwannoma: definition and surgical management. J Neurosurg 2001; 94: 210–215

Definition

- **Leptomeningeal metastases**
  Drop metastases from intracranial tumors: In children, these occur primarily in medulloblastoma and PNETs • In adults, primarily in glioblastoma • Metastases of systemic extracranial tumors occur primarily in breast and bronchial carcinoma, lymphoma, and melanoma • Benign tumors can also produce leptomeningeal metastases (in children) • Predilection for the lumbosacral region.
- **Intramedullary metastases**
  Rare • Most common in bronchial carcinoma, followed by breast carcinoma, melanoma, and lymphoma; rarely in colon and renal cell carcinoma • Predilection for the thoracic spine.

Imaging Signs

- **Modality of choice**
  MRI:
  - Sagittal: T1 with and without contrast, T2, STIR.
  - Axial: T1 with and without contrast, T2.

  Conventional radiographs and CT:
  - Demonstrates associated vertebral metastases.

  CSF examination:
  - Detects malignant cells in leptomeningeal metastasis.
- **Radiographic findings**
  Demonstrates associated bony metastases (lytic and sclerotic lesions).
- **CT findings**
  Used for diagnosing associated bony metastases • Where MRI is contraindicated, CT myelography can demonstrate nodular tumor metastases in leptomeningeal metastatic disease.
- **MRI findings**
  Leptomeningeal metastases:
  - Nodular swellings in the meninges.
  - Agglutinated thickened cauda equina and/or nerve roots.
  - The nodules enhance and images also show diffuse leptomeningeal enhancement resembling icing on a cake.

  Intramedullary metastases:
  - Usually small tumors limited to a single segment.
  - Often located anterolaterally.
  - Circumscribed expansion of the spinal cord.

  Hypointense on T1, hyperintense on T2:
  - Hemorrhage produces an inhomogeneous signal.
  - Marked homogeneous enhancement.
  - Small lesion with disproportionately large amount of associated edema.
  - Metastases to the vertebral bodies.
  - Homogeneously decreased signal on T1-weighted images.

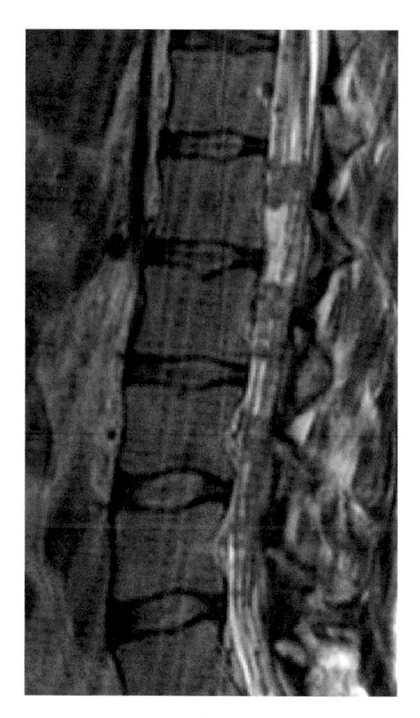

Fig. 5.53 History of surgery for a melanoma in the back a few years ago. The patient complained of increasing conus medullaris and cauda equina symptoms with pain within the last few months. MR image of thoracolumbar region (sagittal, T2) shows nodular deposits on the fibers of the cauda equina.

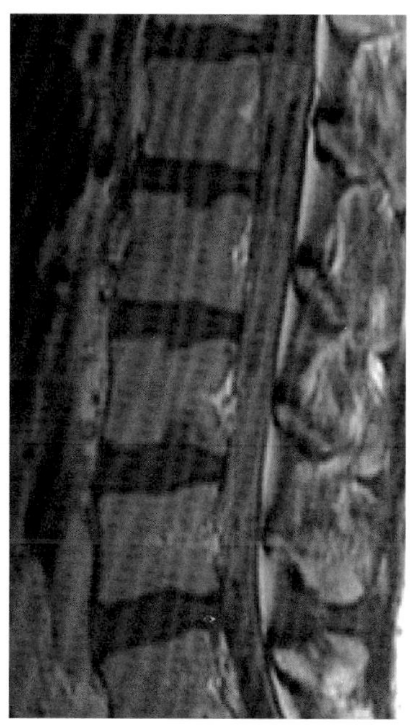

Fig. 5.54 MR image of the thoracolumbar spine (sagittal, T1). Mixed pattern of diffuse and indistinct nodular enhancement along the thickened fibers of the cauda equina. Findings suggest leptomeningeal metastases.

- Increased or decreased signal on T2-weighted images.
- Soft tissue component with disrupted cortex.

Clinical Aspects

▸ **Typical presentation**

Leptomeningeal metastases:

- Asymptomatic for a long time.
- Headache.
- Radicular pain.
- Distal lesions produce cauda equina syndrome.

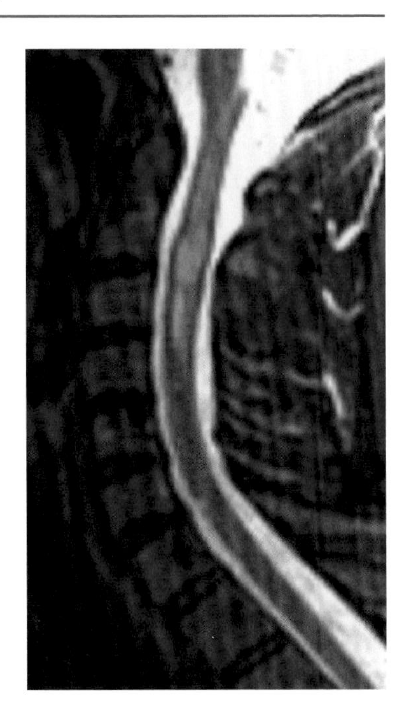

Fig. 5.55 Increasing spasticity in the presence of known breast carcinoma. MR image (sagittal, STIR) shows a hyperintense lesion at the level of C2–C3 with marked edema and a second suspicious lesion at the level of the C6–C7 disk interspace.

Intramedullary metastases:
- Dissociated sensory deficits.
- Flaccid or spastic paresis.

▶ **Therapeutic options**

Leptomeningeal metastases:
- Radiation therapy where CSF flow is obstructed.
- Intrathecal chemotherapy.

Intramedullary metastases:
- Steroids.
- Radiosensitive tumors are treated with radiation therapy.
- Chemotherapy.
- Vertebrectomy.

▶ **Course and prognosis**

Prognosis is poor; mean survival time without therapy is 3–6 weeks.

Differential Diagnosis

Leptomeningeal metastases	– Arachnoiditis – Usually the meninges and fibers of the cauda equina show homogeneous linear enhancement, rarely nodular enhancement – History (surgery, trauma, or infection) – Sarcoidosis, Wegener granulomatosis – Enhancing leptomeningeal lesion usually accompanied by enhancing intramedullary focal lesions (see chest radiograph)
Intramedullary metastases	– Primary intramedullary tumors such as astrocytoma and ependymoma – History (is there a known primary extraspinal tumor?) – Often extends across several vertebral segments
Spinal infarction	– Acute onset of symptoms – Follow-up MRI after 2–3 weeks shows regression of the mass effect and enhancement after contrast administration
Multiple sclerosis	– Follow-up MRI after approximately 4–6 weeks shows complete regression of enhancement in the lesions and no increase in size
Transverse myelitis	– Follow-up MRI after 6 weeks shows decreased spinal cord swelling and intramedullary signal alteration

Selected References

Gamori JM et al. Leptomeningeal metastases: evaluation by gadolinium enhanced spinal magnetic resonance imaging. J Neurooncol 1998; 36: 55–60

Loughrey GJ et al. Magnetic resonance imaging in the management of suspected spinal canal disease in patients with known malignancy. Clin Radiol 2000; 55: 849–855

Schiff D et al. Intramedullary spinal cord metastases: Clinical features and treatment outcome. Neurology 1996; 47: 906–912

Definition

▶ **Epidemiology**
Peak incidence is at 40–60 years • Second most common intradural extramedullary tumor (after nerve sheath tumors) • Increased incidence with neurofibromatosis type II, occurs in younger patients • More common in women than men (4:1 to 8:1).

▶ **Etiology, pathophysiology, pathogenesis**
Benign slow-growing tumor derived from arachnoid cells • Rarely exhibits intradural and extradural or solely extradural growth (5% of lesions) • Predilection for the thoracic and cervical spine.

Imaging Signs

▶ **Modality of choice**
MRI:
- Sagittal: T1 with and without contrast, T2.
- Axial: T1 with contrast, T2.

Conventional radiographs and CT:
- Helpful in evaluating bony destruction with larger tumors.

▶ **Radiographic findings**
Benign erosion of the posterior margins of the vertebral body ("scalloping") • Widening of the neural foramina • Erosion of the pedicles.

▶ **CT findings**
Solid, smoothly demarcated mass isodense to muscle • Calcifications often occur with the psammomatous subtype • CT myelography is useful where MRI is contraindicated.

▶ **MRI findings**
Usually a nodular intraspinal mass develops, plaquelike growth is rare • Tumor compresses and displaces the spinal cord • Broad area of dural contact • Extradural tumors show a hypointense band between tumor and spinal cord • Where both intradural and extradural components are present, the tumor may grow in an hourglass configuration.
T1:
- Isointense to slightly hyperintense.
- Enhancement after contrast administration is variable and inhomogeneous where calcifications are present.
- Adjacent dura enhances with contrast in 5% of cases ("dural tail" sign).

T2:
- Isointense to hyperintense.
- Calcified tumors are hypointense.

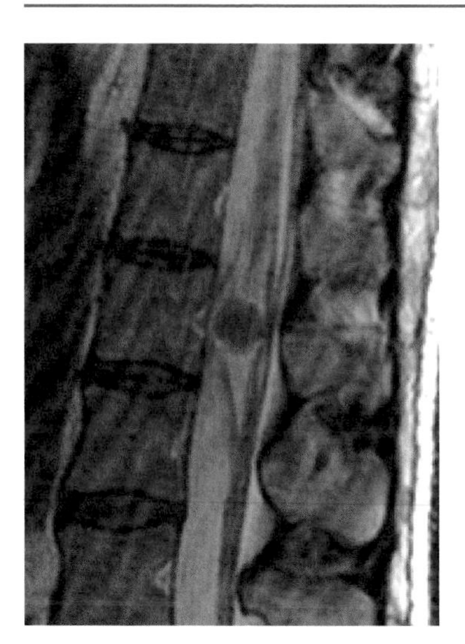

Fig. 5.56 A 67-year-old woman with history of pain for several months. MR image of the thoracic spine (sagittal, T2). Round, hypointense, intradural extramedullary mass.

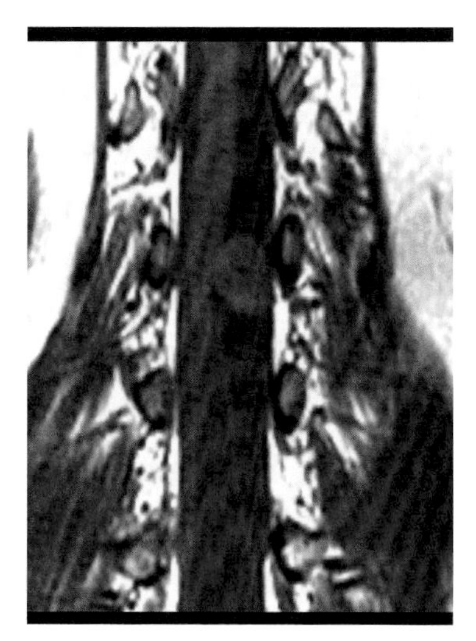

Fig. 5.57 MR image of the thoracic spine (coronal, T1). Intradural extramedullary mass on the left side impressing and displacing the spinal cord.

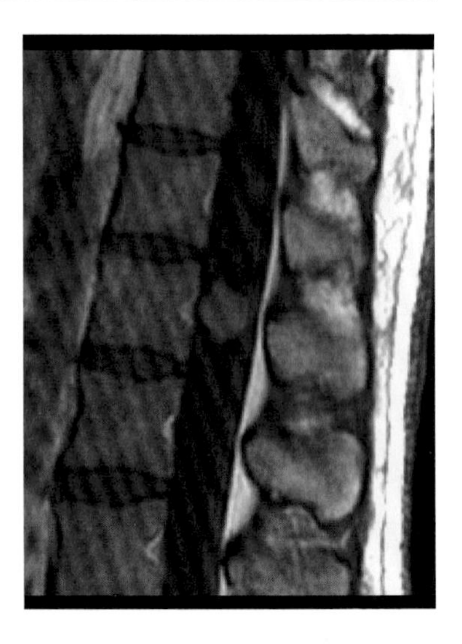

Fig. 5.58 MR image of the thoracic spine (sagittal, T1 with contrast). Mass shows moderate enhancement.

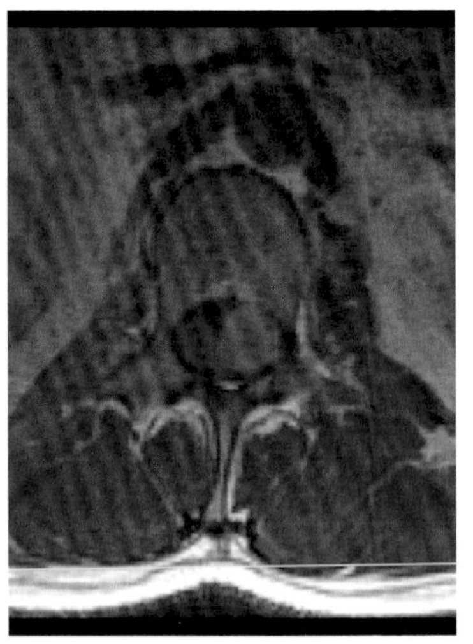

Fig. 5.59 MR image of T11 (axial, T1 with contrast). The mass enhances significantly compared with the spinal cord.

Clinical Aspects

- **Typical presentation**
  Back pain • Motor weakness • Unsteady gait • Sensory deficits • Bladder and bowel dysfunction.
- **Therapeutic options**
  Surgical tumor resection • Tumor may recur following subtotal resection • Supplementary radiation therapy is indicated where total resection is not feasible or with early recurrence of tumor.

Differential Diagnosis

Disk herniation, sequestration	– Associated with degenerative changes in the vertebral bodies – No widening of the neural foramina – Does not enhance
Nerve sheath tumors (schwannoma, neurofibroma)	– Tumor adjacent to or within nerve fibers – Usually hyperintense (schwannoma) on T2-weighted sequences or heterogeneous (neurofibroma) – Cystic components – Different peak age (30–40 years)
Metastases	

Selected References

Gezen F et al. Review of 36 cases of spinal cord meningioma. Spine 2000; 25: 727–731

Kleekamp J et al. Surgical results of spinal meningioma. Acta Neurochir (Suppl) 1996; 65: 77–81

Takemoto K et al. MR imaging of intraspinal tumors-capability in histological differentiation and compartmentalization of extramedullary tumors. Neuroradiology 1988; 30: 303–309

Definition

- **Epidemiology**
Peak age 30–40 years • Most common tumor of the spinal cord and filum terminale in adults (accounting for approximately 40% of intramedullary tumors) • More common in men than women (3:2).
- **Etiology, pathophysiology, pathogenesis**
Arises from ependymal cells of the central canal and terminal ventricle • Associated with neurofibromatosis type II.
Subtypes:
  - *Intramedullary:* Predilection for the cervical spine, less often thoracic spine.
  - *Extramedullary:* Occurs in the filum terminale and conus medullaris (usually myxopapillary subtype).
  - *Metastatic:* Spinal metastasis of intracranial primary tumor.

Imaging Signs

- **Modality of choice**
MRI:
  - Sagittal: T1, T2, blood sensitive sequence.
  - Contrast administration: T1 axial and sagittal.

  Conventional radiographs and CT:
  - Helpful in evaluating bony destruction with larger tumors.
- **Radiographic findings**
Erosion of the vertebral pedicles • Thinning of the posterior margin of the vertebrae • Scoliosis.
- **CT findings**
Visualization of associated bony changes • *CT myelography* (only where MRI is contraindicated): Expansion of the spinal cord, obstruction of CSF flow.
- **MRI findings**
Lesion located in the central spinal cord and exhibiting expansive centrifugal growth • Lesions occurring in the filum terminale show thickened cauda equina fibers and nodular structures but no cysts • Average longitudinal extent is across three to four vertebrae • Often (50% of cases) a large cyst with a small solid component is present • Often associated with syringomyelia • Expansion of the spinal cord.
T1:
  - Usually a hypointense to isointense mass, may also be hyperintense secondary to hemorrhage.
  - Solid tumor components usually show significant homogeneous, irregularly patchy, or nodular enhancement on the cyst wall.
  - Hypointense cysts.

  T2:
  - Hyperintense mass aligned parallel to the longitudinal axis of the spinal cord.
  - There may be a hypointense halo due to hemosiderin deposits (“cap sign”).
  - Hyperintense cysts.

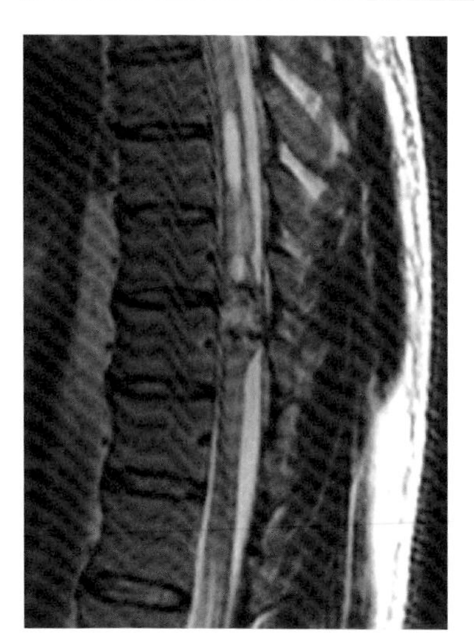

Fig. 5.60 A 40-year-old man with paresthesias in both lower extremities and an unsteady gait. MR image of the thoracic spine (sagittal, T2). Round intramedullary mass with marginal hemosiderin deposits, cysts, and associated syringomyelia.

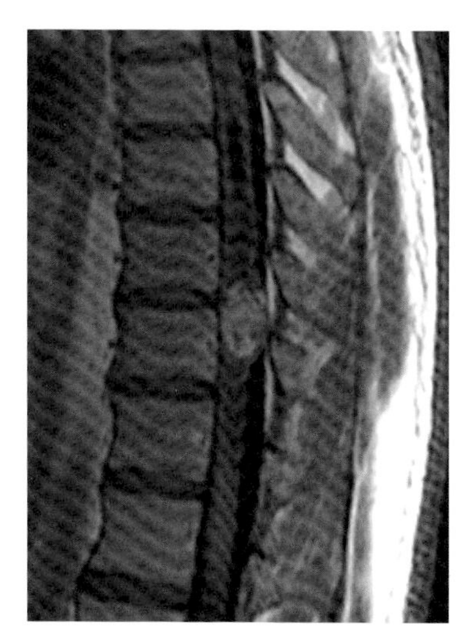

Fig. 5.61 MR image of the thoracic spine (sagittal, T1 with contrast). The tumor shows significant enhancement after contrast administration. The hypointense hemosiderin deposits remain unchanged.

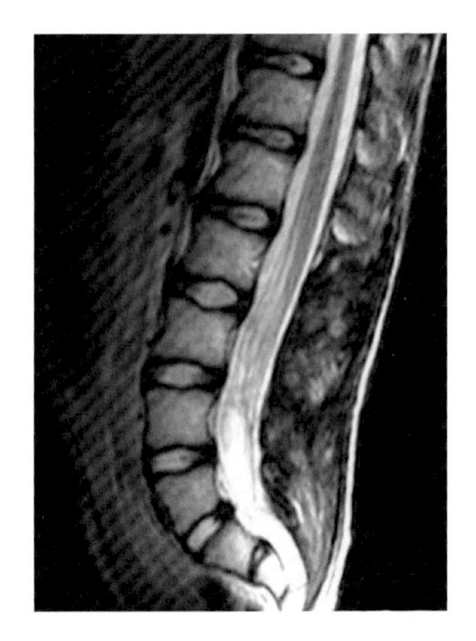

Fig. 5.62 The patient had had increasing, electric-shocklike pain in the lower back and both legs for several months. This was accompanied by difficulty in emptying the bladder, perianal sensory deficits, and weakness in the legs. MR image of the lumbosacral spine (sagittal, T2) shows an irregular pattern of the cauda equina fibers and a large oval mass at the level of L5–S1.

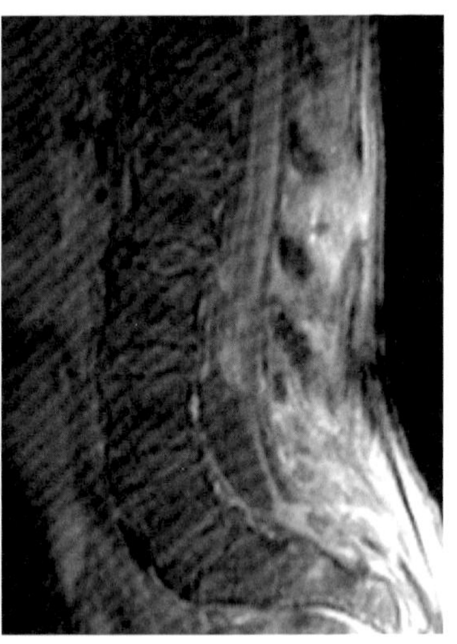

Fig. 5.63 MR image of the lumbosacral spine (sagittal, T1 with contrast). Inhomogeneous at the level of L4–L5. The mass at L5–S1 is hypointense, consistent with a cyst.

Clinical Aspects

- **Typical presentation**
  Progressive neck and back pain • Paresthesias • Motor weakness • Bladder and bowel dysfunction • *Acute paraplegia:* With regressive ependymomas of the filum terminale, bleeding can produce a hematoma with mass effect and subarachnoid hemorrhage.
- **Therapeutic options**
  Laminectomy and radical tumor resection • Postoperative radiation therapy is indicated where only subtotal resection is feasible.
- **Course and prognosis**
  Five-year survival rate is between 68% and 95% • Tumor may recur (5–10% of cases), especially following subtotal resection • Follow-up examinations with MRI.

Differential Diagnosis

Astrocytoma	– Most common intramedullary tumor in children – Rarely in the filum terminale – Eccentric growth with asymmetrical expansion of the spinal cord – Hemorrhaging is less common – Infiltrating – Inhomogeneous enhancement after contrast administration
Hemangioblastoma	– Irregularly patchy, hypointense area due to flow voids – Well-demarcated, significant perifocal edema often present – Often associated with syringomyelia
Metastasis	– Known underlying malignant disease – Higher peak age
Schwannoma (DD: Filum terminale ependymoma)	– Widening of the neural foramina – Arises from the root of the cauda equina (extramedullary intradural location)
Leptomeningeal metastases (DD: Filum terminale ependymoma)	– History (possibly known primary tumor)

Selected References

Fine MJ et al. Spinal cord ependymomas: MR imaging features. Radiology 1995; 197: 655–658

Miyazawa N et al. MRI at 1,5 T of intramedullary ependymoma and classification of contrast enhancement. Neurorad 2000; 42: 828–832

Schwartz TH et al. Intramedullary ependymomas: clinical presentation, surgical treatment strategies and prognosis. J Neurooncol 2000; 47: 211–218

Definition

▸ **Epidemiology**

Peak age 20–40 years • More common in men than women (3:2) • Most common intramedullary tumor in children (up to 90% of cases).

▸ **Etiology, pathophysiology, pathogenesis**

Holomedullary astrocytoma: Lesion extending over the entire length of the spinal cord (rare). Histologic classification:

- Pilocytic astrocytoma (more favorable prognosis).
- Diffuse fibrillar astrocytoma.

Associated with neurofibromatosis type 1 • Predilection for the cervical and thoracic spinal cord.

Imaging Signs

▸ **Modality of choice**

MRI:

- Sagittal: T1 with and without contrast, T2.
- Axial: T2, T1 with contrast.
- Gradient echo sequence.

Conventional radiographs:

Scoliosis • Widening of the spinal canal • Erosion of the pedicles, thinning of the posterior margins of the vertebral bodies

CT:

Visualization of associated bony changes • *CT myelography* (only where MRI is contraindicated): Expansion of the spinal cord, obstructed CSF flow.

▸ **MRI findings**

General:

- Expansion of the spinal cord, usually over several segments.
- Ill-defined border.
- Difficult to distinguish tumor from tumor edema.

T1:

- Isointense to weakly hypointense mass.
- Inhomogeneous enhancement is more obvious in pilocytic astrocytomas than in fibrillar astrocytomas.

T2:

- Hyperintense intramedullary mass.
- Signal inhomogeneities resulting from bleeding, necrosis, or cysts.

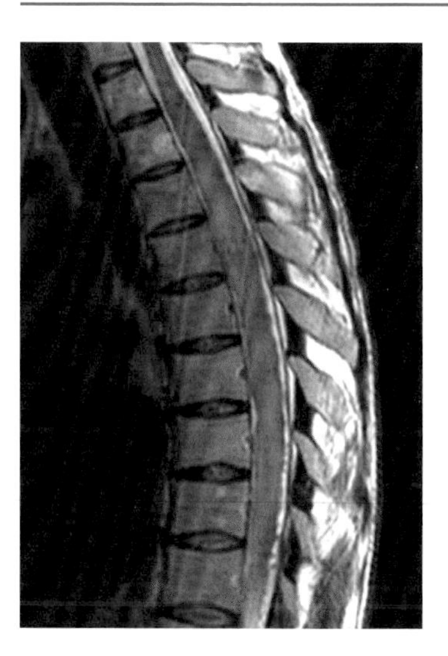

Fig. 5.64 History of increasing gait disturbance over several years. MR image of the thoracic spine (sagittal, T2). The spinal cord is expanded in the middle and lower thoracic regions and appears inhomogeneous and faintly hyperintense. The subarachnoid space is obliterated. A hemangioma is present in vertebra T3.

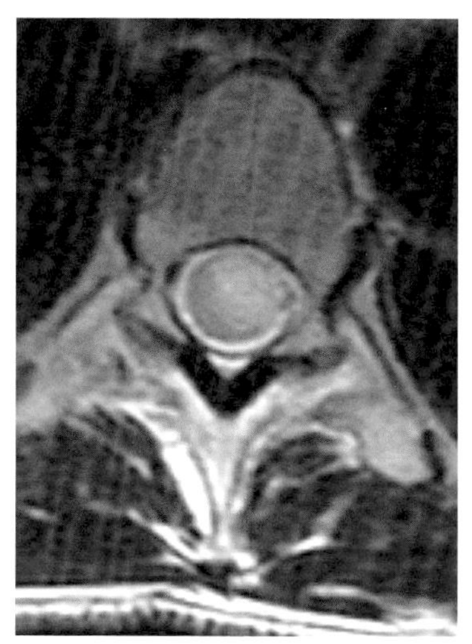

Fig. 5.65 MR image of T10 (axial, STIR). Abnormal signals within the spinal cord.

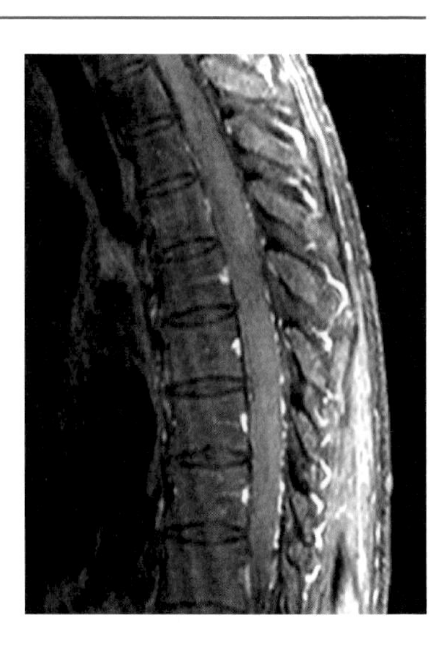

Fig. 5.66 MR image of the thoracic spine (T1 with contrast). Slight diffuse enhancement within the spinal cord.

Clinical Aspects

- **Typical presentation**
  Symptoms progress slowly over a period of months to years • Back pain • Motor deficits • Progressive scoliosis • Cervical lesions produce torticollis • Hydrocephalus • *Brown-Sequard syndrome:* Asymmetric tumor growth produces spastic hemiparesis on one side while reducing pain and temperature sensitivity on the contralateral side • Bladder and bowel dysfunction.
- **Therapeutic options**
  Where tumor progression is very slow with minimal neurologic dysfunction, especially in the infiltrative subtype, one should carefully consider where surgical intervention is indicated • Laminectomy or osteoplastic laminotomy (preferred in children) • Tumor resection and postoperative radiation therapy • Chemotherapy is indicated with subtotal tumor resection and recurrent tumor.
- **Course and prognosis**
  Five-year survival rate is 58%.

Differential Diagnosis

Ependymoma	– Occurs in the center of the spinal cord – More clearly demarcated – Hemosiderin deposits create a hypointense halo on T2-weighted sequences
Metastases	– History (is there a known primary extraspinal tumor?) – Extent of lesion usually limited to one segment
Ganglioglioma	– In children younger than 3 years
Multiple sclerosis	– Follow-up MRI after approximately 4–6 weeks shows complete regression of enhancement in the lesions and no increase in size
Transverse myelitis	– Follow-up MRI after 6 weeks shows decreased spinal cord swelling and intramedullary signal alteration
Spinal infarction	– Acute onset of symptoms – Follow-up MRI after 2–3 weeks shows regression of the mass effect and enhancement after contrast administration

Selected References

Houten JK, Howard LW. Pediatric intramedullary spinal cord tumors: special considerations. J Neurooncol 2000; 47: 225–230

Houten JK, Cooper PR. Spinal cord astrocytoma: presentation, management and outcome. J Neurooncol 2000; 47; 219–224

Lowe GM. Magnetic resonance imaging of intramedullary spinal cord tumors. J Neurooncol 2000; 47: 195–210

Definition

- **Epidemiology**
  Usually manifests itself before 30 years (often at 20–30 years) in the setting of von Hippel-Lindau disease • More common in men than women by a ratio of 2:1 • Accounts for 3–5% of all tumors of the spinal cord, with a predilection for the posterior cervical and thoracic cord.
- **Etiology, pathophysiology, pathogenesis**
  Histologically benign vascular tumor • Seventy to eight percent are idiopathic solitary lesions; 16–25% occur as multiple lesions in von Hippel-Lindau diseased (with retinal and cerebellar hemangioblastomas and abdominal cysts). Associated syringomyelia occurs in 50–70% of cases.

Imaging Signs

- **Modality of choice**
  MRI:
  - Sagittal: T1 with and without contrast, T2.
  - Axial: T2, T1 with contrast.
- **Digital subtraction angiography (DSA)**
  - Preoperative planning.
- **CT findings**
  Enhancing nodules, often adjacent intramedullary cysts.
- **MRI findings**
  General:
  - Small nodule, large cyst.
  - Superficial site in the spinal cord, usually on the posterior aspect.
  - Often diffuse spinal cord swelling because of associated edema.
  - Tumor itself is well demarcated.
  - Larger tumors contain punctate hypointensities on all sequences. These are flow voids produced by rapidly flowing blood.
  - Hemorrhages are common.
  - Associated syringomyelia.

  T1:
  - Isointense to hypointense lesion.
  - Pronounced enhancement.
  - Hypointense to hyperintense cyst, depending on protein content.

  T2:
  - Hyperintense nodular mass.
  - Associated edema is seen and associated cysts are well demarcated as hyperintensities.
- **DSA findings**
  - Hypervascular, sharply demarcated tumor.
  - Visualization of vessels supplying and draining the tumor.

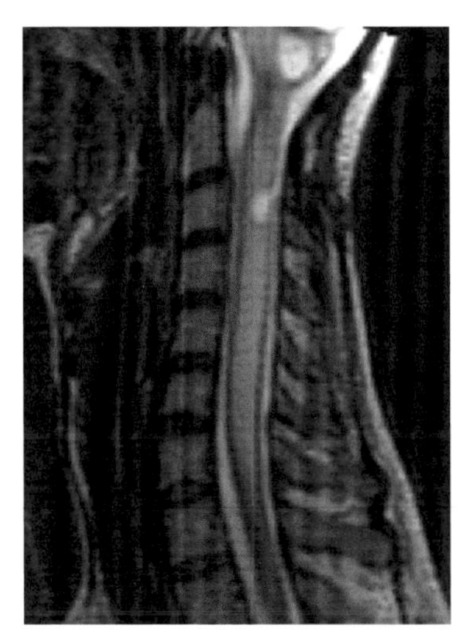

Fig. 5.67 Patient with known von Hippel–Lindau disease and increasing spastic tetraparesis. MR image of the cervical spine (sagittal, T2). The spinal cord appears swollen and hyperintense (associated edema) from the craniocervical junction to C7–T1. At the level of C3 there is a hyperintense lesion with a hypointense halo. There is also a hyperintense mass in the cerebellar vermis. A small hypointense area (flow void) is seen in the center of this mass.

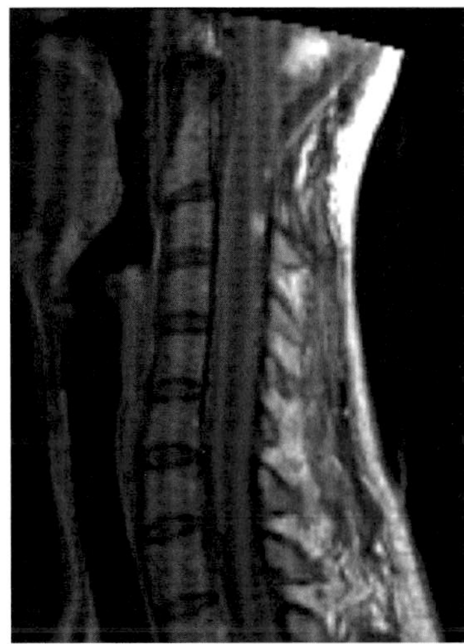

Fig. 5.68 MR image of the cervical spine (sagittal, T1 with contrast). The intraaxial lesions enhance, as do the meninges.

Clinical Aspects

- **Typical presentation**
  Course is insidious; symptoms are exacerbated by associated edema, cysts, and/or syringomyelia • Pain • Scoliosis • Sensory deficits • Paraparesis or tetraparesis • Bowel and bladder dysfunction.
- **Therapeutic options**
  Complete removal of the tumor resection • Preoperative superselective embolization of the vascular feeders may be considered.

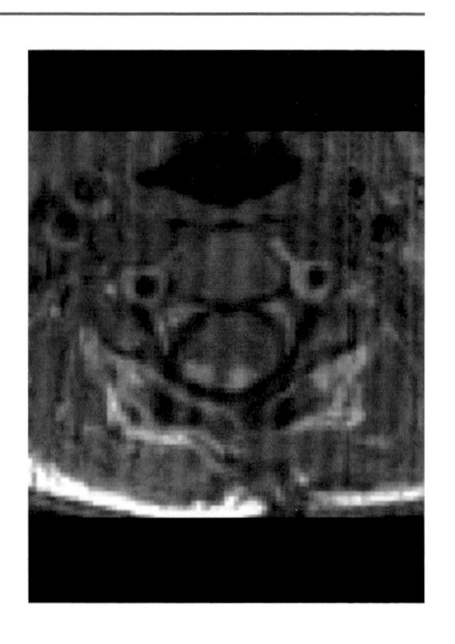

Fig. 5.69 MR image of C4 (axial, T1 with contrast). Enhancing lesions and hypointense signal alterations within the spinal cord. The subarachnoid space is obliterated.

Differential Diagnosis

Astrocytoma	– Isointense or slightly hypointense to spinal cord on noncontrasted T1-weighted images – No flow voids – Enhancement is weak or even absent – Hardly ever cystic – Hemorrhages extremely rare – Poorly demarcated
Ependymoma	– Predilection for craniocervical junction and lumbar theca – No flow voids

Selected References

Baker KB et al. MR imaging of spinal hemangioblastoma. Am J Roentg 2000; 174: 377–382
Lowe GM. Magnetic resonance imaging of intramedullary spinal cord tumors. J Neurooncol 2000; 47: 195–210
Miller DJ et al. Hemangioblastomas and other uncommon intramedullary tumors. J Neurooncol 2000; 47: 253–270

Definition

- **Epidemiology**
  Rare, potentially life-threatening • *Caution:* Distal neurologic deficits • More common in men than women • Peak age for spontaneous occurrence is between 40 and 50 years.
- **Etiology, pathophysiology, pathogenesis**
  Bleeding from the epidural venous plexus • Occurs spontaneously in coagulation disorders and in patients on anticoagulant therapy • Idiopathic (45% of cases) • Posttraumatic.

Imaging Signs

- **Modality of choice**
  Emergency indication for MRI:
  - Sagittal: T1, T2.
  - Axial: T2.
  - Gradient echo sequence.
- **CT findings**
  Hyperdense extradural lesion compressing the dural sac (usually posteriorly).
- **MRI findings**
  Intraspinal, extradural mass that does not enhance • *Sagittal:* Biconvex "teardrop" shape • Increased enhancement of the adjacent meninges (differentiation from an abscess is difficult) • Secondary compressive myelopathy may be seen.
  Posterior epidural hematoma
  - More common.
  - Cannot be differentiated from subdural hematoma.

  Anterior epidural hematoma:
  - "Curtain sign"—hemorrhage is divided into two parts by the membrane of Trolard (not present in a subdural hematoma).

  T1 (according to the age of the hemorrhage):
  - Acute: isointense.
  - Subacute (after 3–4 days): hypointense in the center, hyperintense on the periphery.
  - Chronic: markedly hypointense halo of hemosiderin.

  T2 (according to the age of the hemorrhage):
  - Acute: hyperintense to hypointense.
  - Subacute (> 5 days till several weeks): hyperintense.
  - Chronic: markedly hypointense halo.
  - Gradient echo sequence: better demarcation of the hematoma.

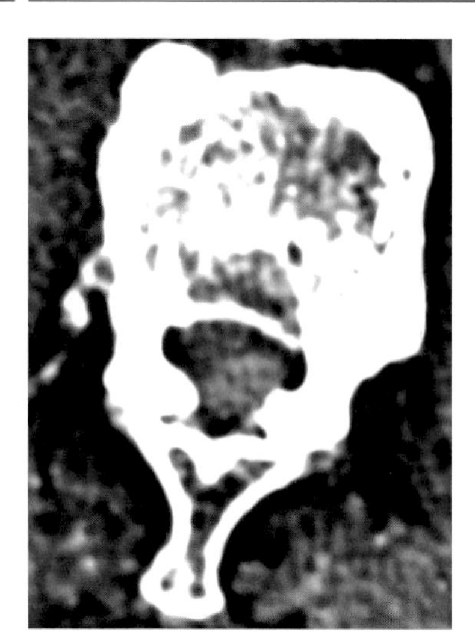

Fig. 6.1 Patient with posttraumatic paraplegia in the legs and sensory deficits distal to the level of vertebra T4. CT of T7 (axial). Left lateral posterior hyperdense oval mass compressing and displacing the dural sac.

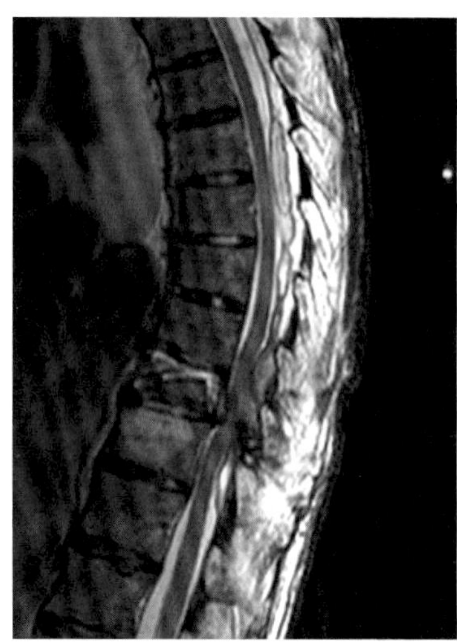

Fig. 6.2 MR image of the thoracic spine (sagittal, T2). Several elongated epidural lesions with contents of varying intensity lying adjacent to the notably hypointense dura. Comminuted fracture of T9 with intraspinal fragments and compression of the spinal cord.

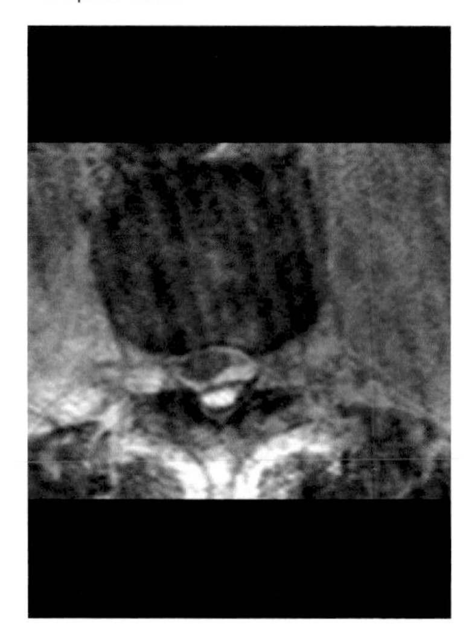

Fig. 6.3 MR image of T7 (axial, T1). Central epidural hyperintense lesion—methemoglobin.

Clinical Aspects

- **Typical presentation**
  Symptoms are identical to those of acute disk prolapse • Severe, often radicular radiating pain at the level of the hemorrhage • Distal neurologic deficits occur within a few hours.
- **Therapeutic options**
  Rapid laminectomy and removal of the hematoma • Delayed decompression will result in neurologic deficits.

Differential Diagnosis

Subdural hematoma	– Concave; anterior lesions that cross the midline are not divided by a membrane
Abscess	– Thickened meninges; associated diskitis or osteomyelitis may be present
Metastases	– Associated pathology in the adjacent vertebral body
Lymphoma	– Homogeneous enhancement
Spinal lipomatosis	– Homogeneous signal intensity, hyperintense on T1 and T2

Selected References

Dorsay et al. MR imaging of epidural hematoma in the lumbar spine. Skeletal Radiol 2002; 31: 677–685
Gundry CR et al. Epidural Hematoma of the Lumbar Spine: 18 Surgically confirmed cases. Radiology 1993; 187: 427–431
Sklar EM et al. MRI of acute spinal epidural hematomas. J Comput Assist Tomogr 1999; 23; 238–243

Definition

- **Epidemiology**
  Intradural arteriovenous malformation (AVM): Usually manifests before 30 years of age • *Spinal dural AV fistula:* Usually manifests after 40 years of age.
- **Etiology, pathophysiology, pathogenesis**
  Abnormal direct communication between an artery and a vein, without a capillary bed between them.
  Classification:
  - *Congenital AVM:* Glomerular (intramedullary nidus), plexiform, or juvenile (complex AVM extending across several vertebral segments), fistulous, (extramedullary intradural) • "High-flow" vascular malformation.
  - *Acquired AVM* (> 60% of cases): Spinal dural AV fistula • "Low-flow" vascular malformation • Spontaneous, posttraumatic, postinflammatory, or postoperative • More than half of all lesions occur in the thoracolumbar spine.

Imaging Signs

- **Modality of choice**
  MRI:
  - Sagittal: T1 with and without contrast, T2.
  - Axial: T2.
  - MR angiography after contrast administration.

  DSA.
- **MRI findings**
  Expanded blood vessels in the spinal canal (intramedullary, intradural, dural), hypointense on T1 and T2 (flow void), hyperintense after contrast administration • Blood breakdown products post hemorrhage and/or rupture • A fistula may be seen • Spinal cord is expanded due to congestive edema (hyperintense on T2-weighted images) • Spinal cord atrophy due to ischemia, bleeding, or chronic compression.
- **MR angiography findings**
  Visualization of vascular structures supplying and draining the malformation.
- **CT myelography findings**
  Visualization of dilated intradural vessels.
- **DSA findings**
  Detailed preoperative evaluation of vascular structures • Differentiation of "high-flow" AVMs from "low-flow" AVMs • Visualization of fistulas.

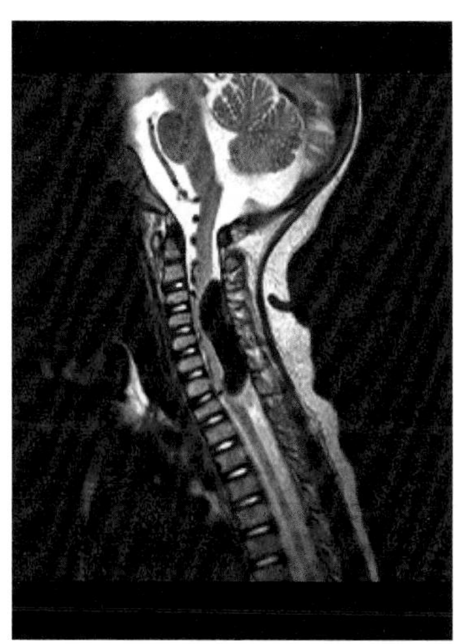

Fig. 6.4 Child with permanent torticollis and progressive spastic quadriplegia. MR image of cervicothoracic region (sagittal, T2). Atypical ectatic vascular structure causing posterior impression of the spinal cord at the level of C4 through T1. Additional abnormal flow voids are seen on the anterior surface of the medulla oblongata.

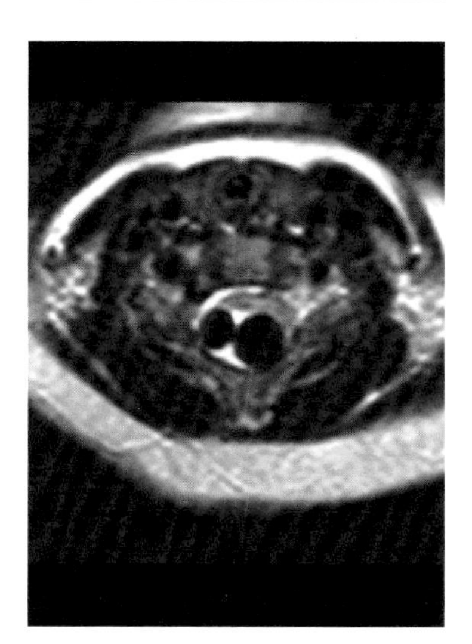

Fig. 6.5 MR image of C4 (axial, T2). Two large vascular cross-sections are present posterior to the compressed spinal cord.

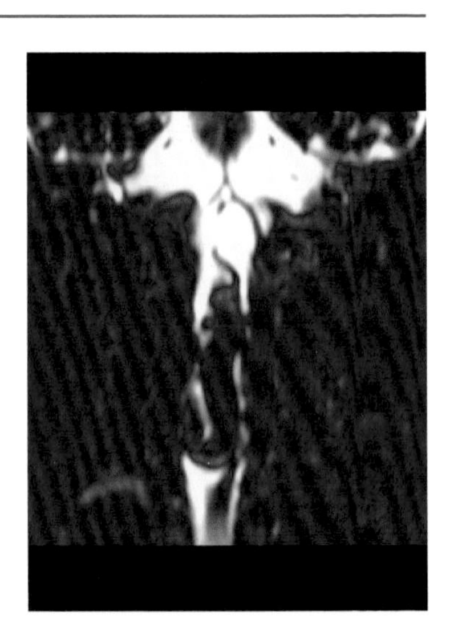

Fig. 6.6 MR myelography (coronal, T12). The vascular malformation is well demarcated against the hyperintense CSF.

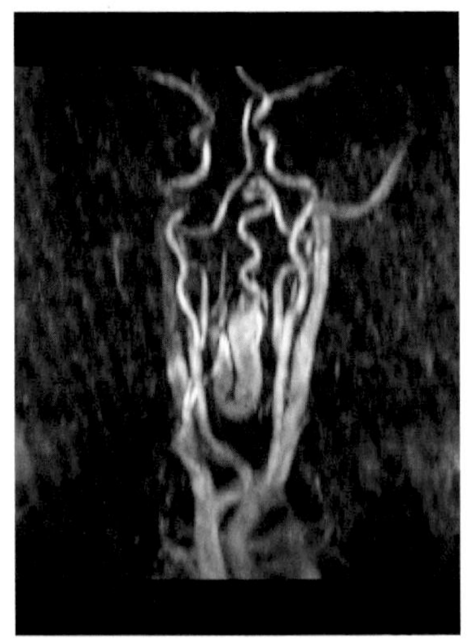

Fig. 6.7 MR angiography (coronal with contrast). Image shows the relationship of the AVM to the vessels supplying and draining it.

Clinical Aspects

- **Typical presentation**

  Intradural AVM
  - Usually manifests itself after age 30 years.
  - *Subarachnoid hemorrhage:* Acute onset of severe headache, meningism, and photophobia.
  - *Intraparenchymal hemorrhage:* Sudden pain, acute neurologic dysfunction.
  - *Mass effect:* Growth of the AVM compresses nerve tissue, leading to neurologic deficits.

  Spinal dural AV fistula:
  - Usually manifests itself after age 40 years.
  - Slowly progressive symptoms over a period of months to years.
  - Progressive weakness in the legs and bladder and bowel dysfunction.
  - Pain that increases with motion or change of position.

  Foix–Alajouanine syndrome (subacute necrotizing myelitis):
  - Extreme course occurs only in a few patients.
  - Characterized by rapidly progressive myelopathy due to venous thrombosis (DD: Intermittent claudication, spinal stenosis).

- **Therapeutic options**

  Endovascular embolization • Open ligation • The two procedures are often used in combination.

Differential Diagnosis

Intramedullary cavernous malformation	– Inhomogeneous signal in the center on T1 and T2 images due to slow-flowing blood. Blood breakdown products of varying age, hypointense halo from hemosiderin deposits on T2-weighted images
Hemangioblastoma	– Significant expansion of the spinal cord, associated cyst or syrinx

Selected References

Cullen S et al. Spinal arteriovenous shunts presenting before 2 years of age: analysis of 13 cases. Childs Nerv Syst 2006; 22: 1103–1110

Koch C. Spinal dural arteriovenous fistula. Curr Opin Neurol 2006; 19: 69–75

Meisel HJ et al. Modern management of spinal and spinal cord vascular lesions. Minim Invasive Neurosurg 1995; 38: 138–145

Thron A et al. Spinal arteriovenous malformation. Radiologe 2001; 41: 949–954

Tomlinson FH et al. Arteriovenous fistulas of the brain and the spinal cord. J Neurosurg 1994; 80: 178–179

Definition

- **Epidemiology**
Rare • More common in arteriosclerosis, aortic dissection, thromboembolic disease, vasculitis, autoimmune disease, syphilis, diabetes mellitus, cardiac arrest, caisson disease, vascular compression due to tumor or trauma, prolapsed disk, iatrogenic cases (aortic surgery, contrast agent toxicity).
- **Etiology, pathophysiology, pathogenesis**
Ischemia in the area supplied by the anterior spinal artery (receives blood from branches of the aorta, supplies the anterior two-thirds of the spinal cord) • Rarely in the area supplied by the posterior spinal arteries • Predilection for the lower thoracic cord and conus medullaris.

Imaging Signs

- **Modality of choice**
Emergency indication for MRI:
  - Sagittal (T1, T2) and axial (T2) slices.
  - DWI, axial and sagittal: Hyperintense signal in the acute stage.

  CSF examination:
  - This can exclude inflammatory and/or infectious disorders of the spinal cord.
- **CT findings**
CT myelography is used where MRI is contraindicated; otherwise CT is not suitable.
- **MRI findings**
DWI:
  - Hyperintense signal immediately after ischemia, very sensitive.

  T2:
  - Acute: Note that the latency period is longer than in cerebral ischemia.
  - Sagittal: Linear signal increase in the spinal cord with slight expansion.
  - Axial: Signal increase in the anterior and posterior spinal cord, primarily in the gray matter (an isolated "owl's eye" sign may be seen in the anterior horn), usually bilaterally in the paramedian region (symmetric or asymmetric).
  - Chronic: Hyperintense glial scar with circumscribed spinal cord atrophy.
  - Associated vertebral infarction: Hyperintense signal alteration in the vertebral body at the same level and supplied by the same artery.

  T1:
  - Subacute: Enhancement is detectable for several weeks.
  - The periphery may appear slightly hyperintense where there is hemorrhagic transformation.

  MR myelography:
  - Conventional angiography shows abnormal vascular structures due to an underlying AVM.
  - Visualization of abnormal vascular structures with the option of embolization.

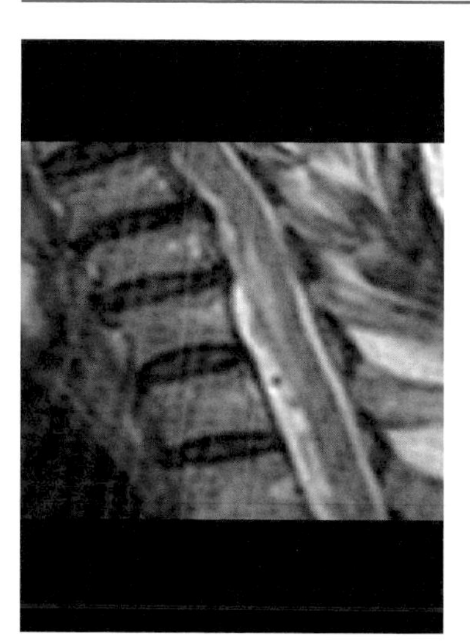

Fig. 6.8 Bilateral paresis in the arms following surgical correction of an aortic aneurysm. MR image of the lower cervical spine (sagittal, T2). Hyperintensity in the anterior spinal cord at C5–C8.

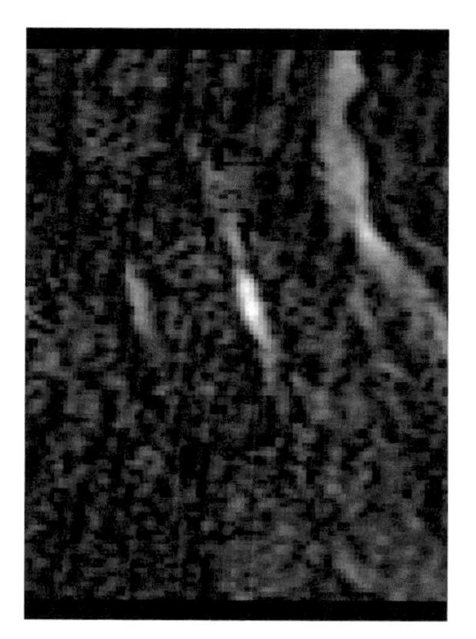

Fig. 6.9 MR image of the lower cervical spine (sagittal, diffusion-weighted): Hyperintensity in parts of the lesion.

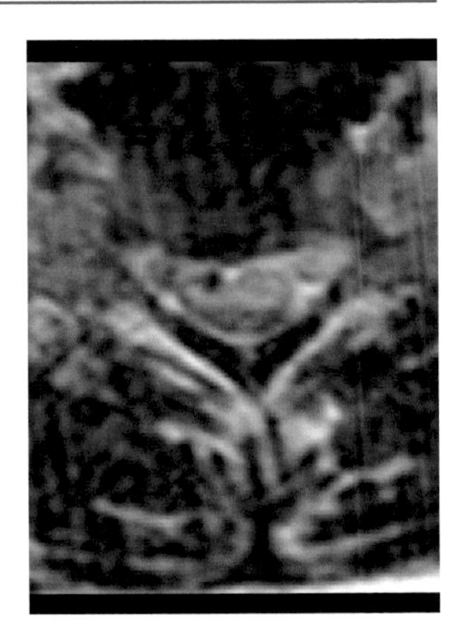

Fig. 6.10 MR myelography of C7 (axial, T2). Hyperintensity mainly in the anterior horns.

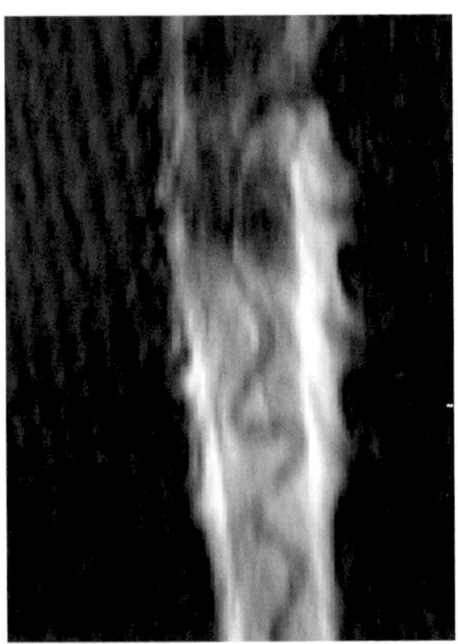

Fig. 6.11 MR angiography (coronal). Atypical tortuous vessel.

Clinical Aspects

- **Typical presentation**
  Paraparesis or tetraparesis, either with acute onset or initially flaccid and then spastic • Usually burning or stabbing pain at the level of the affected segment (80% of all cases) • *Anterior infarction:* Dissociated sensory deficit with loss of sensitivity to pain and temperature caudal to the infarcted level • *Posterior infarction:* Impaired proprioception and sensitivity to vibration • Bladder and bowel dysfunction • *Cervical:* Horner's syndrome.
- **Therapeutic options**
  Medical therapy with aspirin; elimination of vascular compression where indicated • Neurologic rehabilitation.
- **Course and prognosis**
  Permanent neurologic deficits are common • Immobilization promotes comorbidities such as pulmonary embolism and infections.

Differential Diagnosis

Foix–Alajouanine syndrome (subacute necrotizing myelitis)	– Selective angiography to visualize abnormal vascular structures
Spinal cord necrosis due to a thrombosed AVM	– Selective angiography to visualize abnormal vascular structures
Myelitis producing distal neurologic deficits	– Changes in the cord white matter are more pronounced – Inhomogeneous enhancement – Multiple sclerosis – Plaques occur primarily in the lateral spinal cord
Guillain–Barré syndrome (postinfectious polyneuropathy)	– Lacks clinical findings of sphincter dysfunction – Reduced nerve conduction velocity
Vasculitis	

Selected References

Faig J et al. Vertebral body infarction as a confirmatory sign of spinal cord ischemic stroke. Report of three cases and review of the literature. Stroke 1998; 29: 239–243

Loher TJ et al. Diffusion-weighted MRI in acute spinal cord ischaemia. Neuroradiology 2003; 8: 557–561

Weidauer S et al. Spinal cord infarction: MR imaging and clinical features in 16 cases. Neuroradiology 2002; 44: 851–857

Definition

- **Epidemiology**
  This is a common complication of spinal surgery (approximately 41% of cases) • Most common, specific complications include spinal stenosis (lateral approximately 55%, central approximately 15%), recurrent prolapse (extrusion; approximately 15%), arachnoiditis (approximately 10%).
- **Etiology, pathophysiology, pathogenesis**
  Excessive scarring leading to stenosis of the spinal canal and/or neural foramina • Prolonged or new pain, functional deficits, instability.

Imaging Signs

- **Modality of choice**
  MRI:
  - Visualizes the morphologic substrate of the complication.
  - With and without IV contrast agent.
- **Radiographic findings**
  Angulation • Instability (stress views) • Progressive degeneration.
- **CT findings**
  Multidetector CT for multiplanar reconstruction in the sagittal and coronal planes • Bony changes and degeneration • Limited sensitivity in detecting complications in neural structures and soft tissue.
- **MRI findings**
  Axial and sagittal (STIR, T1, T2) • IV contrast to differentiate recurrent extrusion (no enhancement) from scarring (significant enhancement) • In rare cases, recurrent extrusion will also enhance due to reactive inflammatory changes • High specificity for spinal stenosis, recurrent prolapse, arachnoiditis, CSF fistula, and epidural fibrosis.
- **Nuclear medicine**
  CSF fistula.

Clinical Aspects

- **Typical presentation**
  Prolonged and/or increased pain • Limited function • Instability.
- **Therapeutic options**
  Pain therapy (systemic, local interventional, complementary procedures) • Physical therapy • Revision surgery.

Selected References

Kim SS. Revision surgery for failed back surgery syndrome. Spine 1992; 17: 957–960

Markwalder TM. Failed back surgery syndrome. Part I: Analysis of the clinical presentation and results of testing procedures for instability of the lumbar spine in 171 patients. Acta Neurochir (Wien) 1993; 123: 46–51

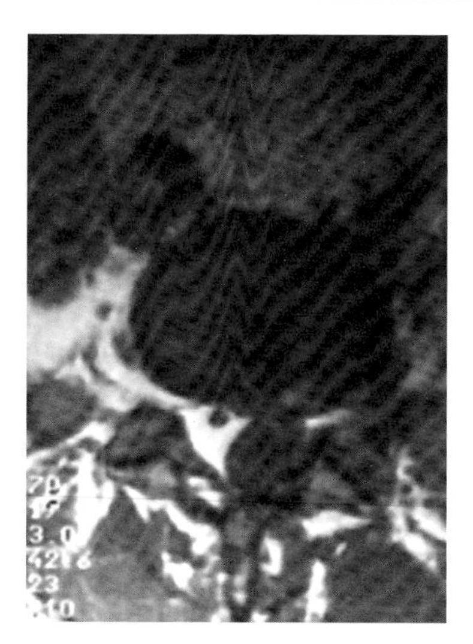

Fig. 7.1 MR image of L2 (axial, T1). Post-disk surgery. There is a left lateral round hypointense mass indenting the dural sac.

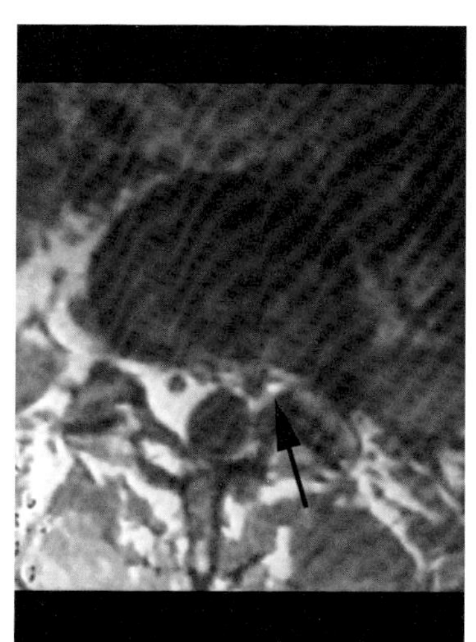

Fig. 7.2 MR image of L2 (axial, T1 with contrast). Significant enhancement of the hypointense area, representing scar tissue with reactive thickening of the nerve root (same patient as in Fig. 7.**1**).

Definition

- **Epidemiology**
  Peak age 20–40 years • Twice as common in men than in women.
- **Etiology, pathophysiology, pathogenesis**
  Spontaneous, secondary to intervention (lumbar puncture, postsurgical), post-traumatic • Loss of intradural CSF volume and pressure • Marfan syndrome (dural defect).

Imaging Signs

- **Modality of choice**
  MRI:
  - Sagittal.
  - Axial.
- **General**
  Thickened dura • Enlarged epidural venous plexus • Extradural accumulation of CSF.
- **CT findings**
  Enlarged venous plexus (hypodense tubular epidural structures) • Arachnoid diverticulum.
- **MRI findings**
  Enlarged venous plexus (signal void) • Extradural fluid accumulation isointense to CSF • Fistula • MR myelography (arachnoid diverticulum) • *Skull MRI:* Signs of cerebral hypotension (thickened, enhancing dura mater; subdural hygromas; caudal displacement of the brainstem).
- **Nuclear medicine**
  Cisternography (sensitivity 60%).

Clinical Aspects

- **Typical presentation**
  Severe occipital headache resistant to therapy • Cranial neuropathy (abducens nerve, optic nerve) • Impaired consciousness • Coma (rare).
- **Therapeutic options**
  Spontaneous remission is common, > 75% of cases • Fluid substitution • Surgical management of the CSF fistula.

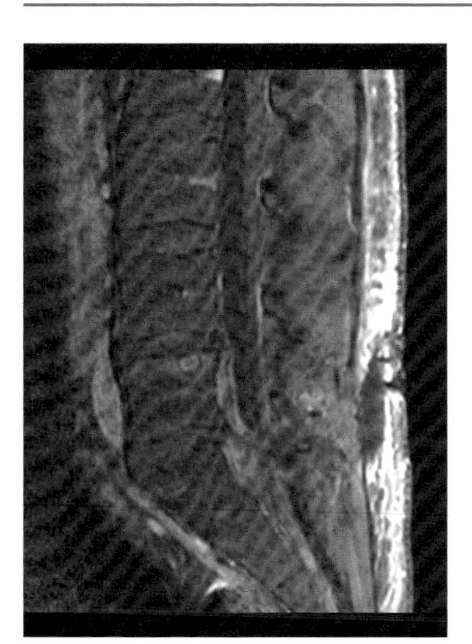

Fig. 7.3 MR image of the lumbar spine (sagittal, T1). Postoperative extradural defect isointense to CSF at L5–S1.

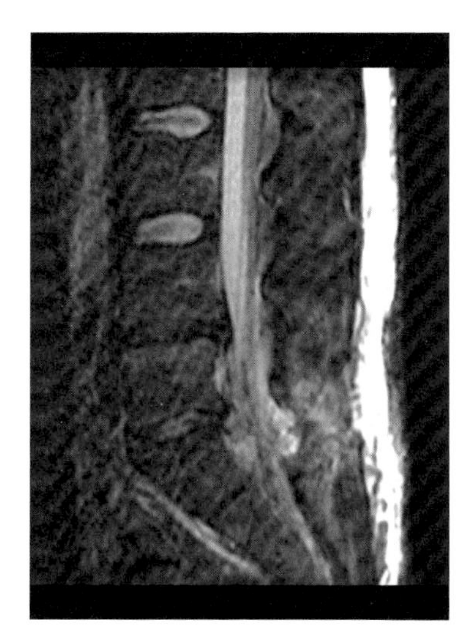

Fig. 7.4 MR image of the lumbar spine (sagittal, T2). Hyperintensity at the surgical site (extradural region). Degenerative disk disease at L5–S1. Posterior disk herniation at L4–L5.

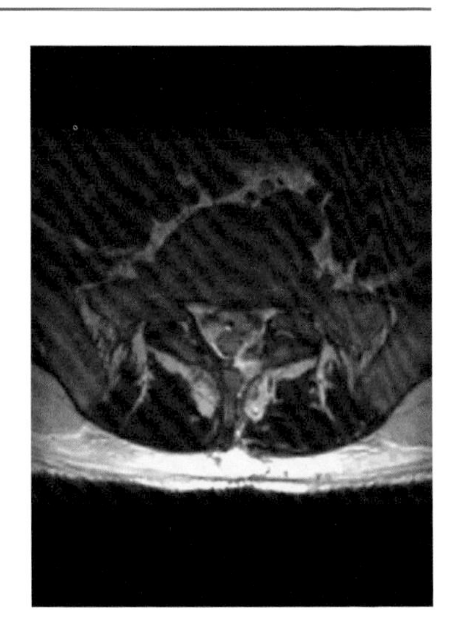

Fig. 7.5 Pain after disk surgery. MR image of L5–S1 (axial, T2). Signal alteration isointense to CSF along the surgical site communicating with the dural sac: a CSF fistula.

Differential Diagnosis

Enlarged venous plexus	– Thrombosis – AVM – Spinal stenosis
Pachymeningitis	– Thickened enhancing meninges – Idiopathic or infectious

Selected References

Black P. Cerebrospinal fluid leaks following spinal surgery: use of fat grafts for prevention and repair. Technical note. J Neurosurg Spine 2002; 96: 250–252

Eismont FJ. Treatment of dural tears associated with spinal surgery. J Bone Joint Surg Am 1981; 63: 1132–1136

Definition

Postoperative scar tissue, which can cause spinal stenosis and/or stenosis of the neural foramina (in approximately 7% of cases) • Physiologic repair mechanism secondary to surgical intervention • The extent of scarring depends on the extent of the surgical intervention and the patient's immune and inflammatory response.

Imaging Signs

- **Modality of choice**
  MRI:
  - Sagittal.
  - Axial.
- **General**
  Enhancing structures that infiltrate the perineural fatty tissue (note that these may have a mass effect).
- **CT findings**
  Enhancing perineural soft tissue structures.
- **MRI findings**
  Perineural soft tissue infiltration • Mass effect is occasionally present (DD: Tumor) • Isointense to soft tissue on T1-weighted images, uncharacteristic findings on T2-weighted images • Enhancement after contrast administration (STIR).

Clinical Aspects

- **Typical presentation**
  Paresthesias • Motor deficit (rare) • Radiculopathy.
- **Therapeutic options**
  Surgical management (lysis of adhesion) • Selective cortisone treatment.

Differential Diagnosis

Tumor – Lymphoma

Disk prolapse

Selected References

Petrie JL. Use of ADCON-L to inhibit postoperative peridural fibrosis and related symptoms following lumbar disc surgery: a preliminary report. Eur Spine J 1996; 5 (Suppl 1): S10–17

Vogelsang JP: Recurrent pain after lumbar discectomy: the diagnostic value of peridural scar on MRI. Eur Spine J 1999; 8: 475–479

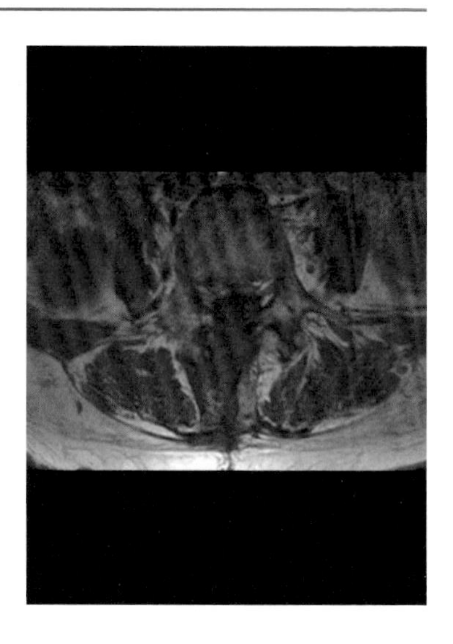

Fig. 7.6 Post right laminectomy. MR image of L3 (axial, T1). Excessive fibrotic scarring (hypointense) leading to spinal stenosis.

Definition

Rapid progressive degeneration of the segments adjacent to the fusion sites • The altered biomechanics in these adjacent segments lead to excessive stresses and segmental overloading • The mechanical overloading causes hypermobility of the segments adjacent to the fusion sites.

Imaging Signs

- **Modality of choice**
  MRI:
  - Sagittal: T1, T2.
  - Axial: T1.
- **General**
  Degenerative disk disease and osteoarthritis of the facet joints, costovertebral joints, and costotransverse joints.
- **Radiographic findings**
  Chondropathy (loss of height in the disk interspaces, disk calcification) • Degenerative disk disease and facet joint osteoarthritis (marginal irregularities, subchondral sclerosis, irregular articular surfaces) • Spondylosis deformans (marginal osteophytes; watch out for stenosis of the neural foramina and spinal canal).
- **MRI and CT findings**
  Dehydration and/or loss of height in the disk interspaces • Modic I–III (MRI) bone marrow changes • Facet joint osteoarthritis (joint effusion, marginal osteophytes, thickening of the ligamenta flava) • Degenerative disk disease and facet joint osteoarthritis (marginal irregularities, subchondral sclerosis, irregular articular surfaces) • Spondylosis deformans (marginal osteophytes; watch out for stenosis of the neural foramina and spinal canal).

Clinical Aspects

- **Typical presentation**
  Rapidly progressive segmental pain • Segmental neuropathy.
- **Therapeutic options**
  Physical therapy (muscle strengthening exercises, proprioceptive training) • osteoporosis therapy.

Differential Diagnosis

Functional segmental fusion (not postoperative condition) with secondary degeneration

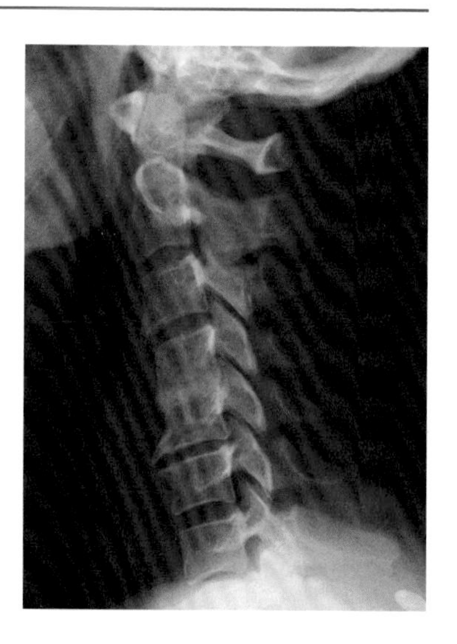

Fig. 7.7 Conventional lateral radiograph of the cervical spine. Spine is extended. Surgical fusion of C4–C5. Degenerative disk disease at C5–C6.

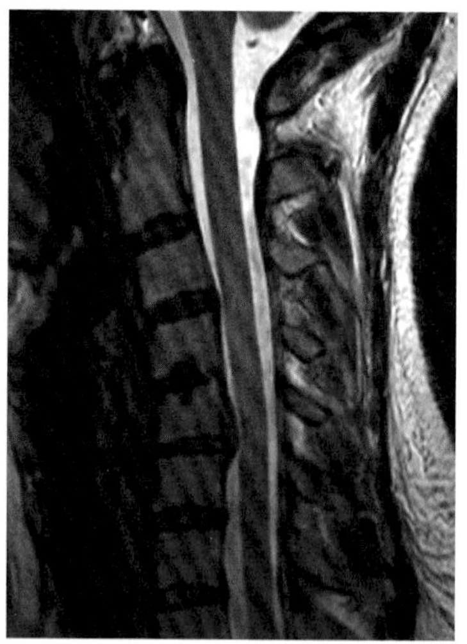

Fig. 7.8 MR image of the cervical spine (sagittal, T2). Marked degenerative disk disease in the adjacent segments after fusion at level C4–C5.

Selected References

Chen WJ. Surgical treatment of adjacent instability after lumbar spine fusion. Spine 2001; 26: E519–524

Eck JC. Adjacent-segment degeneration after lumbar fusion: a review of clinical, biomechanical, and radiologic studies. Am J Orthop 1999; 28: 336–340

Ghiselli G. Adjacent segment degeneration in the lumbar spine. J Bone Joint Surg Am 2004; 86-A: 1497–1503

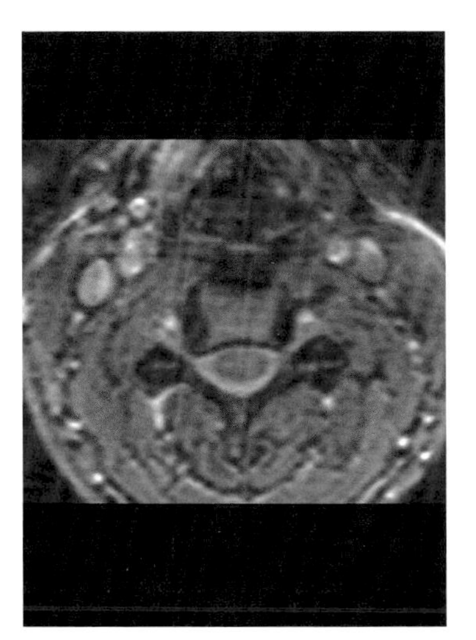

Fig. 7.9 MR image of C4–C5 (axial, T2). Significant posterolateral osteophytes and hypertrophic facet joint osteoarthritis with bony narrowing of the neural foramina.

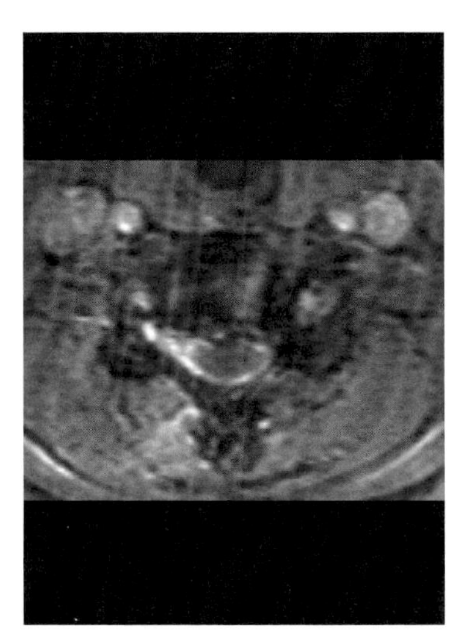

Fig. 7.10 MR image of C4–C5 (axial, T2). Marked progression of the degenerative changes in the same segment as in Fig. 7.**9** 14 months later.

Definition

Segmental stabilization with implants in fractures or spondylolisthesis (pedicle screws, wire cerclage, plate fixation, Harrington rods) and prosthetic disks • The aim is to eliminate diskogenic pain by restricting mobility • *Complications:* Loosening, implant fracture, displacement, accelerated degeneration of adjacent segments • Infection and skin problems • Nonunion or delayed union in patients with osteoporosis, diabetes mellitus, or infections, and in smokers and patients on steroids • Segmental overloading, abnormal stresses (trauma).

Imaging Signs

- **Modality of choice**
  Conventional radiographs.
  CT (MRI for neural structures) • MRI shows artifacts.
- **General**
  Comparison with previous images is helpful in evaluating conventional radiographs (screening studies) • Multidetector CT allows multiplanar reconstruction with significantly reduced artifacts).
- **Radiographic findings**
  Implant fracture, displacement (comparison with previous images is helpful) • Loosening (radiolucent halo, stress views).
- **CT findings**
  Allows evaluation of bony structures and the bone–implant interface in particular (signs of loosening) • Complex and multisegmental stabilization procedures are well visualized • Multidetector CT reduces metal artifacts; multiplanar reconstruction without step artifacts.
- **MRI findings**
  Neural structures (compression) • Soft tissue changes (inflammation) • Spin echo sequences reduce the susceptibility artifacts associated with metal.
- **Nuclear medicine**
  Hot spot (implant loosening, inflammation, pseudarthrosis).

Clinical Aspects

- **Typical presentation**
  Usually asymptomatic • Segmental pain with motion (pseudarthrosis) • Neuralgia.

Differential Diagnosis

Inflammatory changes	– Ill-defined osteolytic areas

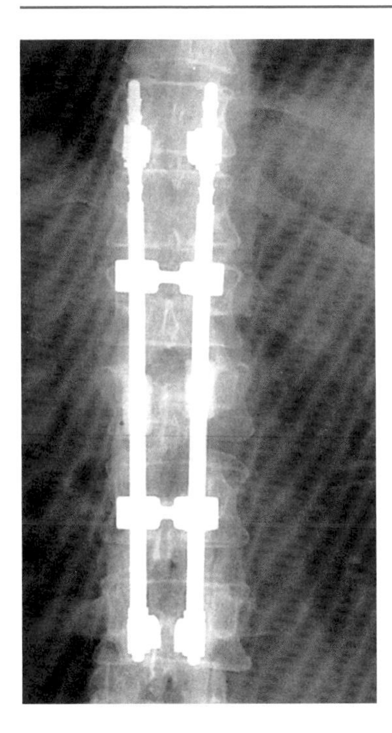

Fig. 7.11 Conventional A-P radiograph of the thoracolumbar spine. Harrington rod in situ after reduction of L1 fracture. Normal findings.

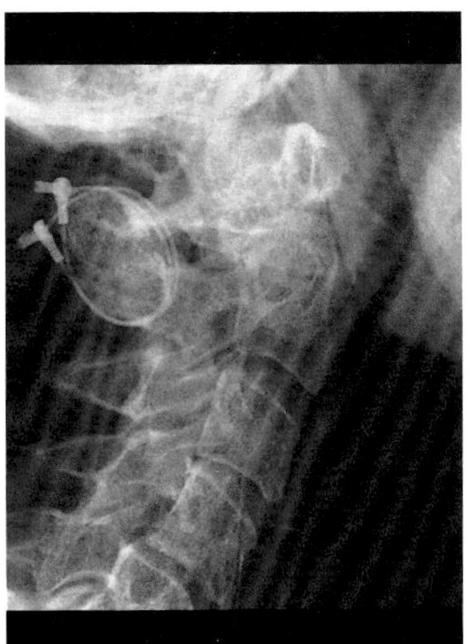

Fig. 7.12 Conventional lateral radiograph of the upper cervical spine. Posterior cerclage wire encircling the spinous processes and bone graft. Normal findings.

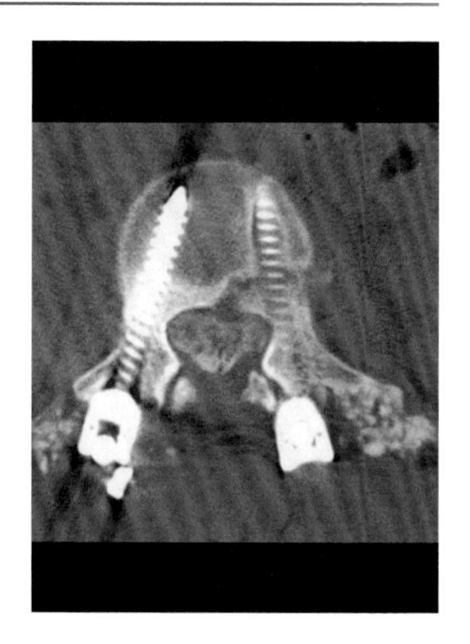

Fig. 7.13 CT (axial). Traumatic avulsion of the left pedicle, treated by open reduction and internal fixation with pedicle screws. The spinal canal is slightly widened. Both screws lie within the cancellous bone. The right screw is surrounded by a widened space with a sclerotic rim indicative of chronic implant loosening.

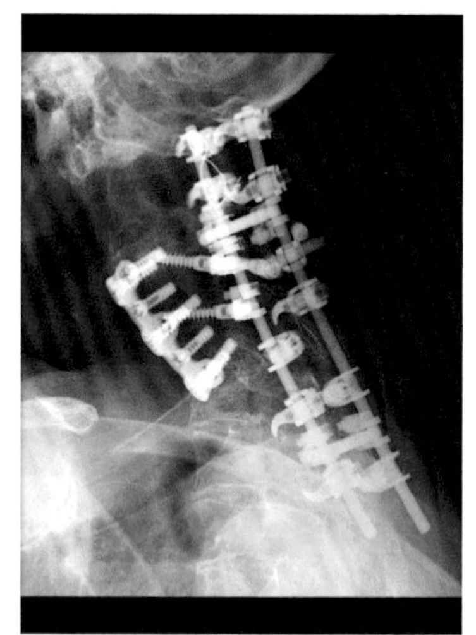

Fig. 7.14 Conventional lateral radiograph of the cervical spine. Multisegmental posterior and anterior stabilization of the cervical spine.

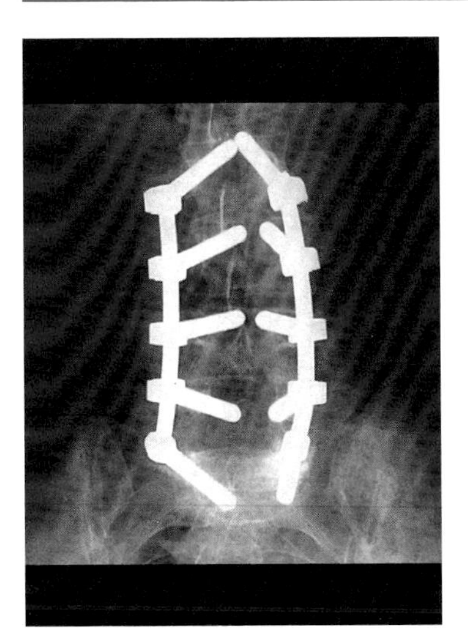

Fig. 7.15 Conventional A-P radiograph of the lumbar spine. Typical position of pedicle screws in lumbosacral fusion.

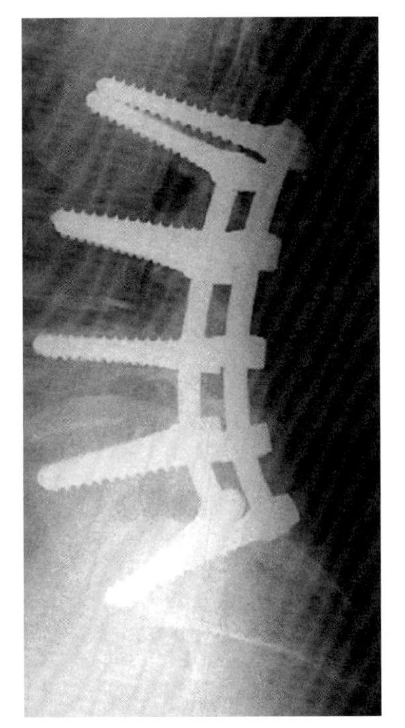

Fig. 7.16 Conventional lateral radiograph of the lumbar spine. The pedicle screws typically lie within the cancellous bone close to the endplates.

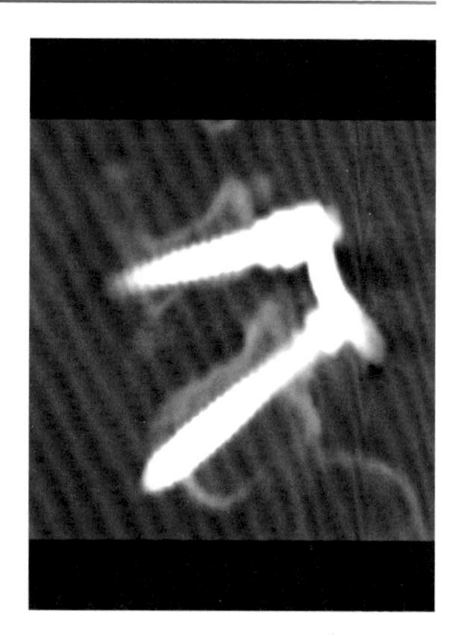

Fig. 7.17 CT of the lumbar spine (lateral multidetector CT). Multiplanar reconstruction with minimal artifacts allowing excellent evaluation of implants in situ. Osteoporotic L4 vertebra with compression fracture. Pedicle screws are too long and extend beyond the anterior margin of the vertebral body.

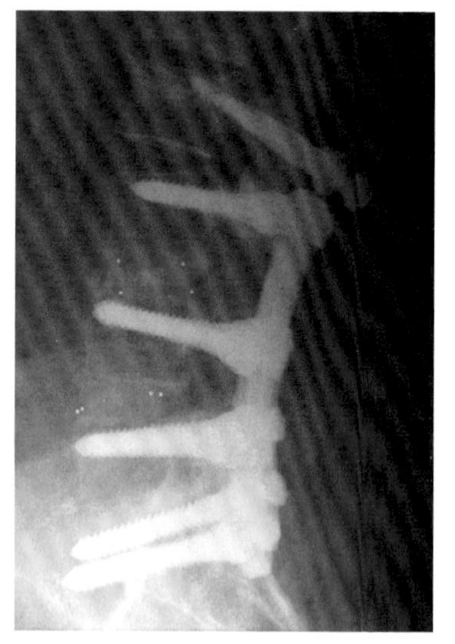

Fig. 7.18 Conventional lateral radiograph of the lumbar spine. Posterior lumbar interbody fusion (PLIF). The superior screw has fractured. This is one of the most common complications of posterior instrumentation.

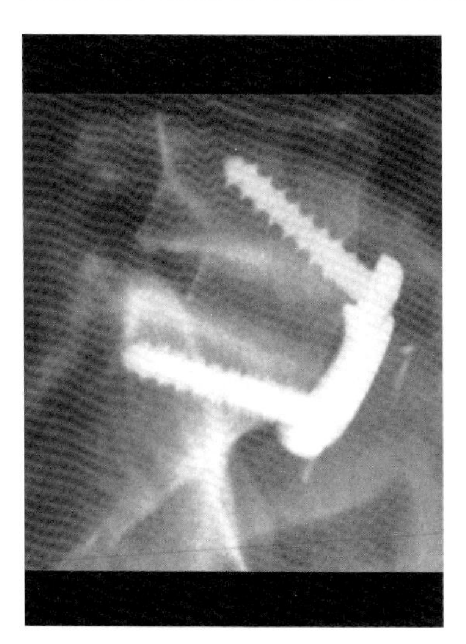

Fig. 7.19 Conventional lateral radiograph of the lumbar spine (detail). Anterior lumbar interbody fusion (ALIF) in disk degeneration. Normal postoperative findings, with the upper screw in an atypical position.

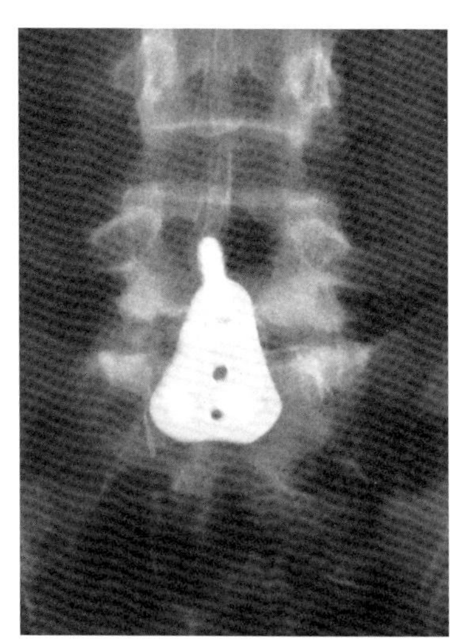

Fig. 7.20 Conventional A-P radiograph of the lumbar spine (detail). ALIF: usual postoperative findings.

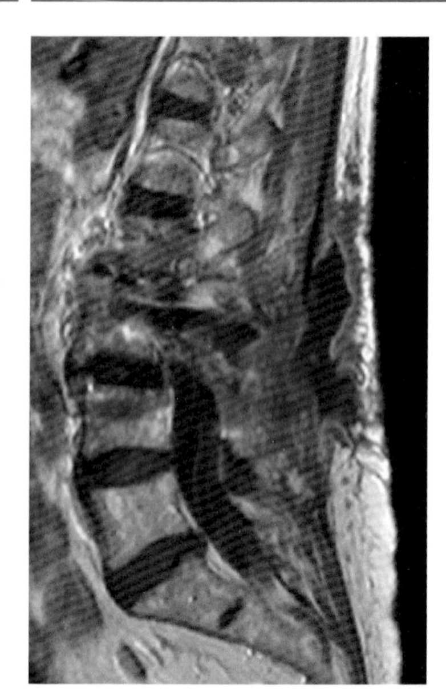

Fig. 7.21 MR image of the lumbar spine (sagittal, T1 with contrast). Abscess secondary to infection following posterior stabilization of L3.

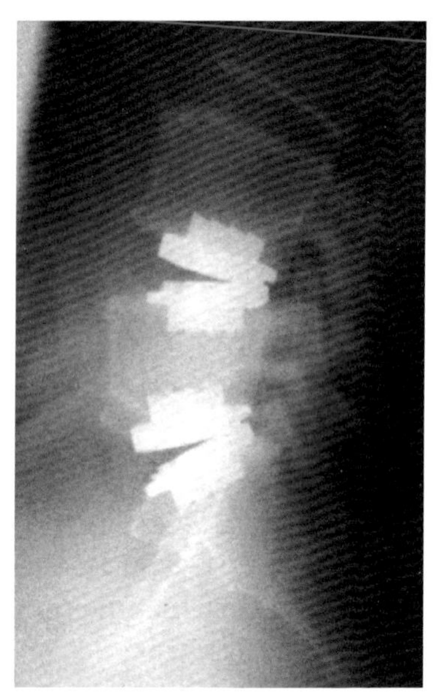

Fig. 7.22 Conventional lateral radiograph. Titanium endplates with prosthetic disks. Cementless implantation. Mobility is maintained, and the patient is free of pain.

Selected References

Lowery GL. The significance of hardware failure in anterior cervical plate fixation. Patients with 2- to 7-year follow-up. Spine 1998; 23: 181–186; discussion 186–187

Slone RM. Spinal fixation. Part 3. Complications of spinal instrumentation. Radiographics 1993; 13: 797–816

Definition

- **Epidemiology**
More common in females than in males (4:1) • Affects 12% of the population • 64% of postmenopausal women have vertebral fractures.
- **Etiology, pathophysiology, pathogenesis**
Metabolic disease with thinning of the trabecular structure and cortex, and reduced bone mass and density • This leads to microscopic and macroscopic insufficiency fractures, fractures as a result of trauma that does not usually cause bony injury • The disorder primarily affects the axial skeleton • Predilection for the thoracic spine • Typical findings include flattened and biconcave "fish" vertebrae • Age-related (senile form), estrogen deficiency, acromegaly, Cushing syndrome, corticosteroids, heparin, calcium phosphate deficiency, alcoholism.

Imaging Signs

- **Modality of choice**
Early diagnosis: Bone density measurement with DEXA
  - T-score: –1 to –2.5 = osteopenia.
  - T-score: < –2.5 = Osteoporosis and fractures.
  - T-score: < –2.5 and fractures = manifest osteoporosis.

  Conventional radiographs:
  - Demonstration of a fracture is diagnostic.

  CT:
  - Reduced bone density is better visualized.

  MRI:
  - In uncertain cases (possible metastases).
- **Radiographic findings**
There is loss of bone mass (> 40%) with greatly increased radiolucency • Thinning of the cancellous bone (loss of secondary trabeculae), cortical thinning • Impression fractures of the endplates (vertebral deformity) • Microscopic and macroscopic fractures (insufficiency fractures) • Compression fractures with or without displacement, spinal stenosis, and biconcave "fish" vertebrae • Kyphosis.
- **CT findings**
Extent of fracture displacement • Q-CT allows quantitative bone density measurement.
- **MRI findings**
Differentiating osteoporotic from metastatic vertebral collapse.
Acute vertebral collapse:
  - Deformation.
  - Diffuse bone marrow edema.
  - Fluid sign.

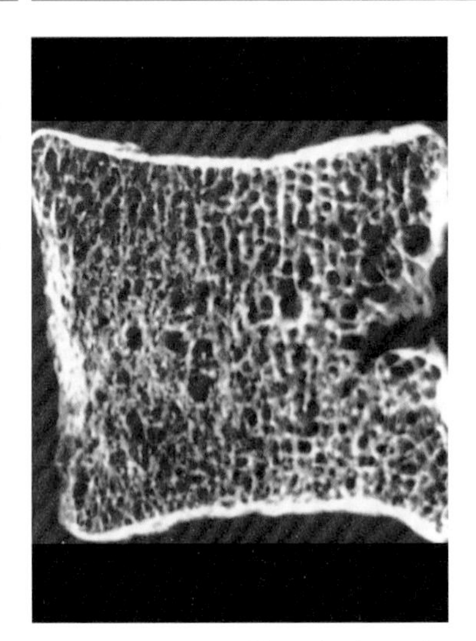

Fig. 8.1 Conventional lateral radiograph of a vertebral specimen showing normal bone structure.

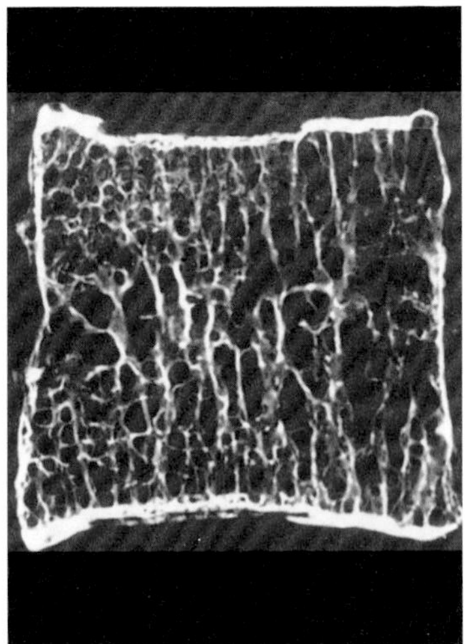

Fig. 8.2 Conventional lateral radiograph of a vertebral specimen showing osteoporotic bone structure (thinning of the cancellous bone with loss of secondary trabeculae emphasizes the longitudinal trabeculae).

Fig. 8.3 Conventional lateral radiograph of the lumbar spine (detail). Vertebral compression fracture with posterior displacement and spinal stenosis.

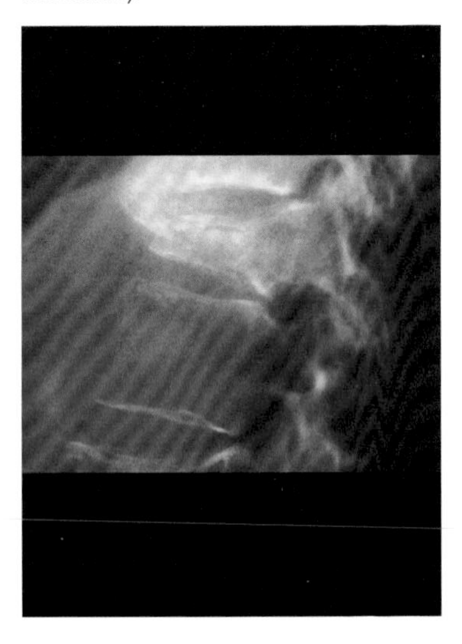

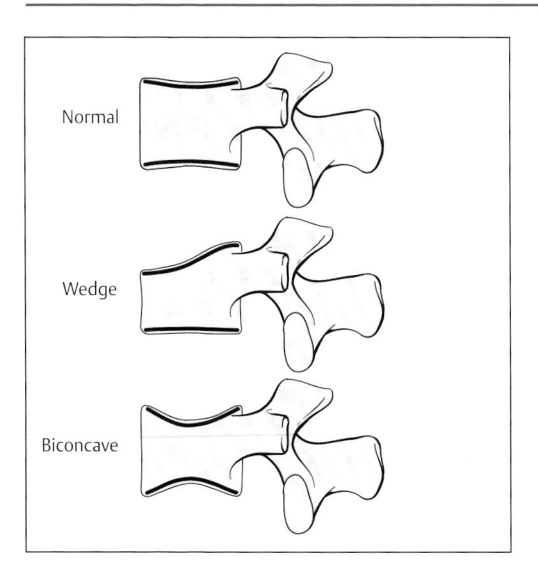

Fig. 8.4 Types of vertebral compression.

Chronic vertebral collapse:
- Osteoporotic: fatty marrow conversion.
- Metastatic: Hyperintense on T2-weighted images, hypointense on T1-weighted images, enhancing.

Diffusion-weighted sequence:
- Increased diffusion coefficient.

Clinical Aspects

▸ **Typical presentation**
Pain • Increasing kyphosis • Neurologic deficits including paraplegia • Increased urinary excretion of hydroxyproline.

▸ **Therapeutic options**
Regular exercise and load bearing (gymnastics etc.) • High mineral and vitamin diet • Bisphosphonate, calcitonin • Osteoprotegerin therapy may be an option in the future • Surgical options include vertebroplasty and correction of kyphosis • *Caution:* Rapid progressive osteoarthritis and/or additional fractures after kyphoplasty or vertebroplasty.

Differential Diagnosis

Hyperparathyroidism	– Clinical findings – Subperiosteal bone resorption and erosion – Schmorl nodes – Fingers affected most severely
Renal osteodystrophy	– Combination of hyperparathyroidism, sclerosis, and osteomalacia – "Rugger jersey" or "rugby shirt" spine (horizontal banding)

Selected References

Damilakis J et al. An update on the assessment of osteoporosis using radiologic techniques. Eur Radiol Nov 28, 2006 [Epub ahead of print]
Grampp S. Radiology of Osteoporosis. Berlin: Springer 2003

Definition

- **Epidemiology**
  Affects 3–4% of adults over 40 years • More common in men than in women (3:2).
- **Etiology, pathophysiology, pathogenesis**
  Synonym: Osteitis deformans • Chronic metabolic disorder (bone remodeling disorder) • Possible viral etiology • Increased familial incidence • More common in the Anglo-Saxon population • Spinal involvement occurs in 30–75% of cases (in order of decreasing frequency: pelvis and spine, femur, and skull • Monostotic or polyostotic • Predilection for lumbar spine • *Three phases:* Lytic or acute phase, mixed phase, and "burned out" or sclerotic phase.

Imaging Signs

- **Modality of choice**
  Conventional radiographs.
  MRI: Only indicated with neurologic symptoms or suspected sarcomatous degeneration (< 1% osteosarcoma and malignant fibrous histiocytoma) • Detects soft tissue tumor, necrosis, and metastases.
- **General**
  Enlarged vertebra with coarse, irregular trabecular structure • Occasionally "ivory" vertebra.
- **Radiographic findings**
  Enlarged vertebra with abnormally coarse structure (early forms include osteoporosis and lysis) • Sclerosis, which may include an "ivory" vertebra • Secondary degenerative changes in the vertebra • Strictly segmental involvement.
- **CT findings**
  Active (lytic) phase with enhancement after contrast administration.
- **MRI findings**
  T1
  - Hypointense irregularity.

  T2:
  - Active lesions (lytic fibrovascular areas) appear hyperintense.
  - In the "burned out" phase, sclerotic and fibrotic lesions appear hypointense. There may also be fatty marrow conversion.

  T1 with contrast:
  - Active phase shows marked enhancement after contrast administration. Intensity of enhancement correlates with disease activity.
- **Nuclear medicine**
  Markedly increased uptake in the lytic (acute) and mixed phases • Uptake correlates with disease activity.

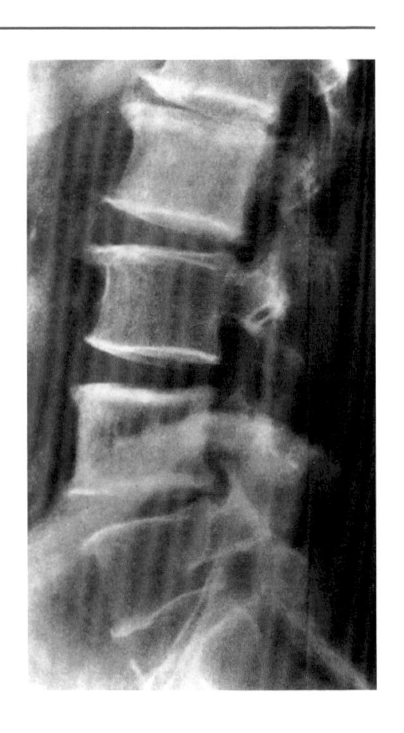

Fig. 8.5 Conventional lateral radiograph of the lumbar spine. L2 is significantly denser and slightly enlarged. It has a coarse trabecular structure.

Clinical Aspects

- **Typical presentation**
  Dull bone pain • Often asymptomatic • Rarely there are associated neurologic symptoms (radiculopathy).
- **Therapeutic options**
  Bisphosphonates and calcitonin.
- **Course and prognosis**
  Prognosis is poor with sarcomatous degeneration, otherwise excellent.

Differential Diagnosis

Vertebra with hemangioma	– Usually no increase in volume
"Ivory" vertebra in lymphoma	– No stranded or striped pattern

Selected References

Freyschmidt J. Skeletterkrankungen. Berlin: Springer 1997

Mirra JM et al. Paget's disease of bone: review with emphasis on radiologic features. Skeletal Radiology 1995; 24: 163–184

Sundaram M. Imaging of Paget's disease and fibrous dysplasia of bone. J Bone Miner Res 2006; 21(Suppl 2): 28–30

Definition

Proliferation of epidural fatty tissue, usually affecting several segments • Causes include obesity, chronic cortisone therapy (steroid abuse), Cushing syndrome, and idiopathic occurrence • Predilection for posterior thoracic spine and anterolateral lumbar spine.

Imaging Signs

- **Modality of choice**
  MRI
  - Sagittal: T1, T2.
  - Transverse: T1, T2.
- **CT findings**
  Proliferation of fatty tissue in the spinal canal with displacement and posterior or occasionally anterior compression of the dural sac.
- **MRI findings**
  Proliferation of structures isointense to fat in the epidural space with deformation of the dural sac and/or spinal cord ("Y" shape) • The nerve roots in the foramina are completely surrounded by extradural fat.
  - T1: Hypointense CSF is replaced by hyperintense fatty tissue.
  - T2: Missing (bright) CSF signal in the compressed dural sac, increased signal in the spinal cord with compressive myelopathy.

Clinical Aspects

- **Typical presentation**
  Radicular pain • Unilateral or bilateral paresthesias • Spinal claudication with spinal stenosis • Cauda equina syndrome.
- **Therapeutic options**
  Weight loss • Reduction or cessation of steroid therapy • Progressive neurologic symptoms are treated by surgical decompression with laminectomy.

Differential Diagnosis

Primary and secondary spinal tumors	– Inhomogeneous enhancement
Epidural abscess	– Associated bony changes – Thickened meninges – Elevated inflammatory markers
Spinal canal lipoma	– Intradural – At least partially encapsulated

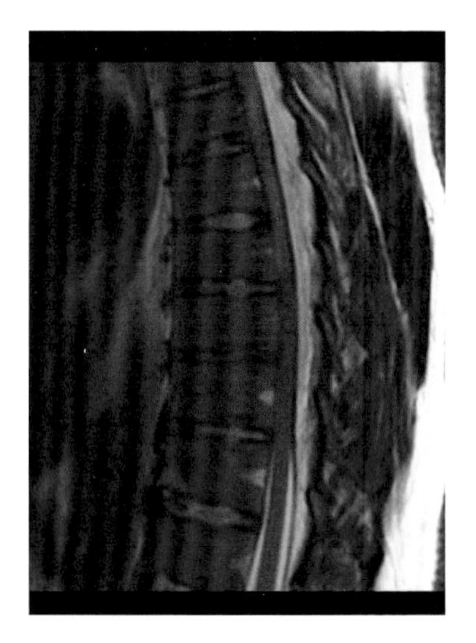

Fig. 8.6 Body builder (chronic steroid user) complaining of increasing weakness in the lower extremities. MR image of the thoracolumbar spine (sagittal, T1) shows a thick layer of epidural fatty tissue.

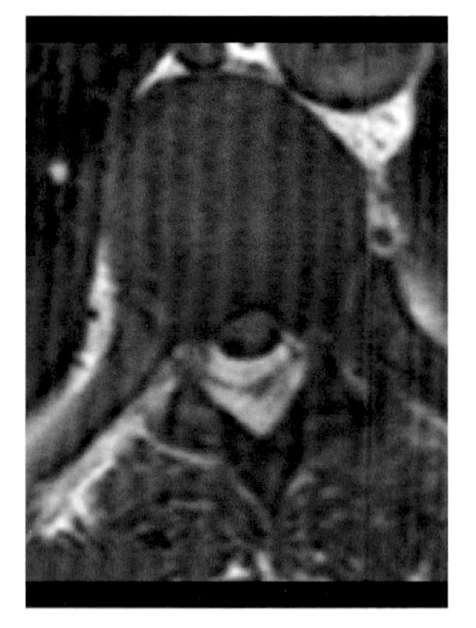

Fig. 8.7 MR image of T12 (axial, T1). Excessive epidural fat narrows the spinal canal.

Selected References

Gero BT et al. Symptomatic spinal epidural lipomatosis without exogenous steroid intake. Neuroradiology 1989; 31: 190–192

Hierholzer J et al. Epidural lipomatosis: case report and literature review. Neuroradiology 1996; 38: 343–348

Robertson SC et al. Idiopathic spinal epidural lipomatosis. Neurosurgery 1997; 41: 68–74

A

abscess
  epidural, *see* epidural abscess
  vs. epidural hematoma 261
  paravertebral 164
  psoas 171
acquired hydromyelia, vs. Arnold–Chiari malformation 3
acute transverse myelitis 182–185
  vs. spinal multiple sclerosis 189
Anderson and d'Alonzo classification, dens fractures 48
aneurysmal bone cyst 204–207
  vs. giant cell tumor 211
  vs. osteoblastoma 200
  vs. osteoid osteoma 197
ankylosing spondylitis 147–151
  vs. diffuse idiopathic skeletal hyperostosis 132
  fractures 154–157
  vs. Klippel–Feil syndrome 28
  and kyphosis 30
  ligament calcification and bamboo spine 152, 153
  vs. psoriatic spondyloarthropathy 143
  vs. Reiter syndrome 146
  vs. Scheuermann disease 35
  stress fractures 83–86
annulus fibrosus 87
  defined 100
anterior lumbar interbody fusion (ALIF) 285
anterior subluxation 73–75
arachnoiditis 178–181
  vs. granulomatous inflammation 177
Arnold–Chiari malformation 1–3
arterial spinal cord infarction 266–269
arteriovenous malformation 262–265
arthritis
  juvenile rheumatoid, vs. Klippel–Feil syndrome 28
  rheumatoid 133–137
    and chronic trauma 138–140
astrocytoma 252–255
  vs. acute transverse myelitis 185
  vs. ependymoma 251
  vs. hemangioblastoma 258
  vs. spinal multiple sclerosis 189
asymmetry, facet joint, vs. malrotation 42
atlantodental subluxation, rheumatoid arthritis 134, 135
atlas, fracture classification 60, 61

B

Baastrup disease 121, 122
bacterial spondylitis
  acute 158–165
  frequency distribution 167
  vs. tuberculous spondylitis 169
bamboo spine 152, 153
Bechterew disease 147
bone marrow inhomogeneity, vs. bone metastasis 221
bone metastases 216–221
breast carcinoma, metastasis 217
Brodie's abscess, vs. osteoid osteoma 197
bronchial carcinoma, metastasis 219
Brown–Séquard syndrome 254
bulge/bulging, disk 100, 101, 103–107
  defined 100
burst fracture 44, 54–57
  vs. Chance fracture 59
  with fissure fracture 54
butterfly vertebra 21

C

calcium pyrophosphate disease, vs. Baastrup disease 122
cartilaginous nodules, vs. Scheuermann disease 35
cavernous malformation, intramedullary, vs. arteriovenous malformation 265
cerclage wire 281
cerebellar tonsils, descent, vs. Arnold–Chiari malformation 3
cerebrospinal fluid (CSF) fistula 272–274
cervical spine
  fat C2 sign 63
  flexion fracture 51–53
  rheumatoid arthritis 134
  trauma, offset sign 61
Chance fracture 58, 59
chondrosarcoma
  vs. chordoma 228
  vs. osteochondroma 203
chorda remnant, vs. disk degeneration 89
chordoma 226–228

classification
  anterior subluxation 73
  spinal cord trauma 66
cleavage fracture 44
cleft vertebrae 21
Codman triangle 229
colon carcinoma, metastasis 218
compression fracture
  vs. Chance fracture 59
  osteoporotic 46, 288
  vs. Scheuermann disease 35
concussion, spinal 66
congenital malformations 1–42
  vertebral, vs. uncovertebral
    osteoarthritis 116
contusion, spinal 66
cord, tethered 9
Currarino triad 13
curtain sign 259
Cushing syndrome 293
cyst
  root canal, vs. synovial cyst 119
  synovial 118, 119

D

degenerative changes, spine,
  vs. rheumatoid arthritis 137
degenerative disk disease 87–89
  and gas release 108
  Modic I 90–92, 98
  Modic II 93–95, 98, 127
  Modic III (spondylosis deformans)
    96–99
  subchondral changes 98
degenerative spinal stenosis
  126–130
Denis classification 43, 58
dens
  destruction, in rheumatoid
    arthritis 135, 136
  fracture 48–50
  rheumatoid arthritis 134
Devic disease 189
diastematomyelia 6–8
diffuse idiopathic skeletal hyperostosis
  (DISH) 132, 143
  vs. ankylosing spondylitis 151
  vs. spondylosis deformans 99
disk bulge, vs. disk herniation
  102
disk calcification 108–110
disk degeneration, *see* degenerative
  disk disease
disk herniation 100–102, 104
  vs. Baastrup disease 122
  definition, American Society
    of Neuroradiology 100
  vs. epidural abscess 174
  vs. meningioma 247
  vs. synovial cyst 119
diskitis
  vs. disk herniation 102
  vs. Klippel–Feil syndrome 28
disk narrowing 160, 161, 168
dislocation, cervical spine 51
disseminated encephalomyelitis,
  vs. acute transverse myelitis 185
distraction injury,
  vs. Chance fracture 59
double railroad track sign 152
drop metastases 240
  vs. tethering 12
dural sac, empty 178, 180
dysraphism, spinal 16
  vs. meningocele 20

E

Edgren–Vaino sign 33
Effendi classification,
  hangman's fracture 63
eggshell appearance 204
Ehlers–Danlos syndrome,
  vs. scoliosis 39
empty thecal sac 178, 180
encephalomyelitis, disseminated,
  vs. acute transverse myelitis 185
eosinophilic granuloma,
  vs. Ewing sarcoma 231
ependymoma 248–251
  vs. astrocytoma 255
  vs. hemangioblastoma 258
  vs. nerve sheath tumor 239
  vs. spinal multiple sclerosis 189
epidural abscess 172–174
  vs. bacterial spondylitis 160
  vs. spinal epidural lipomatosis 293
  vs. tuberculous spondylitis 169
epidural fibrosis, vs. disk bulge 107
epidural hematoma,
  vs. epidural abscess 174

Ewing sarcoma 229–231
  vs. Langerhans cell histiocytosis 214
exostosis 201, 202
extrusion, disk 103

F

facetectomy, partial,
  vs. spondylolisthesis 82, 125
facet joints
  ankylosis 153
  asymmetry, vs. malrotation 42
  degeneration 111–115
  dislocation 73
  osteoarthritis 111
failed back surgery syndrome
  270, 271
fat C2 sign 63
fibrosis
  epidural, vs. disk bulge 107
  peridural 275, 276
fibrous histiocytoma, malignant,
  vs. chordoma 228
filum terminale ependymoma 251
  vs. nerve sheath tumor 239
flexion fracture, cervical spine 51–53
Foix–Alajouanine syndrome, vs. arterial
  spinal cord infarction 269
foraminal stenosis 114
Forestier disease 131
  vs. ankylosing spondylitis 151
  vs. psoriatic spondyloarthropathy 143
  see also diffuse idiopathic skeletal
    hyperostosis
fractures
  ankylosing spondylitis 154–157
  causes 45–47
  classification 43, 44
  vs. facet joint degeneration 115
  insufficiency 138
    sacrum 76–78
  vs. osteoid osteoma 197
  stress, in ankylosing
    spondylitis 83–86
  vertebral
    vs. Modic I degenerative disk
      disease 92
    vs. Modic II degenerative disk
      disease 93
fungal infection, vs. tuberculous
  spondylitis 169
fusion
  physiologic, vs. dens fracture 50
  spinal, surgical 28
  vertebral, acquired 25

G

ganglioglioma, vs. astrocytoma 255
gas release, in disk degeneration 108
giant cell tumor 208–211
  vs. aneurysmal bone cyst 207
  vs. chordoma 228
  vs. Langerhans cell histiocytosis 214
gibbus 30, 31, 34
granulomatous infections,
  spinal cord 175–177
Guillain–Barré syndrome
  vs. arterial spinal cord infarction 269
  vs. epidural abscess 174

H

hangman's fracture 63–65
Harrington rod 280, 281
hemangioblastoma 256–258
  vs. arteriovenous
    malformation 265
  vs. ependymoma 251
hemangioma 190–194
  atypical, vs. Modic I degenerative disk
    disease 92
  vs. Modic II degenerative disk
    disease 93
  vs. multiple myeloma 225
  vs. Paget disease 292
hematoma, epidural 259–261
  vs. epidural abscess 174
hemivertebra, lateral 21
hemorrhage, spinal cord,
  vs. spinal cord trauma 68
herniation, defined 100
histiocytoma, vs. chordoma 228
histiocytosis, *see* Langerhans cell
  histiocytosis
Horner's syndrome 269
hydromyelia
  acquired, vs. Arnold–Chiari
    malformation 3
  vs. diastematomyelia 8
hydrops fetalis 15
hypernephroma, metastasis 218

hyperostosis
flowing 132
skeletal, diffuse idiopathic (DISH) 131–132
hyperparathyroidism, vs. osteoporosis 290

I

impaction fracture 44
infarction, spinal
vs. acute transverse myelitis 185
arterial 266–269
vs. spinal multiple sclerosis 189
infection
vs. Langerhans cell histiocytosis 214
vs. rheumatoid arthritis 137
inflammation
vs. facet joint degeneration 115
vs. osteoid osteoma 197
inflammatory disorders 133–189
instrumentation, complications 280–286
insufficiency fracture 138
sacrum 76–78
intradural tumor, vs. arachnoiditis 181
intramedullary tumor
vs. acute transverse myelitis 185
vs. granulomatous inflammation 177
ivory vertebral body 232, 233, 236, 291, 292

J

Jefferson fracture 60–62
juvenile rheumatoid arthritis 137
vs. Klippel–Feil syndrome 28

K

kissing spine 121, 122
Klippel–Feil syndrome 26–28
Knutsson sign 29, 33
kyphosis 29–32
osteoporotic 30, 32
vs. Scheuermann disease 35
tuberculous 35

L

Langerhans cell histiocytosis 212–214
vs. Ewing sarcoma 231
leptomeningeal metastases
vs. arachnoiditis 181
vs. ependymoma 251
vs. granulomatous inflammation 177
leptomeningitis 175
ligamenta flava, hypertrophy 120, 127
ligament calcifications 152, 153
vs. spondylosis deformans 99
ligament ossification, vs. ligamenta flava hypertrophy 120
lipoma, spinal canal, vs. spinal epidural lipomatosis 293
lipomatosis
spinal, vs. epidural hematoma 261
spinal epidural 293, 294
liposarcoma, vs. Modic II degenerative disk disease 93
lumbarization 4, 5
lumbar radiculopathy, vs. insufficiency fracture of sacrum 78
lymphoma 232–236
vs. bone metastasis 221
vs. chordoma 228
vs. Langerhans cell histiocytosis 214
vs. Paget disease 292

M

Magerl classification, spinal injury 43, 44
malformations
arteriovenous 262–265
congenital 1–42
vertebral 21–25
malrotation 40–42
Marfan syndrome, vs. scoliosis 39
meningioma 244–247
vs. nerve sheath tumor 239
meningocele 16–20
metabolic disorders 287–294
metastases
vs. aneurysmal bone cyst 207
vs. arachnoiditis 181
vs. astrocytoma 255
vs. bacterial spondylitis 160
breast carcinoma 217
bronchial carcinoma 219

vs. chordoma 228
colon carcinoma 218
drop 240
vs. tethering 12
vs. ependymoma 251
vs. epidural hematoma 261
vs. giant cell tumor 211
vs. granulomatous inflammation 177
vs. hemangioma 194
hypernephroma 218
vs. insufficiency fracture of sacrum 78
vs. Langerhans cell histiocytosis 214
leptomeningeal and intramedullary 240–243
vs. meningioma 247
vs. multiple myeloma 225
vs. osteoblastoma 200
osteogenic, vs. spondylolisthesis 82
vs. osteoid osteoma 197
prostate carcinoma 217
vs. tuberculous spondylitis 169
see also bone metastases
Meyerding classification, spondylolisthesis 79, 81, 123, 126
multiple sclerosis
vs. astrocytoma 255
vs. granulomatous inflammation 177
vs. metastasis 243
spinal 186–189
myelitis
acute transverse, vs. granulomatous inflammation 177
vs. arterial spinal cord infarction 269
myeloma, multiple 222–225
myelomeningocele 16–20
vs. kyphosis 29
vs. sacrococcygeal teratoma 15

N

necrosis, spinal cord, vs. arterial infarction 269
nerve sheath tumors 237–239
neurapraxia 66
neuroblastoma, vs. Ewing sarcoma 231
neurofibroma, vs. meningioma 247
neurofibromatosis, vs. scoliosis 39
neuromyelitis optica 189
notochord, persistent 21
vs. hemangioma 194
nucleus pulposus 87
defined 100

O

odontoid process, *see* dens
offset sign, cervical spine trauma 61
onion peel appearance 229
os odontoideum, vs. dens fracture 50
ossification, ligament, vs. ligamenta flava hypertrophy 120
ossified posterior longitudinal ligament, vs. spondylosis deformans 99
osteitis deformans 291
osteoarthritis
facet joints 111
rapidly progressive, after inter-segmental fusion 277–279
uncovertebral 116, 117
osteoblastoma 198–200
vs. aneurysmal bone cyst 207
vs. osteoid osteoma 197
osteochondroma 201–203
osteodystrophy, renal, vs. osteoporosis 290
osteogenesis imperfecta, vs. scoliosis 39
osteogenesis imperfecta tarda 35
osteoid osteoma 195–197
vs. osteoblastoma 200
osteolysis, in bacterial spondylitis 161
osteomyelitis
vs. Ewing sarcoma 231
vertebral body, vs. epidural abscess 174
osteoporosis
vs. bone metastasis 221
fractures, vs. metastatic fractures 46
and kyphosis 30, 32
vs. multiple myeloma 225
senile and postmenopausal 287–290
osteosarcoma
vs. Ewing sarcoma 231
parosteal, vs. osteochondroma 203

P

pachymeningitis, vs. CSF fistula 274
Paget disease 291, 292
pannus tissue, in rheumatoid arthritis 135, 136

parasyndesmophytes, vs. spondylosis deformans 99
paravertebral abscess 164
pedicle screws 280, 282–284
peridural fibrosis 275, 276
plasmacytoma 222
vs. bone metastasis 221
vs. chordoma 228
polyneuropathy, postinfectious, vs. epidural abscess 174
posterior lumbar interbody fusion (PLIF) 284
postmenopausal osteoporosis 287–290
postoperative disorders 270–286
prolapse
use of term 100
see also disk herniation
prostate carcinoma, metastasis 217
prosthetic disks 280, 286
protrusion, disk 103–107
see also bulge/bulging
pseudarthrosis
vs. dens fracture 50
and stress fractures 83–85
pseudospondylolisthesis 81, 82, 109, 123–125, 128
pseudosubluxation, vs. hangman's fracture 65
psoas abscess 171
psoriasis
vs. ankylosing spondylitis 151
vs. Reiter syndrome 146
psoriatic spondyloarthropathy 141–143

R

radiculopathy, lumbar, vs. insufficiency fracture of sacrum 78
railroad track sign 152
Reiter syndrome 144–146
vs. ankylosing spondylitis 151
renal osteodystrophy, vs. osteoporosis 290
rheumatoid arthritis 133–137
and chronic trauma 138–140
juvenile, vs. Klippel–Feil syndrome 28
vs. psoriatic spondyloarthropathy 143
vs. Reiter syndrome 146
subluxation, vs. dens fracture 50
root canal cyst, vs. synovial cyst 119
rotation, with scoliosis, vs. malrotation 42

S

sacralization 4, 5
sacrococcygeal teratoma 13–15
sacroiliitis 144
vs. insufficiency fracture of sacrum 78
sacrum, insufficiency fracture 76–78
saddle anesthesia 128, 179
salt and pepper pattern 191
sarcoidosis 175, 176
vs. arachnoiditis 181
vs. spinal multiple sclerosis 189
sarcoma, *see* Ewing sarcoma
scalloping, vertebral body 237
Scheuermann disease 33–35
and disk degeneration 87
vs. kyphosis 29
vs. scoliosis 39
Schmorl node 33, 87, 88, 110, 127
schwannoma
vs. disk bulge 107
vs. ependymoma 251
vs. meningioma 247
sclerosis, subchondral 109
sclerotic bone islands
vs. osteoblastoma 200
vs. osteoid osteoma 197
scoliosis 36–39
vs. Baastrup disease 122
classification 36
with rotation, vs. malrotation 42
seat belt fracture 58, 59
senile osteoporosis 287–290
sequestration, disk 103, 105
sequestrum, vs. osteoid osteoma 197
shear fracture 44
vs. Chance fracture 59
shock, spinal 66
skeletal hyperostosis, *see* diffuse idiopathic skeletal hyperostosis
spinal cord
granulomatous infections 175–177
severed, vs. spinal cord trauma 68
spinal cord hemorrhage, vs. spinal cord trauma 68
spinal cord trauma 66–68
spinal dysraphism 16
vs. meningocele 20

spinal fusion, surgical,
  vs. Klippel–Feil syndrome 28
spinal infarction
  acute, vs. spinal multiple sclerosis 189
  vs. acute transverse myelitis 185
  vs. astrocytoma 255
  vs. metastasis 243
spinal injury 43–86
  Magerl classification 43, 44
spinal instrumentation,
  complications 280–286
spinal multiple sclerosis 186–189
spinal stenosis 192
  degenerative 126–130
  nondiskogenic
    vs. disk bulge 107
    vs. disk herniation 102
spine, kissing 121, 122
spondylarthritis 111, 112, 114
  and synovial cyst 118
spondylitis
  ankylosing, *see* ankylosing spondylitis
  anterior 147, 149, 150
  bacterial, *see* bacterial spondylitis
  vs. Modic I degenerative disk
    disease 92
  specific, vs. acute bacterial 160
  vs. spondylolisthesis 125
  tuberculous 165–171
spondyloarthropathy
  psoriatic 141–143
  seronegative, vs. rheumatoid
    arthritis 137
spondylodiskitis 158, 159, 161
  aseptic 147, 150
  vs. epidural abscess 174
  vs. Modic I degenerative disk
    disease 92
  vs. stress fractures 83
  tuberculous 175
spondylolisthesis 79–82, 123–126
  Meyerding classification 79, 81
spondylolysis 79
  healed, vs. spondylolisthesis 82
spondylosis, vs. diffuse idiopathic
  skeletal hyperostosis 132
spondylosis deformans (Modic III) 96–99
Sprengel deformity 27
squaring, vertebral body 147, 148, 154
staging classification, sacrococcygeal
  teratoma 13
stenosis
  neural foramina 99, 114
    vs. disk bulge 107
    vs. disk herniation 102
  spinal canal 26, 40, 52, 56, 99,
    120, 192
    degenerative 126–130
    vs. disk bulge 107
    vs. disk herniation 102
Still disease 137
stress fractures, in ankylosing
  spondylitis 83–86
stress phenomena 79–82
subchondral sclerosis 109
subdural synostosis,
  vs. dens fracture 50
subluxation
  anterior 73–75
  atlantodental, rheumatoid
    arthritis 134, 135
  cervical spine 51
  vs. dens fracture 50
  traumatic, vs. rheumatoid
    arthritis 140
surgery, postoperative disorders
  270–286
syndesmophytes 147–149
  vs. spondylosis deformans 99
synostosis, subdural,
  vs. dens fracture 50
synovial cyst 118, 119
syringobulbia 69
syringohydromyelia 69–72
systemic lupus erythematosus,
  vs. spinal multiple sclerosis 189

T

teardrop fracture, cervical spine 51, 52
teratoma, sacrococcygeal 13–15
tethering 9–12
  post-traumatic 71
  recurrent 19
thecal sac, empty 178, 180
tonsils, cerebellar, descent 3
tram tracking 214
transverse myelitis, acute 182–185
  vs. astrocytoma 255
  vs. granulomatous inflammation 177
  vs. metastasis 243
  vs. spinal multiple sclerosis 189

trauma
vs. Baastrup disease 122
chronic, and rheumatoid arthritis 138–140
vs. malrotation 42
vs. spondylolisthesis 125
traumatic subluxation, vs. rheumatoid arthritis 140
tuberculosis 175
tuberculous spondylitis 165–171
tuberculous spondylodiskitis 175
tumors 190–258
vs. aneurysmal bone cyst 207
vs. degenerative spinal stenosis 128
intradural, vs. arachnoiditis 181
intramedullary
vs. acute transverse myelitis 185
vs. granulomatous inflammation 177
nerve sheath 237–239
primary, vs. osteoblastoma 200
vs. sacrococcygeal teratoma 15
vs. spinal epidural lipomatosis 293
vs. syringohydromyelia 72

U

uncovertebral osteoarthritis 116, 117

V

vacuum phenomenon 108–110
vascular disorders 259–269
vasculitis, vs. arterial spinal cord infarction 269
venous plexus, enlarged, vs. CSF fistula 274
vertebra
cleft 25
collapse 289
vs. bone metastasis 221
vs. multiple myeloma 225
vs. spondylosis deformans 99
compression, types 289
fractures
vs. bacterial spondylitis 160
causes 45–47
vs. tuberculous spondylitis 169
fusion
acquired 25
congenital 21, 25
malformations 21–25
waist 25, 27, 28
vertebral body
ivory 232, 233, 236, 291, 292
osteomyelitis, vs. epidural abscess 174
scalloping 237
sequestrum 165
squaring 147, 148, 154
vertebra plana 35, 212–214
von Hippel–Lindau disease 256, 257

W

waist, vertebral 25, 27, 28
wedge fracture, cervical spine 51, 52
Wegener granulomatosis 175, 176

solomon's sword

Clarifying Values in the Church

robert meyners &
claire wooster

Abingdon • Nashville

SOLOMON'S SWORD
CLARIFYING VALUES IN THE CHURCH

Library of Congress Cataloging in Publication Data

MEYNERS, ROBERT, 1922-
Solomon's sword.

Bibliography: p.
1. Decision-making (Ethics) 2. Values. 3. Church work. I. WOOSTER, CLAIRE, 1942- joint author.
II. Title.
BJ1468.5.M49 241 77-9391

ISBN 0-687-39050-8

MANUFACTURED BY THE PARTHENON PRESS AT NASHVILLE, TENNESSEE, UNITED STATES OF AMERICA

ACKNOWLEDGMENTS

We wish to thank Perry LeFevre, Eleanor Morrison, and Robert Willner for their helpful criticisms of this manuscript. We are especially grateful to the students in our classes and to church people in our workshops. They have informed our design and also served as subjects in the testing and validating of the strategies. It is our hope that the usefulness of the result will in part repay these many people for their effort and wisdom.

PREFACE

> And the king said, "Bring me a sword. . . . Divide the living child in two, and give half to the one, and half to the other." Then the woman whose son was alive said to the king, because her heart yearned for her son, "Oh my Lord, give her the living child, and by no means slay it." But the other said, "It shall be neither mine nor yours; divide it." Then the king answered and said, "Give the living child to the first woman, and by no means slay it; she is the mother."
>
> I Kings 3:24-27

The church, like Solomon, faces difficult and puzzling issues of faith and decision. Perhaps this ancient story provides a clue to our problem too.

These pages are an offering to the church, in the belief that pastors and lay leaders long to respond to the need for moral and spiritual direction. This is no easy task in an age when nothing can be assumed about "who believes what," either within the church or without. We cannot depend upon the old ways by which the church might enforce consensus. Nor are many of us prophets, able to arouse the corporate conscience around a clear vision of the will of God for our time. But there are great issues before us on which human fulfillment and even survival may depend. We ignore these problems at our peril.

Solomon established his reputation for wisdom by designing a "values clarification" strategy. This book is our description of a method for dealing with the dilemmas of faith and decision in the church, using the values clarification approach. We have sought to develop and test a model that has these important advantages: (1) respect for the wide range of viewpoints current in the church; (2) flexibility to shape strategies to the uniqueness of local churches and groups; (3) expression of the leader's own convictions without imposing these ideas on the people; (4) clarification of the faith people already hold; (5) consideration of alternative values that may provide possibilities for change or growth; (6) recognition of the emotional as well as the intellectual element in value decisions; (7) analysis of difficult technical and theological ideas with manageable simplicity.

The story about Solomon's sword in the First Book of the Kings ends with these words: "And all Israel heard of the judgment which the king had rendered; and they stood in awe of the king, because they perceived that the wisdom of God was in him, to render justice." That expresses our hope for the church, that the wisdom of God be in our midst, to render justice.

CONTENTS

Preface
I. Dealing with Diversity in the Church *11*
II. Creating and Adapting Strategies *20*
III. The Great Conversation: Christ and Culture *25*
IV. Slippery Sex Roles *48*
V. The Use and Abuse of the Human Habitat *76*
VI. The Right to Life and the Right to Death *102*
VII. Group Goals and Conflict Management *124*
Notes *143*

Chapter I
DEALING WITH DIVERSITY IN THE CHURCH

Today, Christians cannot agree on where the offertory belongs in the Sunday service, much less on questions like busing, abortion, or the guaranteed annual wage. By contrast, when Martin Luther stood before his accusers he knew what the duty of the Christian was. He and his opponents agreed that there could be only one understanding of the faith in that time and place. There was an underlying unity even behind controversy.

The world of conscience in which we live is radically different from Luther's world. First, no underlying unity exists, or, if it does exist, it is so hidden that we cannot depend upon it. The variety of current value assumptions is virtually endless. We call this a pluralistic society, meaning that in contrast to societies in which there is a common set of values, there is in our society a wide range of values and meanings around which people organize their lives.

A second difference in our world of conscience stems from the complexity of the issues we face. To be sure, every generation believes that it faces the most complex problems of all time. Formerly, however, confusion arose out of a lack of knowledge. Ironically, that simplified problems of moral judgment. What people of faith did not and could not know could hardly enter into the calculations of conscience. We, however, are the heirs of an explosion of information. The world has been shrunk suddenly by the technologies of communication and transportation. More people have more contact with one another and do more things that affect more people over a larger space and time span. It can be overwhelming and intimidating to realize that everything I do could be more responsibly decided if I could make my decisions in the light of all relevant and available information.

Conscientious decision is beset then with two opposite threats. On the one hand, I can make my decisions without due regard for the incredible range of technical information available to me. I can choose tonight's menu oblivious of the relation between my diet and world hunger. I can invest in a company without investigating its impact upon the economies of undeveloped nations. On the other hand, I can become paralyzed by the well-meaning desire not to decide or act except on the basis of all the relevant information. Information is available to me in greater amounts than I can ever process. Thus, if I am to act at all, I eventually must choose what kind of and how much information I will consider.

Ponder the enormously complex problem of the ecosystem. It encompasses pollution, population, food, economic growth, industrialization, and world distribution of wealth. These are all interrelated and so complex and fast-moving that even with automated computation we cannot keep up with the data. The mind boggles!

Nostalgia is enticing in the face of such complexity. It must have been great when the church could spend a decade (or a few centuries) discussing the issue and then pass a law forbidding usury, for example. Does it matter that the church was probably wrong about that? Or does it matter that the church has frequently been wrong—on religious liberty, on slavery, on women's right to vote, and on a host of other matters? Would we want the church again to decide these issues? Maybe pluralism is not so bad after all. In any case, pluralism is here to stay and there is little we can do about it. Neither nostalgia for the past nor a utopian dream of the future is likely to alter this hard reality.

How then can the church relate to current human problems in the face of this awesome complexity? One possible answer, of course, is that the church should not try. We could freely admit that the church has no expertise and thus would be better advised to keep a discreet silence than to prattle amateurishly beyond its competence.

However, there is really no way that the church can stay out of an issue like ecology on which human destiny seems to depend. Economic growth, for example, is so much assumed to be a positive value in our culture that it is invisible, like the air we breathe. It is involved in every bite we eat and every item we purchase. It is in every advertisement and every analysis of the economic situation. Yet, if economic growth continues at the present rate, it may eventually become a monster that devours itself. The earth's resources are finally limited. This is not to say that we know what economic value to put in place of "growth" or how we could go about it if we did. But to do nothing and to say nothing is to take a position affirming our present understanding of the importance of economic growth. That may in fact be what many people will decide, but it is irresponsible to make such a decision merely by default—without reflection or conviction.

Moreover, there is ample evidence that these ecological problems involve value questions. Any number of technical and scientific writers have emphasized that there is no solution to our problems unless and until we can develop values that are relevant to the new ecological situation. If the church does not participate in the process by which old values are recovered and new values developed, we may have the blood of our children on our hands.

The problem is that these values cannot be proclaimed by a recognized authority. Nowhere is the authority available to priest or prophet by which the values that might save us could be proclaimed. Theologians and Christian leaders cannot tell the rest of us what opinions we should hold. Even their advice on issues of private morality is less than fully welcome. Questions of sexual morality were once a clear province for ecclesiastical advice. Now, even this issue involves so many technical questions relating to psychological and physical health, world population, hunger, and economic justice that moral pronouncements are strangely inadequate.

This situation should not come as any great surprise to us. No matter how important the church fathers were to the development of a Christian ethos, it was the churches and the people who made up the churches who listened to the gospel, sifted through the conflicting messages, and responded finally with a relatively coherent faith, which became the Christian heritage. If the last fifteen years of social controversy in the churches have taught us anything, it must be that the people in local churches insist on participating in fashioning the faith that is to represent them in the public forum.

Values Clarification

In the light of these considerations the chapters in this book are offered as one model for dealing with controversial issues in the Christian community. What follows is an adaptation of the theory and techniques of values clarification, which had its formal beginning in the work of Louis Raths and his co-workers, Sidney Simon and Merrill Harmin. As a public school educator, Raths faced the problem of pluralism and concluded that while the school could not teach particular values in a pluralistic society, if it did nothing about values, it was neglecting what should be a most important concern of education. He looked at the process of human valuing and described it this way:

1. choosing freely one's beliefs and behavior;
2. choosing from alternatives;
3. choosing after thoughtful consideration of consequences;
4. prizing and cherishing one's beliefs and behavior;
5. affirming publicly when appropriate;
6. acting upon one's beliefs;
7. repeating action in some pattern.[1]

This approach does not try to instill any particular set of values. Rather, it seeks to help people use the seven processes in their own lives. With already formed values, the purpose is to find out what these values are and to see if they have been carefully considered alongside other possible values that might have been chosen.

To accomplish this, a variety of games, strategies, exercises, and simulations are used. Among the many advantages of these strategies is that they are enjoyable. We have long known that education is more effective when it is interesting and enjoyable. Furthermore, in a normal discussion, people are boxed in to their positions as soon as they begin to verbalize them. To agree with a different position is a defeat. The ego is at stake in any possible change of mind or feeling. But in the mood of a game, polarization is forestalled. In many of the strategies people must support views that they do not themselves hold. This helps in understanding the force of feeling and argument that belongs to the other person's position. Sometimes participants will find themselves getting into the role so fully that the values represented in that role become appealing.

Still another great advantage of this approach is the degree to which both thought and feeling can be integrated. Much of what we do in the churches is verbal activity that enlightens the mind. Perhaps we do not think of the church as a highly intellectual place, but it often is. The need for integration of thought and feeling can be clearly seen in a personal matter such as changing sex roles. If I cherish my traditional role as breadwinner or as homemaker, then it may be extremely difficult for me to alter my role in response to my spouse's demand for shared responsibility. I may be intellectually willing, but my acts will not indicate this if I am emotionally unready for change. Clarifying strategies can help uncover such an emotional/intellectual tug-of-war. This may reveal areas where the stress is not so great—where I might be able to meet some of my spouse's needs without negating my own.

The values clarification approach is based on the general civic assumptions of a democratic society. It does not define these assumptions but provides a method for people to refine their democratic understandings for themselves. In the context of the church, we add the further general understanding of God's revealing himself as redeeming love in Jesus Christ. We too, however, do not define these religious assumptions precisely but suggest that by these methods people of the Christian community can refine their own understandings of the nature of this faith and its implications in behavior.

We are always in danger of acting as if the church is a community of sinless saints. Often there is a preconceived notion about what is "Christian," and this is the only view expressed. If, though, we are a community of love, we will provide an atmosphere of freedom and trust within which people can try out the proclamation of who they really are and share the things that matter to them most deeply. We then make a church a place where people can look at choices and consequences and claim their values without fear of condemnation.

At first glance, this atmosphere of freedom may seem uncomfortable for those who understand Christian truth as an authoritative body of knowledge provided by the church and its traditions. Actually, of course, that view is the outcome of a choice these persons have made or are in the process of making, and the same clarifying processes are usefully applied to it. The tension between desire for authority and resistance to authority is an important tactical problem in the churches. Indeed, some people may be threatened by the tacit acceptance of pluralism, preferring to have authoritative answers. There is a great tradition that holds that values are the responsibility of either religious or political authorities. In relation to this emotional issue there are a variety of ways to reduce the threat, some of which are suggested in the next chapter. With reference to the intellectual problem this poses, value clarifying strategies can be used to help sort out the issues of authority in comparison with other ways of determining values. Other ways are suggested in chapter 3.

Clarifying Values in the Church

It may be useful for religious leaders who wish to use the strategies in the following chapters to have before them a statement of the principles of values clarification as we have adapted them for use in the churches. The following ten statements are operational principles intended to be suggestive rather than exhaustive. They will be most useful if leaders revise and complete them for themselves, providing more specific content in the light of their own particular situations.

1. *Emphasize the valuing and deciding process.* If our emphasis is too exclusively on the conclusions to which other people come, the disagreements among us will be destructive and divisive. Sincere Christians are bound to disagree on questions about which the church must provide leadership but on which it cannot provide mandates. Let the emphasis, therefore, be not on judging the conclusions to which other people come but on the valuing process by which persons and groups struggle with their own consciences within the community of faith.

2. *Begin with the faith and values people do in fact already hold.* Persons are not blank tablets on which values can be inscribed. Rather, at every point they have already a core of basic, informing values. In the context of the church some of these values will be biblical and Christian in origin; others will be civic and cultural; still others will be highly individualistic and private. To ignore the values people already hold—to disrespect them—is to court disaster in the church.

3. *Facilitate consideration of alternatives to the values already held.* We are not united because of our agreement on moral or social issues. We are united in a community of faith because we are inspired by a common Lord and share a unique tradition. The love and respect for one another to which we are called by that faith can indeed be the basis for conscientious struggle in mutual support. This struggle may result in accepting alternative values or it may confirm the original values. There may be disagreement and conflict, but it can be creative and redemptive rather than vicious and destructive.

4. *Encourage both emotional and intellectual elements in the valuing process.* Both thought and feeling are important dimensions of the decision-making process. We can find ways of raising and of

respecting both the emotional and intellectual elements while alternatives are freely considered.

5. *Develop methods of group interaction that bring out individual and subgroup concerns and responses.* Teaching, lecturing, preaching, and even group discussion are methods that are overpowering to some people. The authority of the leader, the competence of those who possess much information, the skill some people have in communicating—all of these may override the opinions of those who do not share these qualities. But people are not necessarily convinced when they remain silent or subdued.

6. *It may be more important for people to raise questions than to achieve final answers.* Decisions must be made and elections held, but few important issues are finished with one decision. Values transcend immediate decisions. Faith has to do with lifetime commitments and not with being rid of uncomfortable dilemmas. Premature closure can be an invitation to stop feeling and thinking about the issues.

7. *Provide opportunities for people to proclaim their values.* A value is not a value unless we are willing under appropriate circumstances to publicly affirm what we believe. Witness and testimony have been an important part of the Christian tradition. This expectation has, however, sometimes been restricted to personal devotion and not allowed the richness and breadth of other areas of religious faith. A witness is not something with which others are invited to argue. It is a proclamation. An appropriate response of the hearers is an amen or a nodding of the head—not necessarily in agreement, but by way of saying, "I hear you. I take your witness seriously. I respect your faith."

8. *Encourage action in keeping with values affirmed.* We often preach what we do not act upon. A position or attitude becomes a cherished conviction at the point at which it is acted upon with relative consistency over time. It may be appropriate for the church to support action on which there is general agreement. Otherwise, it may be possible to develop alternative modes of action appropriate to

different views. In any case, it is important to help people get in touch with inconsistencies between their beliefs and actions, not in order to judge them but in order to facilitate their discovering the values on the basis of which they can in fact organize their living.

9. *Claim the right to your own convictions, just as you affirm that right for others.* The process here suggested does not ask leaders to give up their own beliefs or passion. In fact, it requires that leaders reveal themselves. This must be done if only for the sake of objectivity, since the way leaders develop strategies will be influenced by their own bias. There is finally no such thing as complete neutrality. It is neither necessary nor desirable to force our own views on other people, but it is only honest and helpful from time to time to state our convictions and provide a faithful witness. This will also help with the threat that people sometimes feel when the leader's views are hidden. Actually, for most of us the danger is more that we impose our views on others than that our opinions remain too hidden. When it comes to feelings, the opposite may be the case, since many of us find it difficult to reveal who we are on that level.

10. *Expect the graceful event of Christian community.* Christian values are ultimately not individualistic but communal. Leaders may aid in the development of Christian values; individuals may clarify their own convictions; but, the Christian faith is fulfilled in a life together where, in the struggle with one another and with the world, we are as a community called to faith and action. We cannot raise up prophets for ourselves. We cannot by any titanic effort of the will produce agreement or consensus. Only in active expectancy can we wait upon this graceful event, tireless in our efforts to remove the blocks, patient in our hope that it may occur among us, confident in our faith that the promise will be fulfilled.

Chapter II

CREATING AND ADAPTING STRATEGIES

In the chapters that follow we describe strategies that have been created or adapted for use in the church. Each chapter is addressed to a specific controversial issue. Preceding the strategies is a short introduction intended to raise the most crucial elements involved. This includes a statement of the religious values common among us which may be relevant to the issue. Then the exercises themselves are described. Finally, there is a bibliography on the subject intended to provide background reading for either leaders or participants.

Some exercises are presented in detail while others are only sketched in broad outline under Further Suggestions. Most strategies work best if they are adapted by the persons using them to their own needs and the needs of the congregation with which they work. We therefore include here some guidelines to help leaders in their attempts at adapting these exercises or creating their own.

Suggestions for Writing or Adapting Exercises

1. Be clear about your specific purpose before writing or adapting any strategy.
2. Provide a wide range of stances or views in your exercises. Values cannot be clarified if only one side of an issue is presented.
3. In presenting views that are different from your own, try to present them as fairly as possible. Avoid using positive adjectives when describing your position and negative adjectives when describing opposing positions.

4. It is often useful to have people assume roles or support a position that is not their own. Not only do they get a chance to feel the force of another's argument, but this device also keeps them from becoming defensive and too concerned about their own ego. Thus, we frequently suggest dividing people into groups randomly or arbitrarily assigning roles or positions to support.
5. You are not presenting people with scientific tests, and exercises may not come out the way you anticipate. If issues are raised and people become involved in actively sorting out their views and feelings, however, you have achieved a worthy goal. If there is no discussion because everyone agrees, then probably you have made the issues too clear-cut or have loaded the responses in some unforeseen way. Try to learn from such an experience and adapt your exercise accordingly on another occasion.
6. It is important not to make exercises more threatening than your group can handle. Some exercises in this book require a fair amount of trust among the participants to be effective. Thus, it is wise to avoid these exercises in a group that does not have sufficient trust, or to modify them so that people do not have to share those things they might find threatening. Respect people's right to privacy and their need to determine for themselves when to affirm their values openly. When introducing an exercise that people might find threatening, emphasize their freedom not to participate whenever they feel strongly uncomfortable.
7. In spite of careful planning, any exercise may go awry because of unexpected problems. A group may start giving the "religious" responses that they think the leader expects of them rather than their honest beliefs or feelings. They may start arguing with and stop listening to one another. They may even stop responding entirely. If any of these things are happening, people are probably becoming

defensive. It is then best to change to an activity that protects people's privacy. Continual sensitivity to the group's reactions greatly helps in dealing with any of these controversial issues.

8. In some cases in which the instructions are quite complex, it may be easier and more useful to give a demonstration of what is being asked of the group than to give elaborate instructions. Similarly, if a leader feels uneasy about starting out cold using some of these exercises, it may be useful to have a tryout with a few friends or a sympathetic small group.
9. These strategies are seldom sufficient by themselves as an educational medium. (*a*) They assume a certain amount of information about the subjects, but only that involved in regular reading of the newspaper. The process will have failed if it does not encourage people to engage in further reading and discussion. (*b*) The strategies function best as discussion starters or thought organizers. It is a mistake to depend upon them for the entire basis of the consideration of the issues involved. We therefore include the lists of relevant biblical passages and the suggestions for further reading in each chapter.
10. For further guidance, look at the literature of values clarification. We have made the most use of *Values Clarification: A Handbook of Practical Strategies for Teachers* by Sidney Simon, Leland Howe, and Howard Kirschenbaum (New York: Hart, 1972). The exercises are designed for use in the public schools, but many of the formats can be adapted for use in the church.[1]

Suggestions for Writing a Role-play

1. In choosing a situation to role-play, make sure that there are a variety of points of view that people can play convincingly. Have pro and con and mixed positions.

2. It is usually best to have between three and six role-players. More than that number can become too confusing, so that no position comes across clearly. A smaller number may not deal adequately with the complexities of a situation (unless, of course, the situation being enacted is a two-person situation, such as a dialogue between mother and daughter or husband and wife).
3. If the role-play does involve only two people, it may produce undue pressure or stage fright for the players. In that case the whole group can do the role-play in groups of two or in groups of four or five with an audience of only two or three.

Guidelines for Role-playing

Here are some guidelines that are useful for participants to follow when doing role-plays or simulations.

For the players:

1. Be the person you are playing. Respond as spontaneously as you can while imagining what a person with those feelings or beliefs would do.
2. Do not overplay or caricature the role by hamming it up. This breaks the mood and is often unfair to the sort of person being portrayed. Moreover, such overplaying invites the audience to focus on the acting rather than on their reactions to the issues concerning these characters.
3. Ignore the audience as much as possible and concentrate on your role.

For the audience:

1. Restrain comments or excessive laughter. They may distract the role-players.
2. Resist responding to the acting. Instead, think of ways that you might respond in that situation.
3. You may wish to choose one character to identify with and then decide whether you would react as that person does in

the course of the role-play. If not, how would you have responded?

Notes on Guided Fantasies

1. Guided fantasies are most effective in informal groups. People need to be encouraged to get comfortable and to close their eyes so as not to be distracted by extraneous movement. Dim the lights if possible and try to minimize any other potential distractions.
2. Guide the fantasy leisurely, allowing enough time that people may conjure up a picture of what you are suggesting to them.
3. Enunciate clearly so that people are not distracted by straining to understand you.
4. Fantasies can be designed to be relatively undisturbing. However, fantasies that lead people back into their own personal history may be painful. It is important, therefore, to avoid fantasies that might do this if you as leader would feel uncomfortable or inadequately trained to handle such situations. It is also important not to press people unduly to reveal their fantasies since they have the right to determine whom they wish to trust with their pain or joy. On the other hand, such fantasies can present an opportunity for a pastor or leader to be available outside the group to facilitate persons working through issues thus raised.

Chapter III

THE GREAT CONVERSATION: CHRIST AND CULTURE

A many-sided debate about the relations of Christianity and civilization is being carried on in our time . . . publicly by opposing parties and privately in the conflicts of conscience. Sometimes it is concentrated on special issues, such as those of the place of Christian faith in general education or of Christian ethics in economic life. Sometimes it deals with broad questions of the church's responsibility for social order or of the need for a new separation of Christ's followers from the world.

—*H. Richard Niebuhr*

With these words, H. Richard Niebuhr opens his classic description of the historic tension between the authority of the Christian gospel and the social, cultural, and moral values current at any given time and place.[1] The problem is ever present—when we decide to use or not to use national symbols in Christian worship or when we decide to use or not to use religious symbols in public occasions. The tension is at the heart of every debate in which religious ideas are used—in the argument for or against capital punishment, abortion, racial segregation, or prayer in public schools.

There was a time when certain approaches to these issues were more or less characteristic of the various denominations. There were predictable Catholic, Lutheran, or Calvinist ways of sorting out the issues. Today these churches are divided among themselves, and individual believers are torn within themselves. The relation of Christian belief to science, to reason, to education, to personal morality, to politics, is not amenable to simple or permanent solution. The fact is that the issues are not the accidental product of particular situations but represent fundamental dilemmas at the heart of human existence.

Not only theologians argue these issues. Lay persons also do so in boards or committees and in their own consciences. This fact may be hidden by the tendency for the arguments to revolve around concrete issues. The basic relation between the two sources of value and authority are not always sorted out openly. We argue about a question like abortion, using "Christian" reasons for our conclusions, without ever dealing with the authority and function of these religious ideas or their relation to questions of personal and social morality.

Two factors largely account for the murky nature of our typical discussion of the issues of Christ and culture. First is the pluralism of our cultural situation. Culture is never one thing but is, rather, a multitude of meanings, values, symbols, and structures. If that has been a serious problem historically, the values present in American culture today are so diverse as to defy precise identification. If the church has sometimes had difficulty identifying "the culture" to which it is to address itself, the difficulty now is to identify any coherent set of subcultures with which the church and the Christian can engage in active dialogue.

The second factor serving to explain the underground character of the tension between Christ and culture is a crisis in the authority of the Christian gospel. Not only has pluralism divided society, it is also splintering the church. The faith symbolized by the figure of Christ is therefore not one faith but many faiths to many people. Countless Christians experience tension within themselves about the nature of the faith to which they are committed.

Nevertheless, the great conversation goes on, whether openly on precise issues or indirectly on vague issues. People do have convictions. Many people organize a great number of their loyalties around the Christian fellowship and its traditions. Even where this is not the case, our society is one in which many religious symbols are woven into the fabric of public values. The relation of these religious meanings to other values in the social tapestry is a matter of daily attitude and behavior. In these pages, our concern is not with the general problem suggested by this civil religion but with the specific problem for those in the Christian churches who have a deep conviction that the gospel of Jesus Christ has power and meaning in their lives. The relevance of this gospel to a wide range of moral, social, and political questions is a matter of deep and enduring concern.

It should be obvious, however, that there is not available one right and authoritative answer to the problems involved. It may be useful to note briefly H. Richard Niebuhr's description of five ways in which Christians historically have approached the matter.

First, there have been those who pit Christ against culture. In this view the Christian's absolute duty is that of loyalty to Christ and his gospel. All authority from any other source is to be rejected. Medieval monks and radical sectarians have followed this rationale into a drastic withdrawal from the world and its affairs. While this approach is not much in vogue in a society where such isolation is hardly possible, some important dimensions of this attitude still function and must be taken seriously. To some Christians the world seems finally unredeemable, so that the only way to respond to its gross evil is to separate oneself from its infections.

An opposite view has identified the loyalty we have to Christ with the loyalty owed to the social world. The structures and values of culture are the instruments of God's gracious care for the world and his people. There is no great tension to be found between God's revelation of himself in Jesus Christ and his grace available through the ordinary achievements of material, intellectual, and aesthetic progress in society at large. The sacred and secular realms support and enrich each other. Ancient gnostics and modern culture-Protestants have upheld this "Christ of culture" view.

The majority Christian positions through the ages have not been either of these first two extremes but, rather, middle positions that recognize a fundamental tension between Christ and culture while at the same time recognizing an underlying need for dialogue and unity.

Niebuhr describes three such positions, which he calls synthesist, dualist, and conversionist.

The synthesist view, typified by Thomas Aquinas and medieval Catholicism, places the authority of Christ above cultural sources of knowledge and value. There is a kind of hierarchical unity which organizes thought and conduct under divine activity in creation and redemption. There are only apparent contradictions between Christ and culture. They are resolved in principle by God's initiation of both, but are solved in fact by churchly authority. While there are those today who place Christ above culture, there are no longer any grand intellectual syntheses of this nature. Therefore, the modern debate usually revolves around the two final alternatives.

The dualist view holds that the Christian is a citizen of two worlds. In the realm of faith the Christian is called to obedience to God's absolute demands, and, while in our sinful state these are never fulfilled, salvation is available by grace through faith. However, as a citizen of the world, the values and structures of society are the Christian's responsibility. Martin Luther is the major exponent of these two separate moralities. The whole world of human culture is godless and doomed, but God sustains the faithful in the midst of this sickness and calls for structures that will restrain the more destructive tendencies of human sin. Culture cannot be saved or redeemed, but the worst possibilities of chaos and destruction may be contained. The Christian's salvation is, however, beyond these temporal eventualities, in the realm of faith and grace.

Finally, in the conversionist view, Christ enters the cultural world to transform it. To be sure, culture is infected with evil, but culture is a fundamental, not an accidental, aspect of human existence. There is no salvation except as we turn from idolatrous cultural loyalties and recognize God's sovereign rule over all aspects of our life. Augustine and Calvin, who represent this position, were quite skeptical about the possibility of human good. They did, however, believe all things are possible with God. Thus, they expected the transforming power of God in Christ to affect the nature of all institutions and values.

This great conversation, as it progresses in the churches and in the consciences of Christians today, revolves most frequently around variations of these last two perspectives with additional elements from the other three. The basic question seems to be, finally, whether there is to be a separation between religious and cultural values and, if so, how rigid a separation it is to be. Or, alternatively, is there a Christian imperative to bring our religious faith to bear upon the structures and value systems that make up our life together in societies?

There is no one final answer in this conversation. It is not likely or even desirable that some of us should win the debate over others. If the great thinkers in Christian history have not been able to settle the matter, it is likely that God's will for us is not everywhere and at all times the same. The issues emerge in various ways according to the time and circumstances.

In the decade of the sixties and perhaps generally in this century, we have been racked by the tension between church and politics. Conversionists have worked directly and politically for social justice in the name of the church and their faith. On the other hand, those who support a dualist position have emphasized the part of this tradition that places individual morals under the authority of Christian values, while public and political questions have been relegated to the world of dominant cultural values. Thus Christian faith is relevant to private moral questions involving family, children, sexuality, etc. Christian values impinge upon public life primarily in the call to honesty and fairness in business and politics. But the demands of love in the gospel do not have direct relevance to the organization of economic and political life, and these matters are therefore not the concern of the church. Christian people are responsible for those concerns not as Christians but simply as citizens.

The hysteria of these controversies has probably obscured some important dimensions of the problem. The dilemma between Christ and culture is too profound to be resolved by any simple division of personal morality and political organization. For example, children are educated in public schools, and their personal morals are decisively affected by public and political influences. On the other hand, matters assumed to be private may indeed have great political significance. For instance, the church's frequent criticism of the materialism of the American life-style is a critique of personal existence, but it implies a criticism of the economic system that supports materialism. Further, there are often controversial issues that are not clearly either private or public matters. Is abortion, for example, a question of private morality or public policy?

Both dualists and conversionists are concerned, therefore, with new and necessary distinctions between the implications of faith for personal existence and the implications of that faith for public questions. We have not always made these distinctions in appropriate ways. Too often the distinction is overdrawn in the service of self-interest. There is little justification for that in the radical demand of the gospel that we concern ourselves with the welfare of all God's children.

This distinction between private morality and public policy is linked to another one, that between love and justice. A frequent formula addresses Christian love, with its commitment to the welfare of the other, to matters involved in the organization of human intimacy. By contrast, justice is the form the Christian imperative takes when addressed to social and political questions. The Christian is to work for justice in society, seeking to overcome gross injustice and to develop structures that support mutuality and equity.

This, however, is simply another way of stating the problem of Christ and culture. Since justice, or its lack, in the public sphere is a part of culture, the question becomes how the authority of Christ and his love imperative is related to the question of justice.

While the distinction between love and justice is basic to the great conversation, choice and decision are the forms in which the problem of Christ and culture usually come to us. There is not a once-and-for-all choice since we make choices over and over again in our personal lives, in our public decisions, and in our spiritual existence. There are, however, critical experiences in which we are called to make these choices in ways that carry finality and dramatic possibilities for good or evil, apostasy or obedience.

Even Niebuhr's profound analysis does not do justice to the complexity of the Christ-and-culture issue, and our summary above is, of course, yet more seriously oversimplified. Nevertheless, it is in the midst of just such confusion that we live our lives and make daily decisions. We cannot wait upon a definitive analysis of the problem and a decisive statement of the issues. Realistically speaking, we must start with what we have, sort out the approaches that seem most adequate to our perception of the call of Christ and the nature of his church. If we take the fact of sin seriously we will not expect truth to be available to us in simple and obvious form. We will know that in the midst of uncertainty and even deceit we must seek to be obedient to a divine imperative, however dimly perceived or inadequately achieved.

The strategies that follow are intended to focus on some of the issues involved in this great conversation. Some are to be done individually—because everyone finally must do her or his own believing. The pilgrim's is a lonely journey in which the help of others can be sought but not depended upon. Other exercises are to be done in groups within a church—because the obedient response to the call of Christ can take place only in the community of those who understand themselves to be the people of God. This is a gift beyond our deserving, as much a burden as a privilege, a condition marked not by our achievement but by the task and hope to which this community is called. "Christ as living Lord is answering the question in the totality of history and life in a fashion which transcends the wisdom of all his interpreters yet employs their partial insights and their necessary conflicts."[2]

Useful Scriptural References

Leviticus 18:1-5
Daniel 3
Amos 5:21-27
Mark 11:15-19; 12:14-17
John 3:16, 17
Acts 5:27-32; 11:1-8
Romans 13:1, 2
I Corinthians 8:7-13
II Corinthians 6:14-18
I John 2:15-17

Strategies and Exercises

1. Four Churches

Design: This strategy is an imaginative exploration of some Christ-and-culture issues in the context of the local church. There are three stages to the strategy: first, a quick reaction to four different styles of parish life; second, the selection of values to be supported by the church; and, third, small-group discussion of the churches and values.

Method: *Stage I: The Churches.* Duplicate and give everyone a copy of the following descriptions of four churches. Ask people to rank the churches according to which they would prefer for their own. This is a forced choice since they may not find any of the four churches to be their ideal. However, it is like choosing an actual church since it is rarely possible to have one's ideal.

The Descriptions:

Below are brief descriptions of four churches. Read through them quickly. Then rank them from one to four according to how well you like each church. Give a number one (1) to the church you like best and a number four (4) to the one you like least. (This does not mean that your number 1 choice is your ideal church, or that you are being critical of your own church. It merely means that of these four choices, number 1 is your favorite.)

The Church of Christ the Shepherd emphasizes its ministry to individuals, especially those in pain or trouble. Since the church is large, it seeks to develop small groups which will provide a support group to every person in the congregation. One of the ministers has a doctorate in psychology and is a full-time counselor. The entire staff gives high priority to calling and visitation. The educational and preaching programs address problems of personal, family, and vocational life, using the resources of the religious heritage as well as the insights of modern knowledge. The church continues to grow, money is not a problem, and the missionary outreach of the church consists of moderately generous contributions to denominational agencies.

The Church of Christ the Savior is a small church in a working-class suburb. Its emphasis is strongly upon Bible study, prayer, and preaching. Its purpose is first to encourage people to take the gospel message into their own lives in the confidence that when this happens, people will be better persons and better citizens. The church is noted for the warmth of its fellowship, and people are often drawn into the life of the church by its friendliness. The congregation raises money easily for its modest local expenses and it gives generously to foreign missions. There are some people in the church who are no longer comfortable with this practice since they believe the mission board is spending too much money on technical assistance and not enough directly on evangelism.

The Church of Christ the Redeemer is a busy, bustling congregation of moderate size which constantly spins off new programs and ideas. The neighborhood has begun recently to develop new problems. In response, the church has organized an outreach program, including a rehabilitation center for drug users and a pregnancy-testing facility. The minister is regarded as an able counselor and spiritual confidant. There are some small groups in the church which are sharing/caring support groups, and there are a couple of Bible-study groups, and one group of people that is organized around the concern for social issues. There are those who complain that the church does not deal adequately with personal concerns, but others are complaining that the church is not adequately involved in a mission to the world and its problems.

The Church of Christ the King is a small church with an influence out of all proportion to its size. The congregation is very visible in the city and in the denomination, especially in areas that involve social and political issues. The people believe that the churches' witness to Christian love can only be adequately communicated to the world in terms of justice and freedom for all. They believe that the lives of individuals in the congregation are very precious, but this care and concern is chiefly expressed in the deep commitment they share to the struggle for humanizing the society as a whole. There is a strong emphasis upon Bible study and prayer, upon mutual support and encouragement, upon giving money to the mission of the church, but in all of this the ultimate purpose is not personal enrichment and salvation but commitment to the cause of Christ in the world.

Stage II: Values in the Church. When participants have had an opportunity to read and rank the above descriptions, distribute the following sheet for the next stage. Go over the instructions together.

The Sheet:

Here is a list of personal, social, and religious values. How important do you believe each one of these to be? Mark each according to whether you think emphasizing that value is very important (1), important (2), umimportant (3), or actually harmful (4).

moral integrity
spiritual health
knowledge of the Bible
mental health
prayer
racial equality
Christian commitment
physical health
democratic society
forgiveness of sin
good citizenship
economic success
personal salvation
social justice
political freedom
faith in God
belief in life after death
reducing poverty
sexual adequacy
responsible parenthood
personal experience of Christ

Underline those values you believe to be *religious* values. Draw a circle around those values you regard as *social* (as opposed to *personal*) values. Draw a line through those values with which you think the church should *not* be directly concerned. If you considered more than five of the above values to be very important, choose the five that are most important to you personally.

Stage III: Discussion. After most people have finished Stage II, divide the participants into groups of three to five to discuss the churches and the values. Ask them first to share their rankings of the churches and the reasons for their choices. Remind them to be sensitive to one another's feelings about these parish styles and to listen to the reasons expressed.

Next, ask them to spend a few moments comparing their ratings of the churches with the values they selected. Is there continuity between them? Have they selected churches that are concerned with the values with which they believe the church should be concerned? (Note: The purpose is not to induce people to change their ratings, although some may wish to do so. Rather, the idea is to illuminate both the intellectual and the emotional factors in their choices and to practice listening to one another and respecting different views.)

2. Banners and Graffiti

Design: Symbolizing the meaning of the church and the faith it represents can be an important way for people to become aware of the nature of their basic commitment. In a series of meetings on Christ and culture, part of the time can be devoted to designing and making one or more pictures or symbols of the basic ideas emerging in the group. Representations of a symbolic nature, with their verbal and nonverbal messages, can encourage awareness of both our thought and feeling about the faith we are examining.

As the group works together, it is important to identify the core of commonality among the participants, while providing freedom and respect for the range of opinions and beliefs that go beyond the agreement. Making banners, or developing some other form of creative expression, can provide a meaningful way to search for the nature of this common faith.

Method: At first, the planning for such a creation can be very unstructured. For example, a "graffiti wall" can be provided, on which, during the early sessions, people are encouraged to scribble ideas, quotations, jokes, and symbols that come out of the group's interaction or that grasp individuals. From this miscellaneous collection there may gradually emerge certain elements that prove to be especially meaningful to everyone. These can be worked into banners and into songs and liturgies for celebration later on. Affirm and celebrate ideas and feelings that are important to one or two people, even when they do not represent substantial group coherence.

3. A Dream of Saints

Design: This is a guided fantasy that allows people to become aware of the kinds of authority they respect most. Like most exercises, it is useful to mold it to fit the immediate and emerging purposes in the group. The fantasy provides a helpful introduction to a discussion of the nature of religious authority and the differing ways in which it may be perceived. A more systematic analysis may then follow.

Method: Refer to the notes on guided fantasies in chapter 2. Explain to people that the fantasy is an opportunity to let imagination inform our thinking about different ways of understanding religious authority. Suggest taking a few moments to relax quietly and get in a comfortable position. The ellipses (. . .) indicate pauses where people may allow their imaginations to be active. This fantasy will require ten to fifteen minutes.

The Fantasy:

Imagine that you are having a dream. You are tired and a little despondent. . . . You have had a lot of problems recently. You are walking in a woods, enjoying the fresh air and the quiet beauty of the place. . . . You sit down on a log to reflect briefly on your life. . . . Presently you become aware of an old man sitting beside you. He begins to speak with a firm and quiet voice, inspiring your confidence. Pointing to a path in the woods, he tells you there are a number of caves along the way, in each of which dwells a saint. If you walk down the path you may choose one of the saints with whom to spend the day, gathering what wisdom and inspiration you can from the time together. There is only one requirement: You must choose a single question, a most important question for your life, with which to begin the dialogue. Your choices of whom to visit are—

- a mystic, a person deeply attuned to God, able to show others the way to spiritual enlightenment and power. This saint is unconcerned with this world or its comforts but demonstrates a profound satisfaction which remains in the midst of pain or suffering;

- a sage deeply steeped in the wisdom of the Bible, who uses the scholarship surrounding the text to sort out human problems and creative possibilities in daily living and to provide spiritual guidance applicable equally to personal and social existence;
- a hero of the faith who has risked life and personal well-being struggling for the solutions to problems of poverty and injustice in the confidence that obedience to God is its own reward;
- a worldly sage who has learned to make faith eminently practical in daily existence, informing personal life, business, and politics with integrity and Christian devotion;
- a saintly church official who has mediated the authority of the church and its tradition to the people, guiding them through the uncertainties and confusions of the world toward clear and confident answers to basic human problems.

Spend a few minutes choosing which saint you wish to talk with. . . . Now ponder the question you wish to use as your most important question. . . . When you have made your choice, imagine the conversation that goes on between the two of you . . .

Allow a period of silence for people to begin a conversation .. their imagination. Further guidance may be given to facilitate this conversation. When several minutes have elapsed, suggest that they take leave of the saint and return to the group.

Now divide into groups of three to five to discuss the experience. Ask people to report whom they chose, what question they asked, and what interesting or surprising things may have come out of the conversation. Was it a satisfying experience, or was it in any way disturbing? Encourage them to be as open as they comfortably can, but emphasize their right to tell *or not to tell* what they have experienced.

Method II:

An alternative form of this basic exercise may be done without the fantasy. This method is less imaginative but may be more comfortable for a given group or leader. The results, however, are apt to be different.

Place five posters around the room with the name of one of

these saints on each. The posters can be enlivened with a drawing or a symbol. Ask the participants to choose which saint each wishes to speak with and to go to that poster. Have the groups that gather around each poster share their reasons for choosing that saint. If any saint has only one follower, have that person go to another group to express the reasons. When they have done that, ask each group to decide together what question they will ask their saint. Agreement may not be reached, but trying to reach agreement emphasizes listening to, respecting, and compromising with other perspectives. Finally, ask all participants to offer to their small group a one- or two-sentence response to their question.

4. Where Do We Turn for Guidance?

Design: Religious faith may be very important in some areas of our lives and quite incidental in others. This exercise focuses on the functions of religious practice in various situations.

Method: Duplicate and distribute the following sheet. Tell people it is for an exercise in which we ponder the role of religious practice in daily existence:

> As always in these strategies there are no "right" answers. The sheet describes several situations in which a person must make a decision. In each case think about to whom or to what you would turn for guidance in such a situation. For one kind of situation you may find one source important, but for another situation quite other kinds of help may be important to you.

The leader will need to decide in advance whether this exercise will be private or will be discussed in the group afterward. Some people in a church setting may be inclined to give more "religious" answers than they actually feel. If the leader believes this is likely, it will be well to have the exercise be private, perhaps distributed at the end of an evening. The leader may ask to have the sheets turned in anonymously to get more fully in touch with the beliefs and feelings in the group, but everyone should be assured that there will be no discussion of the results.

If no such problem is anticipated, the whole group or small groups can discuss the responses. Follow-up discussion might include these questions:

What are the basic differences between the situations in which religious practice plays an important role and those in which religion plays only an indirect or secondary role?

What religious resources have direct relevance to a problem and which provide a background for important decisions?

What resources do you commonly use in decision-making that are not among the ten listed?

The Sheet

Read each situation and then list in order of importance to you three of the following sources of guidance. Use the numbers given to indicate each resource.

The Resources

1. Pray long and earnestly about the matter.
2. Talk it over with one or two friends I deeply trust.
3. Consult a professional counselor or expert on the subject.
4. Do reading and technical research to get information relating to the problem.
5. Read the Bible in search of inspiration or clues to the answer.
6. Consult official documents of my church to consider the position the church takes on the problem.
7. Consult with my pastor.
8. Spend many hours alone reflecting on the problem and its solution.
9. Read inspirational or other religious literature relating to the subject.
10. Consult with organizations concerned with the matter.

The Situations

A. John, the father of a young family, is offered a job with more money in a distant city away from relatives and longtime friends.___ ___ ___

B. Mary is a twenty-three-year-old professional whose "most serious boyfriend yet" is asking her to live with him to help clarify whether they should be married.___ ___ ___

C. John and Maureen are preparing to retire and must decide whether to stay where they are near their children or to move to a cheaper area with a milder climate.___ ___ ___

D. Charles has a physical condition that may affect his vocational success and is struggling with what vocation to choose.___ ___ ___

E. Jane is a business executive who must decide whether or not to take an action involving great profit to the company but with some possibility of damage to the public interest.___ ___ ___

F. Linda is married and has three children. She has accidentally become pregnant against her own wishes and her physician's advice. She is now considering an abortion.___ ___ ___

G. Walter is a politician who must make a severe budget cut and is deciding between reducing the money to be spent on mental health or on education.___ ___ ___

H. Henry is a foreign policy advisor to the State Department and must make a recommendation regarding the conflicting interests of two nations friendly to our country.___ ___ ___

5. The Mirror of Faith

Design: The purpose of this strategy is to improve communication on matters of faith and commitment. Most of us do not find it easy to express what matters to us deeply; nor are we highly skilled at listening to others. This basic strategy can be used again and again with different subject matter. The subject of interchange may be very broad, such as, What gives my life meaning? Or, the subject can be quite specific, relating directly to some discussion that is to follow or that has already taken place: the meaning of the Bible in my life; the influence of Christ in my daily life; or, more specific yet, what the story of the good Samaritan means to me. The strategy will generally be most useful when the subject is directly tied to ideas and experiences important in the group at the time.

Method: Ask each participant to choose a partner, preferably someone with whom he or she is not intimately acquainted, with whom to have a conversation about the Christian faith. Give instructions using the following or similar words:

> Saying what we believe is not something we do every day. Nor do we have much practice in listening to one another on things that matter deeply to us. For the next fifteen minutes, the two of you are invited to share some of the things you believe as Christians. Sharing requires both speaking and hearing, so the rules will be that when one partner

has made a brief statement (two or three sentences), the other partner reflects back, like a mirror, the gist of what has just been said.[3] The second partner earns the right to make his or her own statement by first reflecting back the statement to the satisfaction of the original speaker. If the first speaker is satisfied with the reflected response, the second partner makes a statement that the first partner then reflects. If either speaker is dissatisfied with a response, the matter should be restated, and the responder tries once again to reflect the statement. A problem in communication can be either in the speaking or in the hearing, or in both.

Note: This is a simple procedure, but there is no simple way to explain it. We therefore suggest that the leader demonstrate a two-sentence interchange with a previously instructed partner. This will save time and reduce anxiety.

6. Role-plays

Design: The practical issues that are raised in the discussion of Christ and culture can be highly emotional and controversial. There is a great need in the church to face these issues in ways that promote understanding and avoid destructive conflict. Role-playing is an important device in moving such discussions forward. People who are expressing the opinions of the personage they are playing are not emotionally involved or directed by their own ego in expressing opinions. They may develop empathy for positions different from their own as the result of representing such opinions. Moreover, there is the possibility of working through feelings and opinions about typical situations that the church inevitably faces, but at a time when the issues do not have to be immediately settled and can therefore be dealt with more dispassionately.

Below are three role-plays that raise Christ-and-culture issues in the context of the local church. These examples obviously may be varied or redone in ways that will make them more useful in a particular situation. It is usually best to avoid role-plays that too obviously replicate current problems in your group or church.

Method: Before beginning, read the guidelines for role-playing in chapter 2. Choose one of the three alternatives below or write your own. Explain the situation to be role-played and ask for volunteers to take the various roles. Give the players separate slips of paper with their roles described in two or three sentences. Include in the description a name and a brief character description. (Stay away from obvious similarities to persons in the group or church.) Consider the following characters: a conservative businessman, two "social-action types" (one who listens to others and one who does not), an elderly person of evangelistic or pious persuasion, etc.

Situation 1: A church member has died and left $25,000 to the church, not intended to go into the regular budget. Three proposals have been made for the use of the money. (1) Finance a five-year program of week-end prayer retreats for members of the parish at the denominational retreat center. (2) Give the money to the Christian Earthquake Relief Committee. (3) Give the money to a local university research project to determine the impact on children of the board of education's busing program. Simulate a committee meeting at which these alternatives are discussed.

Situation 2: The ministerial advisory committee has been asked by the minister to meet with him to help him determine his priorities for his discretionary time. He spends about thirty hours a week in sermon and worship preparation, church administration, and necessary calls on sick persons. He wishes to have advice on how he should spend his remaining time. There are three projects in which he is involved. These are: (1) a program of calling on every member of the congregation once every couple of months; (2) Bible-study groups in the church (there are two now meeting and he would like to organize several more); (3) a joint project with a minister in a nearby community to develop a learning center for school dropouts in the racially mixed neighborhood that lies between the two churches.

Situation 3: A finance committee is meeting to decide what to do about the benevolence budget of the church. There is a total budget of $95,000, of which $17,000 has been tentatively budgeted for benevolences. Have a discussion about the adequacy of this and for what it should be spent.

7. Biblical Round Table

Design: This strategy provides an opportunity to explore imaginatively the conflict between Christian conscience and the dominant culture. The opening chapters of the book of Acts tell the story of the conflict between the disciples and the ruling elders in Jerusalem in the period following the death of Jesus. The elders were responsible for public and religious order and were disturbed by the successful preaching of Peter and John, leading the people into what the elders could only regard as dangerous heresy. The strategy consists of study of the relevant biblical passages and a simulated round-table discussion among several of the principal characters involved in the biblical drama. It is followed by a group discussion.

Method: Suggest to the group that we as Christians are constantly confronting a dilemma between our conscientious beliefs and the values current in our time, even including the laws of the state. Religious objectors to war face this dilemma very dramatically, but we all face it, less poignantly perhaps, when we encounter materialism, immorality in public places, or expectations to act differently in our jobs than conscience would dictate. We will look at these issues as they emerge in the book of Acts to see what light may be thrown on our own dilemmas.

In preparation for the round table, preferably the week before, the leader should ask people to read the first five chapters of Acts, giving special attention to 3:1–4:31 and to 5:12-42. Point out the escalating conflict between the apostles and the Jewish leaders. Emphasize 4:19 where Peter and John are acknowledging the tension. Suggest that people use commentaries and other study aids to reflect on these passages. If only one session is available, give people time to read the essential passages in chapters 4 and 5 before conducting the round table.

The Round Table: Divide the participants into groups of six. Ask each person in each group to assume one of the following roles in the biblical narrative:

the apostle Peter
the apostle John

Annas the high priest
Gamaliel the Pharisee
the lame man who sat beside the gate called Beautiful
Caiaphas of the high-priestly family

Note that while all these persons are male, women in the group may, if they wish, change the gender of the person they represent.

Now ask the groups simultaneously to conduct round-table discussions on the topic "The Responsibility of Citizens to Obey Public Authority." Have the person who takes the role of Peter argue the case as he or she believes Peter might do it, and so on with each of the characters. Suggest that each person in a group make a brief opening statement to be followed by a free discussion among the small-group members. This discussion will ordinarily require a minimum of thirty minutes, but the leader should be alert to bring the whole group back together whenever that seems most useful. If one or two groups seem to have little to say, the leader can join them for a few minutes and take the role of a third apostle or a third high-priestly personage.

The Follow-up Discussion: When the round table has gone on long enough for people to have been excited by their roles and the issues, terminate the round table and bring the entire group back together. Let the emphasis in this discussion be on looking for the ways in which the same issues that plagued the ancient church are present among us today.

Questions might include these:

What conflicts do we feel between our faith and public expectations of us?

Do we know the names of any Christians who are in jail today because of their faith? In this country? Around the world?

Do we personally experience such tensions between our faith and current laws and public morality? If not, is that because the dominant culture is Christian, or is it because our Christian faith has gotten lost in current cultural patterns?

8. Who Owns the Gospel?

Design: One of the ways in which the dilemma of Christ and culture comes to us is in the possibility that the Christian faith has become the possession of certain interest groups. Sometimes the charge is made that Christianity has become the possession of the rich and the powerful or, again, that the faith has been bent to the self-interests of the middle class. Alternatively, there are now theological positions that argue that only the poor and the disinherited are able to understand the depths of this faith. In response to this, some believe that Christianity is relative to time and circumstance and must be relevant to changing needs and problems. Others believe that Christianity is a set of universal truths that transcend the contingencies of different situations and the interests of any groups.

This exercise is a private reflection on these issues. People often do their most serious thinking about value choices after the group session in which the issues are raised. Therefore, it is useful occasionally to distribute a written exercise for people to take with them and ponder at leisure and in privacy. The leader may wish to ask that they be returned anonymously, thus assuring privacy but providing a profile of group attitudes. If such a profile is tabulated, the results should be shared with the group, if that will not reveal any individual responses. The sheets can be distributed with little or no introduction, except it should be emphasized that the sheet is a guide for reflection and not a scientific survey.

The Attitude Sheet:

Consider each of the following statements and think about your own agreement or disagreement. Place a *1* before any statement with which you strongly agree, a *2* before any with which you mildly agree, a *3* before any with which you mildly disagree, and a *4* before any with which you strongly disagree.

___ Christian religious ideas today largely represent middle-class values that are not useful to poor and oppressed people.

___ Christian religious ideas are universal truths and do not represent the biases of any class or group.

___ Christian ideas are deeply influenced by the social and economic condition of those who hold them, but there are elements in the Christian gospel that transcend selfish interests.

___ The poor and oppressed need to develop a Christian theology of their own, independent of traditional ideas that are especially the possession of those who are not poor.

___ Christian ideas have been partly perverted to the selfish interests of wealth and power, and, therefore, for the good of all, we need to reinterpret ideas like freedom and justice in ways that enhance the struggle of those who are striving for liberation.

When you have finished, ponder your reasons. Reflect on the consequences of your opinion. What biases, if any, do you feel you reflect? Would you expect poor people to believe as you do? If not, why? Do your emotions and your ideas go in different directions on any of these statements?

Further Suggestions

1. *I am someone who believes . . . .* This is a commonly used values clarification exercise[4] which is easily adapted to the many issues that arise in relation to Christ and culture. Devise a series of statements, each of which begins with "I am someone who believes." Here are some examples.

I am someone who believes—

that God has a plan for us in this world, and we must seek to form a society reflecting that plan.

that society is too corrupt to be transformed, so we must live as best we can within it.

that because we are human we are sinful, so we must have laws to restrain our sin and corruption.

These statements are duplicated on sheets to be distributed with a place to mark *yes* or *no* after them.

2. *An energy pie.*[5] How should our church be expending its energy in program, time, and money? Have people draw a circle and then divide it into pie slices representing their priorities for the church. Items to be considered may include:

helping people to understand the Bible;
providing retreats so that people can grow spiritually;

trying to increase the community of Christians;
helping people to understand society more, so that they can better perform their Christian duty in it.

3. *I resent . . . I appreciate . . .* Toward the close of a faith exploration, it is useful to have some summing-up experiences, and it is important to facilitate the expression of negative feelings. Since people are rather reluctant to do this, an arbitrary device gives permission. Ask each person first to say something negative about the previous weeks as the price for giving a frank opinion. This provides valuable critical feedback without threatening either the person giving it or the leader.

4. *A simulation based on Acts 15*. This can be designed by the leader using the model found in chapter 4 in the story of Thecla, or an excellent full-scale simulation can be found in *Using Biblical Simulations,* revolving around the Council at Jerusalem.[6]

Further Reading

Benne, Robert. *Wandering in the Wilderness: Christians and the New Culture.* Philadelphia: Fortress, 1972. A plan for parish renewal through "covenant groups" in relation to changing social and cultural needs.

Forel, George, ed. *Christian Social Teachings.* Minneapolis: Augsburg Publishing House, 1971. A collection of classical biblical and historical sources, useful as a reference and for reflection on the issues of "Christ and culture."

Niebuhr, H. Richard. *Christ and Culture.* New York: Harper and Row, 1956. The classic study on which this chapter is primarily based, readable for the concerned lay person.

Shinn, Roger L. *Tangled World.* New York: Scribners, 1975. Based on a television series, this is a popular effort to bring theology to bear on social and cultural problems, raising issues without propounding answers.

Wilmore, Gayraud S. *The Secular Relevance of the Church.* Philadelphia: Westminster Press, 1962. A simply written study of the church and contemporary social problems, with guides for study and discussion.

Chapter IV
SLIPPERY SEX ROLES

For most of human history women have been understood in one of two ways: as chattel at the disposal of males or as subjects of benevolent male authority. Men have been understood in two corresponding ways: as owners of female resources of fertility, labor, and pleasure, or as the benevolent stewards of female resources and guardians of feminine weakness. There is every indication that many women and some men have not been satisfied with even the most benign of these traditional adjustments between the sexes.

The inequities between men and women in our society may be rather less severe than in many other times and places. Nevertheless, there is a gathering storm of resistance to present sex-role arrangements. Every institutional system is now involved in responding to this new situation. Political and economic, educational and religious institutions, are, either under pressure or voluntarily, redefining formal structures as well as informal practices to take account of changing views of the roles of women and men.

All these changes impinge upon the church, directly and indirectly. The role of women in the leadership of the church long ago departed from Paul's literal instructions to silence, but now the change is from minor roles of leadership in acceptably feminine offices to major policy offices, both volunteer and professional. Every major decision-making body is under pressure to have substantial or even proportional female representation.

Leadership changes, however, may be only the outer layer of profound changes taking place in the lives of the people who make up religious communities. The churches are largely organized around the traditional family. Now there are many families with working mothers who are both too tired and too sophisticated to do what they have always done at home and in the church. At the same time their jobs release different expectations in them. The church is called to provide creative and sensitive guidance to persons struggling with these issues. Value questions, whether personal, social, or political, are interlaced with technical questions. Therefore, the church must pick through the complex issues in search of the value choices on which its tradition may provide wisdom. We can state these choices in the form of three basic questions.

Some New and Difficult Questions

1. *Biology*. Are our social arrangements between the sexes based primarily upon biology, or are they to a significant extent based upon social learning? If they are rigidly biological, changes may be impossible or disastrous. If sex roles are based on socialized attitudes, then they may be subject to creative change.

On the basis of scientific investigations, it is not precisely clear what sex differences are biological or genetic. Many of the characteristics we have long assumed to be biological in origin turn out to be learned so early and so subtly that we are largely unaware of their origins. Emotional attitudes revolving around sex, parenthood, the vocations of homemaker and breadwinner, do not seem to have any direct biological base. The virtues of tenderness, compassion, and intuition, as well as the contrasting characteristics of initiative, aggressiveness, and rationality, increasingly appear to be more rooted in social attitudes than in biology.

What then are the appropriate social arrangements by which male and female carry on their life together? Biological research cannot answer that question alone. We must decide for ourselves what relevance biological data have for the values we hold. What is the significance of physical stature, hormonal balances, and reproductive structures? On an average and statistical level these differences are fairly clear, but what they imply about behavior is a matter of judgment. These judgments were once quite universal in our society, but now they are subjects of discord and controversy, influencing judgment on each of the successive difficult questions.

2. *Family.* What functions does the family serve in the birth and nurture of children, and how can these be met without placing undue burdens on one sex? Biology has dictated that the responsibilities of childbirth fall on women. Traditionally, society also has placed the responsibility for nurturing children primarily if not exclusively on women. Probably the greatest impetus for change in the role of women has come from the development of contraception, which makes childbirth avoidable and thus increases the range of freedom available to women. Economic changes make large families a liability where once they were an asset. In addition, world population problems are contributing to an ethos in which children are coming to be regarded more as a personal choice than as a social duty. Many responsibilities for children have been shifted from the family to public institutions, as in the case of education.

The result is that women are not tied to the home by grim necessity, but when they remain in the home, many of the satisfactions and much of the respect formerly surrounding their homemaking have disappeared. While many women remain content with the role of wife and mother, others are struggling for a way of life that permits power and autonomy either through financial and vocational independence or through redefining their relationship to husband and children. Men are also divided. Some, probably most, as special beneficiaries of the traditional system, prefer that things remain as they have been. Others, although they feel no need of their own, nevertheless respond cooperatively to the desire of women to redefine relations between the sexes. Still others enter the dialogue for new understandings, not only in response to the agitation of women but out of their own sense of dissatisfaction. Not all men are comfortable being vocationally ambitious and sexually aggressive, rational rather than emotional, analytical rather than sensitive. Believing themselves pressed into such uncomfortable expectations, they are exploring new ways of understanding their existence as men.

3. *Exploitation*. How can relations between the sexes be ordered so as to facilitate the legitimate concerns of all who are involved? It is surely no secret that women in large numbers, and not just militant liberationists, feel themselves frequently exploited and subject to personal and social discrimination. This exploitation has two basic elements.

(a) Women as sex objects. Women who are young and attractive frequently feel themselves objectified in public media and subjected personally to the seductionist approaches of male acquaintances. A society that fails to prevent the drastic increase in rape is a matter of deep disquiet among women and men sensitive to female vulnerability. Women who do not find themselves the idealized object of the cult of youth and beauty nevertheless are objectified by a culture that expects physical attractiveness or nothing from women.

(b) Women as dependents. Women take the names of the men they marry. Many experience this as a symbol of transferring dependence from one household to another. Credit restrictions under which they have long suffered represent not only economic dependence but a broad cultural resistance to female independence. Changing rules and expectations are making it easier for single and married working women, but the difficulty of married women who remain in the home is virtually unchanged. What in industry would be regarded as serfdom is tolerated in marriage—work without payment in the form of power-conferring resources. The discomfort of this situation is intensified by the instability of marriage in this society. Many women feel the humiliation even of alimony laws, which presume them to be incompetent and unable to take care of themselves without male patronage.

Feelings of dissatisfaction about all these questions are far more general than any agreement upon the appropriate responses. There are political dilemmas on the one side and intimately personal quandaries on the other. Not many of us are sure we have the answers. Does Christian faith have resources on which we may call in sorting out faithful ways to respond to these issues? Let us call to mind some of the historic values of Christian faith that may relate directly to the question of how we order relations between men and women.

Male and Female in Christian Perspective

From tribal Judaism to contemporary Protestantism the role of women has been at issue. Many believe that relevant models for appropriate behavior are difficult to find. Nevertheless, behind the centuries of humankind's tragic disobedience to the divine covenant, there can often be found the basis for a finer response to God's gracious gift in creation of sexual difference.

1. *Creation and redemption.* In the two stories of creation, two different moods are expressed so far as male and female are concerned. In Gen. 1:27 there is an equity described from the beginning. "So God created man in his own image, in the image of God he created him; male and female he created them." Both woman and man are made in the image of God. However, in the second story, in Gen. 2:18 and 22, there is the hint that woman exists for the sake of man. "Then the Lord God said, 'It is not good that the man should be alone; I will make him a helper fit for him.'" "And the rib which the Lord God had taken from the man he made into a woman and brought her to the man."

In the third chapter, in the story of the temptation, it is Eve who first succumbs to the serpent. Some women theologians regard these passages as the beginning of centuries of prejudice against women of which the Judeo-Christian tradition has been guilty. Others believe that the stories describe the goodness of God's creation in creating male and female for each other, but the "fallen character" of human nature in both men and women is constantly fracturing the beauty and goodness of each other. The curse resulting from their sin falls upon them both. Therefore, the relationship between men and women, like all other aspects of creation, is in need of redemption.

How should these passages be interpreted? What other biblical passages would throw light on our understanding of men and women? Who are some important women in the Bible? What accounts for the fact that there are so few heroines in the biblical record?

2. *Justice and love*. The biblical story tells of God's demand that everyone be treated with justice and love. This emphasis, everywhere apparent, reaches its height in the Prophets. "I will betroth you to me in righteousness and in justice, in steadfast love, and in mercy. I will betroth you to me in faithfulness; and you shall know the Lord" (Hos. 2:19). The requirements of justice and love are the marks of faithfulness to God. Whatever social and personal arrangements there are between men and women in society, they must conform to justice and be redeemed by love. The one requires fairness, equity, balance; the other is the response of mercy when these arrangements break down, as they inevitably do. Yet the passage is only secondarily a statement of the divine command, while it is first of all a statement of God's dealing with his people.

There is a gentle irony in choosing this quotation from Hosea, rather than Mic. 6:8; Amos 5:24; Isa. 30:18; or any of dozens of passages in which the requirements of righteousness and mercy are laid down. Hosea here uses his experience of an unfaithful wife, whether personal or fictitious, to illustrate Israel's unfaithfulness to God. Israel is, of course, made up of both men and women. Does the book hold only the women of Israel responsible for the nation's faithfulness? Certainly not. Harlotry may have been a powerful analogy ready at hand for Hosea, but the analogy itself may be a mark of the incompleteness of even the prophet's vision of the nature of love and justice. Even the grandest vision of human faithfulness is nevertheless human and therefore always imperfect. Unfortunately, it is all too often the already disadvantaged who are further maligned by our imperfect vision.

It is important therefore to note that the biblical understanding of justice and love has a peculiar bias on behalf of the disadvantaged. Given our history, that bias must include women. The Bible is filled with injunctions for fair treatment to the fatherless, the widow, and the stranger at the gate. In Jesus' parable of judgment, the elect are those who minister to the hungry, the thirsty, the stranger, the naked, the sick, or the prisoner. There is a kind of compensatory justice that emerges in these passages. Does that have some relevance for the reordering of relations between men and women?

3. *Vocation and worth.* Pauline Christianity frequently describes conversion to this faith as a calling to which the Christian is to respond and remain faithful. At the same time, every person possesses gifts which are to be faithfully dispatched. Protestant Christianity has taken this biblical idea as the basis for understanding Christian responsibility in the world. Thus, we are expected to perform the function of a vocation as a divine calling. As in the New Testament, differences in vocation denote differences in function and, in theory at least, not differences in worth. In fact, the calling in Christ neutralizes differences in value. The grandest statement of this comes from Paul when he writes to the Galatians: "There is neither Jew nor Greek, there is neither slave nor free, there is neither male nor female; for you are all one in Christ Jesus" (Gal. 3:28).

The Christian understanding of vocation does not imply differences in value. If women are called to certain vocations and not to others, that can imply no difference in value. However, that may be a statement more honored in the breach than in reality. In our society, at least, people are judged more by their vocation than by any other single characteristic. Persons are introduced to one another by the job they do. One consequence is that the worth of persons is determined by their job. And by that criterion, women in our society have lesser status. It is no wonder then that many women seek to establish their own worth independently of any man and on the basis of a calling that is significant and prestigious.

What relevance does the Christian understanding of calling have for our ordering of male and female roles? Does it require that we change society so that people will be regarded equally no matter what their job or function is? Or does it require that women join the ranks of men in the competition for jobs that carry high social value? Are there other ways of understanding the roles of men and women so that invidious distinctions are not involved? These are some aspects of the Christian heritage to have in mind as we ponder the possible values to use in defining sexual distinctions. What other aspects of this tradition are important and relevant to this reflection?

Useful Scriptural References

Genesis 1–3
Judges 4, 5
the book of Ruth
Isaiah 3:11-12
Amos 5:21-24
Luke 10:38-42
I Corinthians 12:4-26
Galatians 3:23-29

Strategies and Exercises

1. Biblical Round Table

Design: This strategy provides an opportunity to explore imaginatively various depictions of women in the Bible as intensively as time and the inclination of the group permit. It can be an interest and awareness stimulator or an alternative way to do an in-depth study of women in the Bible.

Method: Suggest to the group that one way to understand better the roles of women in the Bible is to reconstruct imaginatively the situations of various biblical women. To do this you are going to divide into small groups of two to four people. Each group will choose one person to play the biblical woman their group is assigned to research. (It can be open for men to play these roles as well as women.) The others in the group will help this person develop a response to the topic of the round-table discussion, How I See My Role as a Woman.

Below is a list of women who might be assigned to the various groups. You may reduce or extend this list. It would be useful, however, to include in your selection some women who followed the traditional role of wife and mother and some who participated more fully in the public life of Israel or the early Christian church, so that a dialogue might emerge.

After assigning each group a woman, give each the relevant biblical references to research the likely position and views of its woman. In an hour-long session, only about twenty minutes should be spent in group preparation. If you have a longer session or are spreading the round table out over a couple of sessions, then each group can also consult various biblical commentaries or interpretations for more in-depth study.

Call the groups back together and have the people who are representing the women gather around a table or in a circle. Ask one to begin the discussion of how she sees her role as a woman. In an hour session this discussion can last only about twenty minutes. If a longer time is available it may be pursued longer, providing *at least* fifteen minutes is left for follow-up.

After stopping the round table, have people drop their roles and discuss how it felt to play these parts. Did they identify with their part, or did they have a hard time keeping in the role? Ask the others how they felt. Did they feel unsympathetic to some of the women? Then explore how the experience of twentieth-century women compares to the experience of these women. What relevance, if any, do these women in the Bible have to women today, and to the discussion of changing sex roles?

List of Possible Women to Include in a Biblical Round Table:

Sarah: Gen. 12:10-20; 16:1-7; 17:15-21; 18:1-15; 20; 21:1-14

Rachel: Gen. 29:12-35; 30:1-36
Deborah: Judg. 4:4-16; 5
Miriam: Exod. 15:19-21; Num. 12
Mary, mother of Jesus: Matt. 1:18-25; 2:8-11; Luke 1:26-56; 2:4-7, 15-20
Mary and Martha: Luke 10:38-42; John 11:1-40; 12:1-8 (Both of these women should be played if one is.)
Mary Magdalene: Matt. 27:55-61; 28:1-10; Mark 15:40-41; Mark 16; John 19:25; 20:1-18

2. Autobiographical Exploration of Sex Roles

Design: A starting point for many discussions about sex roles can be an exploration of the roles to which members of the group have been socialized. In the following exercise people are asked to complete a number of statements about the role expectations they learned from various sources and to make some judgments about them.

Method: The following exercise can be duplicated and given to people to complete privately. Answers may be as brief or as lengthy as the individual wishes, but spontaneous replies should be encouraged. Afterward, participants can divide into small groups to discuss the notions that molded their ideas about sex roles, their feelings about these, and their hopes or fears for sex roles in the future. Remind people that while significant sharing greatly aids the exploration of the issues, no one should feel compelled to share more than he or she is comfortable revealing.

The exercise:

Complete the following statements for your own sex.

My parents told me that boys/girls should . . .
The school told me that boys/girls should . . .
The church told me that boys/girls should . . .

My parents told me that a man/a woman should . . .
The school told me that a man/a woman should . . .
The church told me that a man/a woman should . . .

My greatest joy in being a man/a woman is . . .
My greatest pain in being a man/a woman is . . .
My greatest anger in being a man/a woman is . . .

The thing I would most like to change about my sex is . . .
The thing I would most like to change about the opposite sex is . . .

3. Who Should Be Able to Be a ______________ ?

Design: This exercise is designed to be done with the one following, Roles in the Church. Putting exercises into cycles is often an effective way of getting people to look at an issue from a number of viewpoints and to see how coherent their value responses are. These two exercises can reveal whether people have a set of expectations within the church different from outside the church. Are people more or less willing to change church roles than secular roles?

Method: Give all persons a sheet with a list of occupations on it. Have them check whether they think men only, women only, or both sexes should be able to do each job. Tell them you would like to make a profile of how the group feels about these occupations, so they should *not* put their names on their papers. Instead, have the papers turned in anonymously or put in a ballot box. At this point the group might take a break while some volunteers tabulate the results. After the results are tabulated and posted, people can discuss their reactions to the group profile. If there are some occupations that a number of people feel only men or only women should do, the reasons for this sex differentiation can be explored.

Suggested Occupations List:

Check the *M* column by each occupation that you feel only men should have. Check the *W* column by each occupation that you feel only women should have. Check the *B* column by each occupation that you feel both men and women can have.

Occupations	**M**	**W**	**B**
professor	—	—	—
corporation executive	—	—	—
nursery/preschool teacher	—	—	—
janitor	—	—	—
nurse	—	—	—

Occupations	**M**	**W**	**B**
cook/chef	__	__	__
counselor	__	__	__
army combatant	__	__	__
social worker	__	__	__
farmer	__	__	__
lawyer	__	__	__
chemist	__	__	__
doctor	__	__	__
pilot	__	__	__
homemaker	__	__	__
construction worker	__	__	__
plumber	__	__	__
electrician	__	__	__
truck driver	__	__	__
secretary	__	__	__

4. Roles in the Church

Design: This is an exercise on attitudes toward women in leadership roles in the church. It most usefully follows the preceding exercise or a discussion of changing sex roles. People are asked what sex-role changes they personally are willing to accept in the church. A group profile is made, which lets participants see how closely their feelings correspond to those of the group as a whole. More importantly, a comparison of the group's profile with the current practice of their church opens the way for a discussion of whether the group's responses reflect the acted-on values of the church or not. In conjunction with Who Should Be Able to Be a __________? the opportunity is also presented to compare the reasons given here to limit or to expand equal employment in the church with the reasons given in relation to secular employment.

Method: Give everyone a copy of the chart below. (The nomenclature can be changed to reflect your church more accurately.) Explain that this chart offers a chance to express anonymously whom they are willing to have fill each of the listed positions in their church. If they want men only in a given position, they are to check the *M* column, if women only, the *W* column. If they are willing to have either a man or a woman (or both men and women) in a given position, then they are to check the *E/B* column. Make a group profile as suggested in the preceding exercise.

Once the profile is completed and posted, go down the list as a group and mark which sex actually does each job in their church—men only, women only, or both. It is useful to put the number of men and the number of women on the various committees. A group discussion can then begin, letting people express how they feel about their own position in relation to the group's responses as a whole and exploring the unity (or lack of it) between the group's response and the church's practice. Is the church practicing traditional role assignment while the group is willing to accept departure from this? Or, has the church departed from traditional role assignments and is the group unhappy about this? Can the group think of reasons for these discrepancies and see any way to make their values the acted-on values of their church? If done in a cycle with Who Should Be Able to Be a ______ ? discussion can conclude in an exploration of whether the group wishes to treat the sexes differently inside and outside of the church. If so, why?

Suggested Chart of Church Positions:

Who would you be willing to have fill the following jobs in your church?

Position		**M**	**W**	**E/B**
senior minister		—	—	—
associate minister		—	—	—
finance committee (e.g., trustees)	—chairperson	—	—	—
	—member	—	—	—
policy committee (e.g., elders)	—chairperson	—	—	—
	—member	—	—	—

Position		**M**	**W**	**E/B**
pastoral support committee (e.g., deacons)				
	—chairperson	___	___	___
	—member	___	___	___
Sunday school teacher	—preschool	___	___	___
	—elementary	___	___	___
	—high school	___	___	___
minister/director of Christian education		___	___	___
choir director		___	___	___
secretary		___	___	___
custodian		___	___	___
ushers		___	___	___
coffee hour/social function workers		___	___	___

5. Who Gets the Boot?

Design: In this strategy a small business firm must choose whom to fire. It is designed to be a lively way to show us how we consider sex in relation to such values as age, seniority, competency, and economic need. It is a good strategy to use in an intergenerational group—both young and old can enjoy it. It also gives people a chance to identify with a perspective that may not be their own, and thus develop a more sympathetic understanding of the other person.

Method I: Relate the situation to the group and brief them on the list of employees. Then divide into smaller groups of three to six persons, and tell each group that it is an advisory board that must recommend to the businessman, using his criteria, whom he should fire.

Method II: Relate the situation to the groups and assign or ask for volunteers to play each of the employees. Each of these people should then argue for his or her own self-interest, that is, why he or she should stay and someone else should be fired. Those not assigned a role may assume the role of the businessman and ask for further justifications or clarifications or offer rebuttals to

various people. At the end, all participants should cast ballots listing the people they would fire.

The Situation:

Due to worsening economic conditions and a severe cutback in orders, the owner of a small business must reduce his staff from ten to five persons. He is concerned about the profitability of his business, but, at the same time, he wishes to be sensitive to humanitarian values. His employees are:

1. A very competent married middle-aged woman who works because she enjoys the job and likes having some money she can call her own.
2. A very competent single young man who joined the firm about ten months ago and looks as if he could go far.
3. A divorced woman in her thirties with three children, aged three to seven, who is working to support herself and her young family. She clearly works because she needs the money and is absent frequently because of the children's illnesses.
4. A man in his thirties who has a wife and two children he must support. He clearly does not have his heart in his job—it is just a way to earn money.
5. A young single woman who was hired just shortly before the competent young man described above. She, too, is very able and could go far.
6. A fifty-eight-year-old married man who has been with the firm for twenty-five years. At this point, he has something of a drinking problem, causing him frequently to be late or absent.
7. A fifty-five-year-old widow who is very pleasant, but not terribly efficient. The job keeps her from becoming too lonely, as well as supplementing her otherwise meager income from her late husband's estate.
8. A middle-aged married man whose wife has a good job and whose two children have left home. They could live on his wife's salary.
9. A middle-aged married man whose wife also works and who has one child in high school and two in college.
10. A middle-aged married woman who works to help make ends meet while she and her husband put their son through college.

6. Male/Female Communication[2]

Design: This strategy is an effective way to develop a dialogue between the men and women in a group on their respective perceptions and assumptions about the opposite sex. It usually reveals a number of generalizations about men and women that do not hold up in the ensuing dialogue and often makes people more aware of both the advantages and disadvantages of current sex roles.

Method: Divide into small, same-sex groups of three to six persons. Give each of the groups four large sheets of paper with one of the following questions at the top of each sheet. Make sure the male groups get the questions for men, the female groups the questions for women. Tell the groups which question to look at first and when to move on to the next question. Five minutes per question is usually sufficient. During this time, the group is to list all the responses to the given question on which they generally agree. (If, for example, only one person in a group feels a certain way, that response should be omitted unless a way is found to phrase it so that others agree.)

Suggested Questions:

Questions for Men

1. What are the advantages of being a woman?
2. What are the disadvantages of being a woman?
3. What makes me feel like a man?
4. What makes a woman feel like a woman?

Questions for Women

1. What are the advantages of being a man?
2. What are the disadvantages of being a man?
3. What makes me feel like a woman?
4. What makes a man feel like a man?

When all four questions have been completed, each male group should exchange lists with one female group. After looking at the other group's lists, the two groups can then come together and address themselves to such questions as:

How accurate were the perceptions of the other?
Were there any surprises? What feelings did the lists arouse?

Were there any overall feelings about the nature of male vs. female lives (for example, men have the advantage professionally, women personally)?

Were there any positive or negative feelings about what made people feel like a man or like a woman?

7. Sex-Role Reversal Dramas:

Design: This strategy involves role-playing in which the roles of men and women are reversed. Apparently equitable situations may be revealed by this device to be far from such an abstract ideal. The extent to which the reversal seems ludicrous indicates the gulf between our reality and the ideal. In fact, these reversals are often useful for getting people in touch with just how much equality they really want.

Method: Refer to the guidelines for role-playing in chapter 2. Tell people you would like to do some role-playing to explore the issue of sex-role equality and ask for volunteers. Describe the role-play situation. Give the actors a little time to consider their parts, then begin. When they have played out the given situation, stop and give them the reverse situation to play.

After they have finished, have them react to the situation. Did they find the situation particularly difficult to play one way or the other? Did it seem absolutely ludicrous to them one way? Why? What about the audience? What different responses did the situation and its reverse arouse in them? Did anybody feel that they would have responded very differently than the role-players? Would they like to play out the situation? (Frequently someone in the audience does respond differently and wants to do this.)

Role-play 1: Husband and wife are both young professionals. The husband is offered a much better job in a city five hundred miles away. He comes home and starts trying to persuade his wife to move. (The group can decide what jobs both people have and otherwise flesh out these characters.)

The reversal: The entire situation is kept the same, except this time it is the wife who gets offered the much better job five hundred miles away and tries to persuade her husband to move.

Role-play 2: The policy-making board of the church has eight men and two women. They are in the midst of a discussion of whether to nominate more women in a conscious effort to secure equal sex representation on the board. (Ask people to assume various viewpoints in discussing this issue.)
The reversal: The board is made up of eight women and two men. The same perspectives now should be represented in relation to the opposite sex.

8. The Trial of Thecla and Paul[3]
Introduction:
In the New Testament Apocrypha there are several stories about women who assumed active roles of leadership in the early church. Of these, probably the story of Thecla is the most important. It is included in the apocryphal book the Acts of Paul and is one of only two parts of this book that has survived in full. Its survival has been attributed to the fact that the story of Thecla was often related independently of the rest of the Acts of Paul as an inspiration for women wishing to enter monastic orders in the fourth and fifth centuries. The story of Thecla was probably a local historical legend related to Paul. It was written before A.D. 190 and is referred to by Tertullian.
This story raises many of the sex-role issues that are currently confronting people in the church. It touches the issue of women's rights in relation to marriage, authority, ordination, and the apostolic mission.
Purpose of the Simulation:
A full-scale simulation of this kind is intended to help people come to an understanding of the story by actually participating in a re-creation of the original events. The simulation also illustrates a methodology that might be used in exploring other situations in the Bible or in the history of the church in which a conflict occurred that is still pertinent today.

In a simulation, people play out the significant features of a given event. They are asked to immerse themselves fully in the event and to feel the force of the situation as the original participants might have: to feel the limitations and the freedoms, the struggles and the decisions. It is hoped that, in the course of doing this, the event might come alive in a way that normal biblical or historical study often does not.

The simulation is neither pure drama nor pure scientific reproduction. Participants should begin by trying to portray as accurately as possible the significant features of the original situation, but once the simulation is under way, and people are feeling the force of the original events, they may go where the force leads them. A discussion period follows the simulation to let people express how they were affected by the experience and to explore the reasons for any differences between their re-enactment and the actual event.

The Simulation Situation:

Everyone is gathered at the trial of Thecla and Paul. Thamyris, Thecla's fiancé, has brought Paul and Thecla before the Governor because Paul's teachings concerning asceticism and Christianity have made Thecla unwilling to fulfill her betrothal vow. Thecla has said she wants to follow Christ instead of marrying Thamyris. Thamyris feels Thecla should be punished for breaking her vow, and that Paul should also be punished for encouraging women to break their betrothal and marriage vows. The Governor, Castelius, must decide who, if anyone, is guilty.

Simulation Preparation:

Before attempting the simulation, leaders or facilitators should make themselves thoroughly familiar with the material here.

When the group assembles, the facilitator should explain what a simulation is and give the above background information. Then the group should be divided into four subgroups and assigned one of the following roles:

1. Thecla and her supporters
2. Paul and his supporters

3. Thamyris and his supporters
4. Castelius and lesser judges (his advisors)

Each group should then be given copies of the simulation situation, the background notes for their particular group, and the text printed below from the Acts of Paul. These will be their aids in preparing for the trial scene. They should be asked to study these materials, to choose the person who will play Paul, Thecla, Thamyris, or Castelius, to select a note-taker for their group, and to develop a good defense (or offense) for their person. If time permits, the three groups appearing before the judges might also discuss their strategy about what witnesses they would call to support their case and assign people within their group to play these roles. In any case, a minimum of half an hour will be needed for groups to formulate adequately their positions. If a group meets regularly it could prepare the simulation one week and enact it the following week. The simulation can be made as elaborate or as simple as is desired.

During the group preparation time, the facilitator should be prepared to assist people in any way necessary—providing further materials or references, clarifying the nature of the task, and helping any group having difficulty understanding their task.

Text to be distributed to each group:[4]

From the Acts of Paul, II: The Story of Paul and Thecla

5 And when Paul entered into the house of Onesiphorus, there was great joy, and bowing of knees and breaking of bread, and the word of God concerning abstinence and the resurrection; for Paul said:

Blessed are the pure in heart, for they shall see God.

Blessed are they that keep the flesh chaste, for they shall become the temple of God.

Blessed are they that abstain, for unto them shall God speak.

Blessed are they that have renounced this world, for they shall be well-pleasing unto God.

Blessed are they that possess their wives as though they had them not, for they shall inherit God.

Blessed are they that have the fear of God, for they shall become angels of God.

6 Blessed are they that tremble at the oracles of God, for they shall be comforted.

Blessed are they that receive the wisdom of Jesus Christ, for they shall be called sons of the Most High.

Blessed are they that have kept their baptism pure, for they shall rest with the Father and with the Son.

Blessed are they that have compassed the understanding of Jesus Christ, for they shall be in the light.

Blessed are they that for love of God have departed from the fashion of this world, for they shall judge angels, and shall be blessed at the right hand of the Father.

Blessed are the merciful, for they shall obtain mercy and shall not see the bitter day of judgement.

Blessed are the bodies of the virgins, for they shall be well-pleasing unto God and shall not lose the reward of their continence, for the word of the Father shall be unto them a work of salvation in the day of his Son, and they shall have rest world without end.

7 And as Paul was saying these things in the midst of the assembly in the house of Onesiphorus, a certain virgin, Thecla, whose mother was Theocleia, which was betrothed to an husband, Thamyris, sat at the window hard by, and hearkened night and day unto the word concerning chastity which was spoken by Paul: and she stirred not from the window, but was led onward by faith, rejoicing exceedingly: and further, when she saw many women and virgins entering in to Paul, she also desired earnestly to be accounted worthy to stand before Paul's face and to hear the word of Christ; for she had not yet seen the appearance of Paul, but only heard his speech.

8 Now as she removed not from the window, her mother sent unto Thamyris, and he came with great joy as if he were already to take her to wife. Thamyris therefore said to Theocleia: Where is my Thecla? And Theocleia said: I have a new tale to tell thee, Thamyris: for three days and three nights Thecla ariseth not from the window, neither to eat nor to drink, but looking earnestly as it were upon a joyful spectacle, she so attendeth to a stranger who teacheth deceitful and various words, that I marvel how the great modesty of the maiden is so hardly beset.

9 O Thamyris, this man upsetteth the whole city of the Iconians, and thy Thecla also, for all the women and the young men go in to him and are taught by him. Ye must, saith he, fear one only God and live chastely. And my daughter, too, like a spider at the window, bound by his words, is held by a new desire and a fearful passion: for she hangeth

upon the things that he speaketh, and the maiden is captured. But go thou to her and speak to her; for she is betrothed unto thee.

10 And Thamyris went to her, alike loving her and fearing because of her disturbance, and said: Thecla, my betrothed, why sittest thou thus? and what passion is it that holdeth thee in amaze; turn unto thy Thamyris and be ashamed. And her mother also said the same: Thecla, why sittest thou thus, looking downward, and answering nothing, but as one stricken? And they wept sore, Thamyris because he failed of a wife, and Theocleia of a child, and the maidservants of a mistress; there was, therefore, great confusion of mourning in the house. And while all this was so, Thecla turned not away, but paid heed to the speech of Paul.

11 But Thamyris leapt up and went forth into the street and watched them that went in to Paul and came out. And he saw two men striving bitterly with one another, and said to them: Ye men, tell me who ye are, and who is he that is within with you, that maketh the souls of young men and maidens to err, deceiving them that there may be no marriages but they should live as they are. I promise therefore to give you much money if ye will tell me of him: for I am a chief man of the city.

12 And Demas and Hermogenes said unto him: Who this man is, we know not; but he defraudeth the young men of wives and the maidens of hubsands, saying: Ye have no resurrection otherwise, except ye continue chaste, and defile not the flesh but keep it pure.

13 And Thamyris said to them: Come, ye men, into mine house and refresh yourselves with me. And they went to a costly banquet and much wine and great wealth and a brilliant table. And Thamyris made them drink, for he loved Thecla and desired to take her to wife: and at the dinner Thamyris said: Tell me, ye men, what is his teaching, that I also may know it; for I am not a little afflicted concerning Thecla because she so loveth the stranger, and I am defrauded of my marriage.

14 And Demas and Hermogenes said: Bring him before Castelius the governor as one that persuadeth the multitudes with the new doctrine of the Christians; and so will he destroy him and thou shalt have thy wife Thecla. And we will teach thee of that resurrection which he asserteth, that it is already come to pass in the children which we have, and we rise again when we have come to the knowledge of the true God.

15 But when Thamyris heard this of them, he was filled with envy and wrath, and rose up early and went to the house of Onesiphorus with the rulers and officers and a great crowd with staves, saying unto Paul: Thou hast destroyed the city of the Iconians and her that was espoused unto me, so that she will not have me: let us go unto Castelius the

governor. And all the multitude said: Away with the wizard, for he hath corrupted all our wives. And the multitude rose up together against him.

16 And Thamyris, standing before the judgement seat, cried aloud and said: O proconsul, this is the man—we know not whence he is—who alloweth not maidens to marry: let him declare before thee wherefore he teacheth such things. And Demas and Hermogenes said to Thamyris: Say thou that he is a Christian, and so wilt thou destroy him. But the governor kept his mind steadfast and called Paul, saying unto him: Who art thou, and what teachest thou? for it is no light accusation that these bring against thee.

17 And Paul lifted up his voice and said: If I am this day examined what I teach, hearken, O proconsul. The living God, the God of vengeance, the jealous God, the God that hath need of nothing, but desireth the salvation of men, hath sent me, that I may sever them from corruption and uncleanness and all pleasure and death, that they may sin no more. Wherefore God hath sent his own Child, whom I preach and teach that men should have hope in him who alone hath had compassion upon the world that was in error; that men may no more be under judgement but have faith and the fear of God and the knowledge of sobriety and the love of truth. If then I teach the things that have been revealed unto me of God, what wrong do I, O proconsul? And the governor having heard that, commanded Paul to be bound and taken away to prison until he should have leisure to hear him more carefully.

18 But Thecla at night took off her bracelets and gave them to the doorkeeper, and when the door was opened for her she went into the prison, and gave the jailer a mirror of silver and so went in to Paul and sat by his feet and heard the wonderful works of God. And Paul feared not at all, but walked in the confidence of God: and her faith also was increased as she kissed his chains.

19 Now when Thecla was sought by her own people and by Thamyris, she was looked for through the streets as one lost; and one of the fellow-servants of the doorkeeper told that she went out by night. And they examined the doorkeeper and he told them that she was gone to the stranger unto the prison; and they went as he told them and found her as it were bound with him, in affection. And they went forth thence and gathered the multitude to them and showed it to the governor.

20 And he commanded Paul to be brought to the judgement seat; but Thecla rolled herself upon the place where Paul taught when he sat in the prison. And the governor commanded her also to be brought to the judgement seat, and she went exulting with joy. And when Paul was

brought the second time the people cried out more vehemently: He is a sorcerer, away with him! But the governor heard Paul gladly concerning the holy works of Christ: and he took counsel, and called Thecla and said: Why wilt thou not marry Thamyris, according to the law of the Iconians? but she stood looking earnestly upon Paul, and when she answered not, her mother Theocleia cried out, saying: Burn the lawless one, burn her that is no bride in the midst of the theatre, that all the women who have been taught by this man may be affrighted.

Background Notes for Thecla and Her Supporters:

You are a young woman who has been betrothed to Thamyris. In your society, this means that he already has virtually all the rights of a husband over you. Thus, most people feel your fiancé is justified in his anger at you for failing to fulfill his rights. You were betrothed before you heard Paul preach, however, and now you wish to become a follower of Christ. You know that a man would rarely be prosecuted for breaking his betrothal vow. You feel you have as much right as any man to become an active follower of Christ. From what you have heard, the surest way for you to become a true follower is to remain a virgin and pursue the ascetic life. Devoting yourself fully to Christ has become your main desire. You do not know whether Paul will personally support you at your trial, but you know what you feel you must do if you are to follow his gospel.

Background Notes for Thamyris and His Supporters:

You feel betrayed by Thecla and are very angry with Paul. In your society, once a man is betrothed he has virtually all the rights that a husband has over his wife. You support your society's belief that a woman's place is in the home and feel that Paul is threatening the primacy of the home with his teachings. In your opinion, Paul is a destroyer of marriages, and you want him dealt with by the authorities accordingly—after all, he seems to have taken Thecla away from you. Furthermore, you would like Thecla punished for her waywardness. To this end you determine to bring both of them before the Governor, Castelius, to seek justice.

Background Notes for Paul and His Supporters:

You have been preaching in Iconium for several days and suddenly find yourself arrested and accused of taking men's wives away. When asked what you teach, you tell the Governor, but you do so in rather general terms. Your defense is that you preach the word of God and the hope for all in salvation. You do not directly support Thecla at the trial. Sometimes your position concerning women may seem somewhat ambiguous. (Remember that elsewhere you say wives should be subject to their husbands.) You may rely on the text given here entirely, or you may use other texts to support your belief in the importance of forsaking corruption and assuming the ascetic life for salvation.

Background Notes for Castelius an His Advisors:

You have been asked to judge whether Paul is guilty of making women break their marriage vows. You have also been asked to issue judgment on Thecla's refusal to marry Thamyris. She is betrothed to him, and in your society this means that she is under obligation to fulfill the marriage vows. Breaking such a vow is a serious offense. It is also, of course, a serious offense to encourage others to break their betrothal or marriage vows. After hearing Thamyris' charge, you question first Paul and then Thecla about their response to Thamyris' accusations. You are a curious judge and want people to explain themselves fully.

The Simulation: After the preparation period, have the groups reassemble. Arrange a courtroom setting, or have the four main characters sit around a table with the rest of their groups seated behind them. (Groups should have easy access to their speakers so they can caucus or otherwise support them.) Ask Castelius to begin by stating the purpose of the trial and calling on Thamyris to make his accusation. Castelius may ask any questions he desires to clarify the issues. After the defendants present their cases, he may wish to offer a chance for one response from Thamyris and one rebuttal from each defendant. Then the case could be voted on by the judges as a group, or there could be more cross-examination if time permits. A half hour should be sufficient for a simple simulation. If a more elaborate simulation is enacted, then the witnesses would appear after the initial statements as part of the rebuttal and cross-examination period.

The Follow-up Session: At this point the leader should assume control again. The actors should drop their roles, and the leader should tell the rest of the Thecla story, since it is unfamiliar to most people. Briefly, it is as follows:

> At the trial, Castelius has Paul scourged and sent from the city, but Thecla he condemns to be burned at the stake. The flames, however, do not touch her, and she is released. Immediately she goes searching for Paul. She finds him and announces her determination to become a preacher. Paul does not say she cannot, but he does say that she must undergo a temptation if she is to become worthy of an apostolic mission. Accordingly, he immediately sets up such a situation by abandoning her to the local prince of another town who wants her as his concubine. In her attempts to resist the prince, she knocks the crown off his head. This is interpreted as an act of treason, and she is brought before another court on the grounds of assaulting the Crown.
>
> At this trial, the women of the town band behind her, and a shouting match ensues between the men who uphold the supremacy of the state and the women who feel lawless attack by men on women must be stopped. Once again Thecla is condemned to death, and this time faces a series of unusual punishments in the arena. Again, however, she miraculously escapes death. As the result, she proclaims herself as one of God's anointed, baptizes herself, and gives herself the right to baptize others. When she encounters Paul again, she already has a band of followers, and he agrees that she has proved she has a charge to baptize and a commission to preach.

Remind the group that this story was an inspiration for many women in the early church. Thecla was particularly important to women who wished to enter monastic orders instead of marrying. She was referred to in many prayers and eulogized for making the role of virgin acceptable.

At this point, it is useful to get group reactions to the simulation and to the story of Thecla. What kind of feelings did the simulation arouse? Did people expect the Governor to make the decisions he did at the first trial? Were they aware of any stories about women's participation in the early Church? Do any of the issues in the Thecla tale have parallels today? How does the notion of vocation relate to the issue of sex roles?

Further Suggestions

1. Explore the creation story in Genesis and what the Fall means in terms of the present views of man and woman by doing the simulation "What Happened in the Garden?" in *Using Biblical Simulations,* Donald Miller, Graydon Snyder, Robert Neff (Valley Forge: Judson Press, 1973).
2. Ask people to bring magazines and newspapers they no longer want. Let everyone thumb through them and cut out pictures for collages representing the views of male and female common in these media.
3. Look at various denominational statements on human rights or women in church and society. Have a discussion on changing sex roles in which participants must represent several different denominational perspectives. You may then wish to explore in depth your own denomination's perspective on changing roles.
4. Role-play a pulpit search committee's meeting in which the possibility of hiring a woman minister is under discussion. She might be in competition with a man with slightly inferior credentials. Have a wide range of viewpoints represented on the committee: someone who believes strongly that it is time for the church to witness to equality by hiring a woman; someone who believes equally strongly that a woman's place is in the home; someone who personally believes in equality but does not think the church is ready for female leadership; someone who has reservations about many women but thinks this particular one would do a good job, etc.
5. Explore Paul's statements concerning male and female. How can these various statements be reconciled? Resources that might be used for such a discussion are:

Scriptural passages: I Corinthians 7; 11:1-16; 12; 14:26-40; Galatians 3.

Constance Parvey, "The Theology and Leadership of Women in the New Testament," in *Religion and Sexism,* ed. Rosemary Ruether (New York: Simon and Schuster, 1974), pp. 117-49.

Robin Scroggs, ''Paul and the Eschatological Woman,'' *Journal of the American Academy of Religion,* XL (1972), 283-303.

Further Reading

Hardesty, Nancy, and Scanzoni, Letha. *All We're Meant to Be: A Biblical Approach to Women's Liberation*. Waco: Word Books, 1975. A readable and well-researched book which analyzes afresh Old and New Testament views of women and attempts to draw implications from this re-analysis for the liberated Christian woman.

Harkness, Georgia. *Women in Church and Society*. Nashville: Abingdon, 1972. A statement on the status of women using historical and biblical resources by a theologian with a long-standing reputation.

Mollenkott, Virginia Ramey. *Women, Men, and the Bible*. Nashville: Abingdon, 1977. An evangelical author takes a close look at sex roles in the Bible and develops a theory of total personhood based on a fresh understanding of the biblical message.

Money, John, and Ehrhardt, Anke. *Man and Woman, Boy and Girl*. New York: New American Library, 1974. A rather technical book reporting on twenty years of gender research at Johns Hopkins Medical School and the implication this research has for the biology-vs.-cultural-conditioning argument concerning sex roles.

Ruether, Rosemary, ed. *Religion and Sexism*. New York: Simon & Schuster, 1974. A collection of essays on the images of woman in the Judeo-Christian tradition—indispensable for this subject.

Russell, Letty. *Human Liberation in a Feminist Perspective: A Theology*. Philadelphia: Westminster Press, 1974. A moderate view stating the special contributions to human liberation available through the unique experience of women.

Chapter V
THE USE AND ABUSE OF THE HUMAN HABITAT

Have you ever sat beside a pond on a summer afternoon and pondered the mystery and miracle of life in that small ecosystem? There are organisms discharging what others need and receiving in turn what they require. The whole exists in a delicate balance by which the conditions of life are sustained. Now by some gigantic feat of imagining we are required to make the leap from the pond to a cosmic biosphere. We ourselves live in such a balanced habitat, as wide as the world and wider. Humankind is an endangered species. Our survival is called into question by three basic threats.

Hazards to the Ecosphere

First, there is the *race between food and mouths*. It took thousands of years for world population to reach its first billion in 1850. Only eighty years were required to reach the second, thirty-one to reach the third, and now only fifteen years to reach the fourth. While the population increase is tapering off in the wealthy industrial areas, the rest of the world's population is doubling every quarter century. Even if a zero-population-growth rate were to be achieved by the year 2000, in another fifty years there would be another doubling in population.

Starvation is already rampant. One third of the world's population is malnourished, with 20 percent on or over the edge of starvation. The food available per capita worldwide has not increased in forty years, and has actually decreased in the last decade. A tragic irony is that the worst population increases are unlikely to be realized since available food supplies will not support doubling populations. The people who would be having babies die when they are babies.[1] If food production were significantly increased, this would result in higher population-growth rate, thus maintaining a constant state of misery and hopelessness.

To increase per capita agricultural food production, the amount of land under cultivation and its yield must increase. About half the world's arable land is currently under cultivation. The other half might be developed but would require tremendous capital expenditure. Even so, population would someday surpass land requirements, probably by the year 2000.[2]

Both increased agricultural use of land and the employment of "miracle seeds" require greater use of water and chemicals. Only half the necessary amount of water would be available naturally; the only source for the remainder would be sea water, which requires desalinization. This process involves large expenditures of energy and unknown climatological side effects. Chemicals used to increase food production may introduce into the ecosystem imbalances that deplete the microorganisms in the producing soil, reduce the oxygen-producing capacity of lakes and rivers, and finally move up the food chain until they become harmful to humans.

There are other lines of hope for food production to be sure. Marine fish currently provide 15 percent of the world's animal protein. But dragnet techniques that have been employed to scrape the ocean floor destroy for many years the algae beds where the fish feed and lay their eggs. Fish-pumping techniques have, for the present at least, virtually destroyed the anchoveta fishery, which formerly accounted for 20 percent of the world's fish catch. More visionary are the hopes for synthetic foods, microbiological protein production, and, perhaps, a genetic breakthrough permitting the crossing of plant and animal organisms.

All these possibilities for solving the twin problems of population and food involve *environmental stress,* the second basic threat to the survival of humankind. Every approach to the increased production of food has involved the withdrawal of resources from the biosphere and the introduction of others into the system, thereby placing strains upon the natural systems. We are left with the hideous possibility that the means by which we feed the hungry have endangered the earth.

The major disruptions to the environment have, of course, not been the result of feeding billions at a minimum standard; nor are future hazards likely to be so. Rather, the strains on the environment have been more a function of affluence. If American eating habits were applied worldwide, present agricultural output would feed only 1.2 billion instead of the 4 billion persons who must be fed.[3] In the industrial nations, production has been increasing at a rate of 7 percent a year, thus doubling every decade. At that rate, annual resource extraction would be thirty-two times larger in fifty years, and a thousand times larger in a century.

We do not really know the extent of the earth's resources, but what we do know is far from encouraging. There is the possibility of an improved technology for extracting trace elements from land and sea, but such a process will require vast expenditures of energy, the sources for which are not immediately obvious.

Every North American is aware that industrial production involves the emission of undesirable elements. We drive to work inhaling the exhaust of the cars in front of us, pass smokestacks belching pollution, give up old fishing streams because the fish have died. We dismiss these discomforts as among the costs of economic growth, but they may be the source of a pressure upon industrial growth comparable to that of starvation upon population. Even if the earth escapes the immediate pressures of this pollution, there could be another crisis in two hundred years when global thermal pollution may embroil the earth. The outer limits of industrial growth finally depend upon the capacity of the ecosphere to absorb the heat produced or transferred.

Let us suppose that all these problems were to be solved:

population tapers off soon after the year 2000; per capita food production increases to match that population; strain upon the environment is reduced to tolerable limits. The tragic fact is that we would be living in a grossly unfair world. The poor would be poorer than they are today. Vast populations would be doomed to miserable existence watching the luxury of the wealthy.

This results in the third basic threat to the survival of humankind, the threat of *nuclear war*. It is a perennial problem to try to achieve at least minimal justice in the face of forces of greed and disdain. Cruel inequities have a way of erupting into rebellion and war. Historically, rebellion has more often brought defeat to the rebels than redress of their grievances. That fact, however, is not a dependable deterrent. Poor nations may hope to lessen their misery by "wars of redistribution," to use Robert Heilbroner's phrase; the use of nuclear power in such wars threatens terrible devastation. At best, the spectacle is one of decades of threat; at worst, there is the vision of nuclear war.

A Question of Values

This recitation of the ecological problems confronting us may sound as if they are best left to experts. What enlightenment can the church and Christian faith bring to such issues? To be sure, we do need to be aware of the technical complexity of the problems we face. That is not enough, however, since there are basic questions of value involved in every proposal for solving ecological problems. The major scientific studies addressed to these issues since 1970 all include statements of the social, moral, and even religious values regarded as necessary for ecological salvation.

E. F. Schumacher, an economist seeking to address the problems of industrial growth, affirms the classical virtues of prudence, justice, courage, and temperance as the requirements for human survival.

By contrast, Robert Heilbroner expects that authoritarian political structures will be the price of human survival. In predicting the elements of a postindustrial order, he projects a view of production and consumption that is frugal rather than prodigal. Science will play a reduced role; the work ethic will wane; and, society will turn in the direction of the exploration of inner states of experience. "Tradition and ritual, the pillars of life in virtually all societies other than those of an industrial character, would probably once again assert their ancient claims as the guide to and solace for life."[4] Heilbroner further expects the struggle for individual achievement to give way to communally ordered goals. Thus he offers a moral, even theological, prediction.

The second report to the Club of Rome (*Mankind at the Turning Point*) is based on computer scenarios manipulating variables in the ecosphere, but the conclusions of the report are statements about values. Short-term considerations are subordinated to long-term possibilities. Narrow nationalism is replaced by global, concerted action. Cooperation rather than confrontation is held up as the model for successful policy. The recommendations further include "a new ethic in the use of material resources" and an attitude toward nature based on harmony rather than conquest.[5]

Whatever responses are made to the hazards facing the human habitat, questions of value are involved. It should be obvious then that there is in fact no way the church can remain aloof from the dilemmas posed by ecological crisis. The Christian's response to the crisis will involve the entire range of religious beliefs and practices that inform the view of the self, the world, and God. However, some elements in the tradition may have a direct relevance to ecological dilemmas, and it will therefore be useful to have some of these specifically in mind.

Christian Faith and Ecological Values

Understandings of nature in the Judeo-Christian tradition. Many observers have concluded that the ecological crisis is related to the disrespect and exploitation of nature. Accordingly, they believe the renewal of reverence for nature is an important clue to the solution of the crisis. The question, therefore, is, Have the understandings of nature in Christian history been a part of the problem or a clue to the answer? In response to this question there are three elements in the Christian understanding of nature that need to be considered.

1. *The earth is a divine creation.* The stories in Genesis reveal a view of nature that can be distinguished from two other ancient alternatives. Nature was often regarded as sacred—to be treated with awe and wonder and, indeed, worship. The alternative was to experience nature as demonic—something to be feared and placated. The Jewish religious spirit, however, responded to nature as God's creation. Thus, creation is good but is neither the ultimate source of meaning for human life nor a final threat to human well-being. In the first creation story the refrain after each day's creation is "And God saw that it was good." This litany culminates after the creation of man and woman with the words "And God saw everything that he had made, and behold, it was very good" (Gen. 1:31).

2. *Humankind is given dominion over the earth.*

> So God created man in his own image, in the image of God he created him; male and female he created them. And God blessed them, and God said to them, "Be fruitful and multiply, and fill the earth and subdue it; and have dominion over the fish of the sea and over the birds of the air and over every living thing that moves upon the earth." (Gen. 1:27-28)

The Bible is unequivocally human-centered. The earth is the locus of the drama of salvation, the place where God is saving persons and peoples.

3. *The earth remains a divine possession.*

> The earth is the Lord's and the fulness thereof,
> the world and those who dwell therein;
> for he has founded it upon the seas,
> and established it upon the rivers. (Ps. 24:1-2)

Humankind is the steward of the earth and not its owner. The earth and its resources may not be disposed of at will. The world is valued in and of itself as a divine creation and possession and not simply because of its usefulness to us.

Some people see these ideas as the religious basis of a sound ecological ethic in which the earth is a gracious gift of God to be used with restraint and respect. Others see these biblical ideas as supporting an exploitative attitude toward nature. It may be that science and technology have been aided in Western civilization by cultural attitudes that make nature an appropriate object of study and manipulation. The question now is, Does such an attitude make inevitable an exploitation that leads to ecological destruction?

The historical arguments are technical and complicated, but what may be more important presently is the forging of theological and ethical positions consistent with cherished values, while providing an adequate basis for living in a world of limited resources.

The dignity of work. From the Genesis story, in which God took man and put him in the garden of Eden "to till it and keep it," to Paul, the tentmaker who outlined the Christian understanding of divine "calling," there has been a religious basis for work and productivity. Protestantism has especially emphasized this point of view, now often called the Protestant Ethic. For some ecological critics, there is not likely to be a solution to our problems unless we reject the personal and social obsession with production, which inevitably involves consumption. For others, the ethic of work and responsibility is a ground for hope, since it represents the religious motivation for solving human problems.

The gospel of love and the ethic of responsibility. There are two very difficult dilemmas at the heart of ecological problems. One is the paradox of self-interest. The ecological situation is filled with horror stories, which presumably might motivate us on the basis of self-interest and self-preservation to change course, to make the necessary sacrifices, and to learn to live on a less consumptive level. It is entirely possible, however, that just such self-interest is what has gotten us where we are, and acting out of self-interest will hasten disaster.

A second dilemma is the tension between the need of the rich for total consumption to be reduced and the need of the poor for their lot to be improved. Policies adopted on the basis of the self-interest of the rich may result in disastrous conflict with the self-interest of the poor.

It is precisely the weakness of self-interest to which the ethic of love addresses its power. We are called as Christians to love our neighbor. Global ecological crisis is stretching the definition of the neighbor to include persons far removed in time and space. The horizons of our responsibility now extend to the farthest corners of the earth and to generations yet unborn. Self-interest cannot deal with responsibility so remote. In the religious understanding of life there is not a one-to-one correspondence between action and reward but, rather, a basic confidence that a response of gratitude for the love which is first freely given to us provides an ultimate reward. The specific nature and meaning of this grateful response must now be explored anew, just as every generation has had to determine the nature of its own grateful response.

The Christian hope. Analysts of the present crisis are having a very difficult time avoiding cynicism about a human future. There are technological optimists who assume that since science has shown itself so inventive, it will provide the solution to the problems it has created. That seems a hollow hope to those who see technology as the problem rather than the answer. There are moral optimists, too, who assume that human moral fiber is sufficient to undertake the titanic changes necessary for survival. Both kinds of optimists have a heavy task to convince people overcome by despair in the face of present predictions. The response has sometimes been a furious cynicism, but more frequently a quiet despair, which concluded, "There is nothing I can do."

The Christian hope has always transcended the immediate historical threat. Our faith is not in technology, and certainly not in our own moral health. We know ourselves to be sinners, people of fragile faith, with uncertain goals and unworthy motives. We know, too, that we are precious in God's sight and that he loves us in spite of our unworthiness. The risk of faith is to act as if what we hope for is already present.

Toward the end of *An Inquiry into the Human Prospect,* Heilbroner writes:

> If then by the question: "Is there hope for man?" we ask whether it is possible to meet the challenges of the future without the payment of a fearful price, the answer must be: No, there is no such hope . . . with the full spectacle of the human prospect before us, the spirit quails and the will falters.[6]

That is the kind of situation for which the Christian hope is made, forged as that faith was in the fires of the destruction of previous ages and civilizations. It is not hopeless, surrendering to disaster. Neither is it naïvely optimistic about a future that cannot be. It does not escape into other-worldly irresponsibility, since it is *this* world that we have so far been given by a gracious God. Rather, it is completely devoted to the survival of this world, *its* people and *its* grandeur, while the hope in which it finally rests is beyond the power of an ecological disaster to destroy.

Useful Scriptural References

Genesis 1, 2; 9:1-7
I Chronicles 29:1-6
Psalms 24:1-6; 104
Isaiah 51:6
Matthew 6:19-21, 25-34; 25:14-46
Acts 17:22-31

Strategies and Exercises

1. Views of Nature
Design: There are many ways to view nature and our relationship to

it. The following exercise presents a series of statements with which people are encouraged to agree or disagree. Coupled with follow-up discussion it can enable participants to clarify their own understandings about nature and humankind's relationship to it.

Method: Duplicate and distribute the following sheet. Go over the instructions together. When everyone has completed the sheet, have a discussion over such issues as:

What are the main views of nature represented in these statements?
What are the chief responses to nature suggested in these statements?
Which statements can be supported by biblical passages?
Which best reflect the needs of the world today?
Can these statements be reconciled with a Christian view of nature?
Did the statements that I agree with show any consistency or pattern?

The Sheet:

There are many ways to view nature and our relationship to it. With which of the following statements do you agree? Check the *A* column where you agree with the statement. Check the *D* column where you disagree with the statement.

A	D	
___	___	All living things are creatures of God and deserve our protection.
___	___	Nature is inherently good, but we frequently destroy or corrupt it.
___	___	All nature should be treated with reverence as one of God's gracious gifts.
___	___	Nature is neither good nor bad in itself, but is made by God to be used for our purposes.
___	___	We must use our higher gifts to subdue nature or become subject to an inhuman world ruled only by the natural laws of survival.
___	___	We were made by God to take control of and to subdue nature.
___	___	We are a part of nature and therefore must use it wisely, or destroy ourselves.
___	___	We have been given control over nature, but we must still exercise wise stewardship over it.

A D
___ ___ We both transcend and are a part of nature, which means that we must balance control of nature with responsible action toward it.
___ ___ Nature is sacred and must be treated with reverence.

2. The Budget Pie

Design: It is virtually impossible to measure qualities like love or benevolent concern. However, we can examine how we use or apportion limited resources—such as time or money—in supporting those things for which we say we care or have concern. In this exercise, people must decide how they would apportion a church's limited benevolence budget to take care of various possible Christian concerns. This may aid reflection on how ecological issues figure in these priorities.

Method: Tell the group that they are now going to have the opportunity to decide how a church should spend its limited benevolence budget. They will have a pie before them, which represents the total benevolence budget, and a list of various projects that the church could support. They must divide the pie according to how much of the total budget they would like to give to any particular project. They may add any project they would like to see the church support and refuse to budget for anything on the list they feel does not merit the church's concern. They can give half or more of the pie to one item if they think it is particularly important (see diagram, p. 87). When most people have finished, the following issues can be discussed:

How do your priorities relate to ecological concerns?

Do you want to put more emphasis on projects with long-term or on those with short-term goals?

Do you want to concentrate on aid at home or abroad? (If you have discussed some of the proposals of Schumacher, Heilbroner, or the Club of Rome, you can discuss the group's priorities in relation to their proposals. For example: Are your benevolence concerns consistent with the Club of Rome's notion that the U.S. must concentrate on development abroad and reduced consumption at home?)

The Budget Pie:

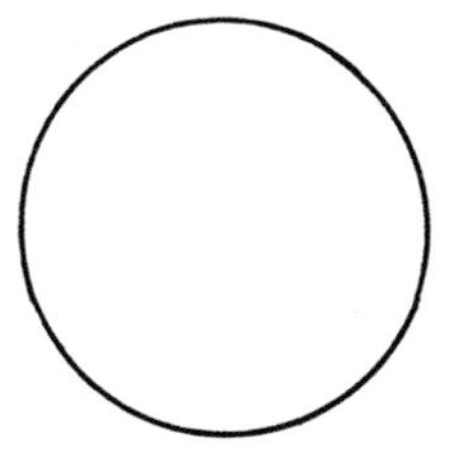

Here is a pie that represents a church's total benevolence budget. Divide it into portions that represent the amounts you think should go to:

domestic hunger programs
food for the world's hungry
birth-control assistance
agricultural technology for the Third World
industrial technology for the Third World
education programs to decrease consumption in the U.S.
world health improvement
housing assistance for American poor
homes for the aged
evangelistic missions in the Third World
educational missions abroad
aid for the development of solar energy
any other project(s) you would like to see supported

3. The Individual vs. the Church[7]

Design: This strategy allows individuals to witness to where they stand on various ecologically related issues and to what stance they feel the church should take. People do not always feel that the church should take the same stand that they as individuals do. The follow-up discussion can explore the reasons for some of these differences. It can also provide the opportunity for people to express some of the fears and anxieties they might have had when they found themselves standing alone on a given issue.

Method: Before the group meets, print the statements on the next page on large sheets of paper and display them on opposite walls in the order shown. When you are ready to do this exercise,

The church should keep out of this.

The church should actively oppose this.

The church should help individuals sort out their personal stand on this.

The church should provide guidelines but not offer active support or opposition.

The church should actively support this.

This should be supported by appropriate legislation.

This should be supported by informal, nonlegal means.

This should be discouraged by informal, nonlegal means.

This should be opposed by appropriate legislation.

This is not a matter for individual decision; it should be left to religious, political, or scientific experts.

explain that this strategy will provide a chance to affirm publicly some of our ecological values. If the church honors both charity and witness, then it should provide the opportunity at times for people to express their beliefs without fear of judgment and condemnation.

Point out the statements lining the two walls. Tell them that you will read a number of controversial proposals for dealing with the ecological crisis. First they are to move to the statement that most closely reflects what they personally feel should be done about this measure. While they are standing in front of their chosen statement, ask them to talk to others also standing there. Do they have similar or different reasons for making this choice? In a couple of minutes ask them to move to the other side of the room and stand in front of the position they feel the church should take on this measure. Again, ask them to talk to others standing in front of the same position. Continue in this fashion by reading another proposal and again having the participants first take a stand as an individual and then one for the church. Adapt or choose those measures out of the suggested list that relate to what your group is studying. Four to six proposals are usually sufficient.

While doing this exercise, be sensitive to people who end up standing alone before a given statement. At the end, you can ask the group how it felt to stand alone or to be part of the herd; how it felt to see someone else stand alone or everyone else grouping around a single statement. Is it hard to affirm one's stance in such situations? Was there any consensus about what the church should be doing?

Suggested Ecological Proposals:

1. Free contraception for all who want it (provided by the government).
2. High taxes on luxury goods (e.g., hi-fis, cameras, high-performance autos, furs, etc.).
3. Greater restrictions on industrial discharge into the air.
4. Gas rationing.

5. Making certain plastic products illegal (e.g., plastic cups, bags, cutlery, etc.).
6. Sterilization of those with three or more children.
7. Redistribution of wealth.
8. Greater control of chemical use (i.e., in insecticides, fertilizers, food additives, etc.).

Note: A list like this one will need to be altered as technological changes occur.

4. Goals for America and for Other Countries

Design: This strategy is designed to make people more aware of the various self-interests involved in ecological decisions. Participants choose possible national goals from different given perspectives and then explore the reasons for and results of different choices.

Method: Divide people into four groups. Give each person a list of possible national goals. Tell group 1 that they are to choose the three goals they think are most important for *America in the short term*. Tell group 2 they are to choose the three goals that are most important for *America in the long term*. Tell group 3 they are to choose the three goals that are most important for *an underdeveloped country in the short term*. Tell group 4 they are to choose the three goals that are most important for *an underdeveloped country in the long term*. Group members should try to agree on these choices.

After fifteen or twenty minutes, have the groups report their choices. Explore how compatible the American and the underdeveloped country's goals are with each other. Raise the question of how the concept of economic justice fits in with ecologic conservation. Consider the reasons for differences between short-term and long-term goals. What should be the Christian response to these various sorts of self-interest?

Suggested List:

Possible National Goals

economic growth
industrial development

military defense
population control
conservation of energy
development of new sources of energy
solving the problem of domestic hunger
solving the problem of world hunger
increasing average life expectancy
higher standard of living
increasing the standard of living of American poor
increasing the standard of living of the poor of the world
scientific and technological progress
increased food production
replacing economic growth with economic stability
developing simpler life-styles
developing values which conserve resources
international security, world peace
education and knowledge
(any others you think are important)

5. The Year 2050

Design: A variety of methods are presented here to show the types of activities that can be done with a simple list of issues or values that need attention. In this case the list contains a number of statements that might be true in the year 2050.

Method I: Duplicate the list of statements and have people rank them according to which they think would most likely be true in the year 2050.

Method II: Have people choose the three statements they think are most likely to be true. Divide into small groups and have each person tell the other members of his or her group which statements they chose and why. The object would be to hear others' views—not to outargue each other.

Method III: The list of statements can be cut apart and put into a hat or box. Each person then draws one statement out of the hat and is given one or two minutes to present all the reasons as to why that statement is likely to be true. After hearing all these arguments, the group as a whole could try to pick the three most likely predictions.

Method IV: Various of these statements can be used to support religious, scientific/technological, or political views of the future. Accordingly, people can be divided into three groups, with one group supporting a view that science will conquer all, another arguing that the powerful will win out, and a third saying that religion will save humanity. These groups can then try to convince each other of the validity of their position.

Suggested Statements:

In the year 2050 . . .

Science and technology will have solved the problems of hunger, energy, population, and natural resources.

Starvation and economic collapse will be rampant.

Free economy systems will have solved the problems of resources, energy, and food.

Religion will have replaced greed with sharing.

War will have solved the problems of hunger and exhaustion of resources by destroying most of the population.

God is the Lord of history and will preserve the human race.

The rich nations will survive, but poor peoples will have perished.

Democracy and free enterprise will have proved inadequate in solving ecological problems, and chaos and disaster will be general.

The poor nations will have overcome Western civilization and will dominate the world.

Christian values that revere the earth and support a simple life will be the popular standard.

Totalitarian governments will be in control and will engineer population and resource control.

God has promised another destruction of the world, and it will have taken place.

6. Personal Life-style and the Ecosystem

Design: This strategy has three stages. In stage I everyone is asked to react to a variety of family life-styles. In stage II each person ranks the relative seriousness of factors that might destroy the ecosystem. In stage III participants compare their life-style choices with the rankings of the potentially harmful factors and try to reach consensus in small groups as to which family described is leading the most ecologically destructive life-style. In the course of this strategy people may come to realize that their likes and their intellectual judgments are not always consistent.

Method: *Stage I.* Duplicate the stories below and distribute them to all participants. Tell them to read and rank the stories according to which family's style appeals to them the most. Their first choice may not be a style they actually like, but it should be the one they like most out of the given styles.

The Stories:

Here are some descriptions of families who have chosen differing life-styles. Read and then rank them according to their appeal to you. That is, put a *1* by the family whose life-style you find most appealing, a *2* by the one you find next most appealing, and so on, with a *5* by the one that you find least appealing.

Bob considers himself to be a "self-made man." He is proud of the fact that the factory he started fifteen years ago now grosses several million a year and is still growing. He will happily quote facts and figures about its success and expanding production to anyone who shows the slightest interest. But, beyond this, he likes to think of himself as a good family man and provider for his wife and two sons. He is glad that his wife, Janet, does not have to work as hard as his mother did.

Janet enjoys doing volunteer work at the hospital once a week, as well as participating in several women's organizations, a church group, and a couple of bridge clubs. She always sees to it, however, that she is home in time to prepare a good hearty dinner for her family, and she likes to send them out in the morning with a breakfast steak under their belts—she feels there is no better way to start the day.

They are both proud of their two teen-aged sons and hope to give them the best education that money can buy. They are grateful that they have been able to give the boys the material things that neither of them were able to have as children. They have also been able to afford a large home in a good suburb. The one real luxury they see themselves as indulging in is expensive vacations. They always take a Christmas holiday together in the Carribean, and in the summer they let the boys choose to spend a month as they most desire—whether that means sending them to a dude ranch in Texas or accompanying them on a trip to Hawaii.

John is a successful corporation lawyer and his wife, Linda, runs a smart little boutique. They have two teen-aged daughters and a twelve-year-old son. John encouraged Linda to start the boutique business when their son entered school and she became very restless and dissatisfied staying at home alone.

Because they feel it is important to do things together as a family, and they like the idea of their children getting out of their urban environment, they have bought a place in the country to go to most weekends. In the summer they go swimming, sailing, fishing, and, now, water-skiing with their new fiberglass outboard. In the winter they go snowmobiling and skiing. They have two snowmobiles, but they are thinking of getting a third so that they can all go out together. They sometimes feel that this might be a bit extravagant, but then they remind themselves of their belief that the main cause of juvenile delinquency today is the collapse of the family unit. By doing these good, wholesome activities together they are seeing that their family stays together. The sports that they share not only help build physical fitness—they help bind the family together.

Steven is a teacher in a community college, and his wife Ann also teaches part-time in the local schools. They have a large family, six children ranging in age from six to sixteen. Ann resumed teaching because they felt they needed the money to cover some of the little things that they really could not afford on Steven's salary—such as camping trips in summer or the extra special Christmas or birthday present that one or another of the kids always wanted. Now that she has been back at the job for a couple of years, however, and the children have begun to assume more responsibility around the house, she finds that she really enjoys the stimulation of an outside job as well as coming home to her ever-active family.

During the week the family mainly eats convenience foods, but on weekends Ann enjoys preparing steaks or roasts and lovely homemade desserts. Sunday dinner, in particular, is treated as a special occasion where they share with one another their current activities, joys, and concerns. At these times Ann and Steve forget their occasional financial pinch and really enjoy their large family.

Richard and Carol know that some of their friends think they are rather peculiar. Two years ago Richard gave up his well-paying job with a market research firm when he got fed up with the restrictiveness of his working hours and the questionable ethics he felt were involved in many of the jobs he did. They sold their suburban house and moved farther out in the country, where they bought a large old farmhouse and some land with another couple.

The two couples have been working hard restoring the old house, and it is now beginning to look like quite a period piece. They have had a large enough garden these first two years to freeze and can enough vegetables for their own use for the entire winter. By next year they hope to expand enough to sell some produce in the local farmer's market. They have been doing a lot of reading about organic gardening as they would like to use as few pesticides and chemical fertilizers as possible. By combining two households, they have been able to sell off a dishwasher, a washing machine, a dryer, and two cars. They have found that sharing upkeep on such items has cut their living expenses considerably. Richard has been doing some free-lance market research to help make ends meet, but because of their reduced income needs, he has been able to refuse the jobs he thought were questionable and has had more time to put into the projects around the farm that he enjoys.

George and Helen have two children, a boy aged seven and a little girl aged four whom they adopted. George works in a social agency—which is what prompted them to adopt a second child rather than have one of their own. They felt that they would be happier, and of more service, in helping the plight of a human already in unhappy circumstances than in bringing yet another being into existence.

Helen has also become interested in working in a social agency, so she is currently attending a local college. Their little girl goes to nursery school, and George helps with dinner and puts the children to bed so that Helen can have time for her studying. While she is studying in the evenings, he frequently is working on some woodworking project—he has made most of the furniture for both the children's rooms.

Weekends they usually try to do some activity that the children would enjoy—such as going to a park, zoo, or museum—and they try to set aside some time for each other. Their time together may be spent just lolling in bed, or they may spend it talking and catching up with each other after a busy week. When they can find the time, they like to make wine, garden, and listen to music. With so many things to do and ways to enjoy themselves, they wonder how anyone can ever be bored.

Stage II. After most people have finished Stage I, give each person a copy of the factors listed below. Go over the instructions together.

The List:

Potentially Harmful Factors

Here are some factors that are frequently cited as leading to an ecosystem crisis. Rank them according to how harmful you think each is. Number 1 should be the factor you think is most harmful, number 11 the one you think is least harmful. You may add any factor you consider to be particularly destructive.

overpopulation
too much reliance on animal (particularly beef) protein
air and water pollution
destruction of nonrenewable natural resources—minerals, etc.
overproduction of nonessential consumer products
excessive energy consumption
overindustrialization
destruction of agricultural land
failure of people to adopt different value systems
failure of people to reduce living standards
unequal income distribution, producing starvation for some, overabundance for others.

Stage III. When nearly everyone is finished, ask people to compare their rankings of the factors with their story rankings. Did the couple they like best lead the most ecologically nondestructive life-style? What other values influenced their rankings?

Ask them to rerank the stories now according to how ecologically destructive they think each family's life-style is. Number 1 should be the family leading the *most harmful* life style, number 5 should be the one leading the *least harmful* life-style. Then have everybody get into groups of three and try to reach consensus within the groups on these rankings. Fifteen or twenty minutes should be allowed for this. Encourage people to listen to one another's reasoning and to work hard at devising a ranking acceptable to all.

7. The Protestant Work Ethic

Design: John Wesley once said, "Make all you can, save all you can, give all you can."[8] That in a nutshell expresses what is often called the Protestant work ethic, although it has become an important element in technological society and not the unique characteristic of Protestanism. It involves the religious belief that one is called by God to be productive in society, frugal in the use of resources, and benevolent in relation to others. Some people are now questioning an ethic that fosters production at a time when we must become more conservative of the world's resources. This exercise explores the implications of this ethic for ecological responsibility.

Method: Introduce the notion of the Protestant work ethic and the concerns that some people are expressing today. After some discussion, have all persons list all the advantages they can think of for continuing to live out this ethic. Then have them list all the disadvantages they can think of. Ask them to evaluate these advantages or disadvantages they have isolated. What would they like to change? Can they list any courses of action that might be taken to change these things? These considerations may be shared in the whole group or in small groups.

8. Life-style Changes I Could Make

Design: This exercise is designed to be taken home after a discussion on ecological issues. It gives people a chance to reflect privately on what changes they personally could make to become more ecologically responsible.

Method: A discussion of the human ecosystem is not complete

without some reference to what we as individuals might do to become ecologically more responsible. Even if we as individuals cannot make much impact on the total system, do we not still have some responsibility to be sensitive to these issues and not to create more ecologic havoc than necessary? If we make changes in our life-styles, must we all make the same changes? Might it not be easier for me to give up one thing and you to give up something else? These are the kinds of issues that should be discussed before handing out the sheet (shown on p. 99) for private reflection.

9. Role-plays

Design: Two role-playing situations are presented below to exemplify the various ways in which role-playing can be used to explore ecologically related issues and the church's response to them. In the first situation, a church is being asked to support actively a clean-water campaign in its neighborhood. In the second one, a developed and an underdeveloped country vie for funds from the World Bank. The costs of economic justice and the development of more ecologic technology are pitted against each other.

Method: Refer to the guidelines for role-playing in chapter 2. Relate the situation you would like to role-play and solicit volunteers. After giving people the descriptions of their parts, allow a little time for considering the roles.

Upon completion of the role-play, ask the actors to drop their roles and to react to the experience. Did they find the roles difficult or easy to play? Ask the audience for their reactions. With whom did they empathize? Which parts did not elicit sympathy? Were there any roles other persons would have played differently? What insights were gained from the experience?

Situation 1:

A local citizens' action group has been fighting hard to stop two area industries from discharging pollutants in a small river that runs through the neighborhood. They have approached your church, since it serves

Life-style Changes I Could Make

Below are some changes that individuals could make in their life-styles in response to the grave ecologic situation. Rate yourself as to how difficult it would be for you to make any of these changes. Place yourself at point 1 if the change would be very easy for you to make, point 2 if it would be fairly easy for you to make, point 3 if it would be somewhat difficult to make, point 4 if it would be very difficult to make, and point 5 if it would be virtually impossible for you to make.

	1	2	3	4	5
1. substitute chicken and fish for beef	•	•	•	•	•
2. become a vegetarian	•	•	•	•	•
3. buy fresh foods rather than convenience foods	•	•	•	•	•
4. recycle paper, glass, and metal	•	•	•	•	•
5. refuse to buy any more small appliances	•	•	•	•	•
6. agitate for more efficient large appliances	•	•	•	•	•
7. reduce chemical fertilizer and pesticide use	•	•	•	•	•
8. join a car pool	•	•	•	•	•
9. replace present car with a smaller one	•	•	•	•	•
10. buy nonphosphate detergents	•	•	•	•	•
11. share large appliances with a friend	•	•	•	•	•
12. (list your own ideas)	•	•	•	•	•
13.	•	•	•	•	•
14.	•	•	•	•	•

this area, and asked that the church actively support them in their fight for cleaner water.

At the church meeting when this issue comes up, there are present:

1. a person who thinks it is the church's role to preach the gospel and to keep out of secular matters;

2. a woman who worries about her two young boys playing in the river, and who would like very much for the church to support her concern for cleaner water;

3. a man who is an executive in one of the companies concerned and thinks he is balancing larger issues of costs, etc., with local environmental concerns—he does not think the church has the expertise to enter this discussion;

4. a man who thinks the church really exists only when it acts out in the world the word it preaches—he wants to support a citizens' group.

Reenact the meeting. (At the end you can take a vote as the members of this church to decide which course of action to pursue.)

Situation 2:

A developed and an underdeveloped country both approach the World Bank for financial aid. The bank officials must choose between these two projects—they cannot fund both. Divide people into three groups representing the bank, the developed country, and the underdeveloped country. Let the two countries argue their cases before the bank and have the bank make its decision. (This could be a full-scale simulation if the groups researched the positions thoroughly.)

Notes for the Underdeveloped Country: You wish to construct a traditional plant to build engines for tractors and small machinery. Your country badly needs the jobs that such a project would offer, and you would like very much to be more self-sufficient.

Notes for the Developed Country: You want to develop the technology for a more energy-efficient ore-extracting plant. This will be a very expensive process, but holds great hope for extending the life of various natural resources.

Notes for the Bank Officials: You are concerned with the financial responsibility and economic benefit of proposals that come before you. You try to be as objective as possible in making your decision.

Further Suggestions

1. Stage a mock political campaign in which one party stresses industrial growth and the other party stresses ecological responsibility.

Devise slogans, party platforms, etc.
2. Ask people to survey the waste they throw out each week. Estimate its worth, its usefulness to someone else, its weight, or its volume.
3. Explore an issue that has numerous ramifications and is of interest to your church or community. Brainstorm all the ways this issue might be resolved and the courses of action that might be taken to remove various barriers or obstructions.
4. Write your own role-play on an ecological issue of interest or relevance to your church. Include enough viewpoints to cover the arguments, both pro and con. Some issues that might be considered are: pollution caused by PCBs; current asbestos levels in industry; the use of nondegradable or slowly degradable pesticides; the building of a nuclear power plant; rezoning of prime agricultural land for a housing development; etc.

Further Reading

Barbour, Ian G., ed. *Earth Might be Fair: Reflections on Ethics, Religion and Ecology*. Englewood Cliffs, N. J.: Prentice-Hall, 1972. Contains incisive chapters by philosophers, scientists, and theologians exploring ecological values.

———. *Western Man and Environmental Ethics: Attitudes Toward Nature and Technology*. Reading, Mass: Addison-Wesley, 1973. A series of essays by persons representing a wide range of interests and disciplines, including some highly critical of Christian perspectives as being ecologically destructive.

Derr, Thomas Sieger. *Ecology and Human Liberation: A Theological Critique of the Use and Abuse of Our Birthright*. Geneva, Switzerland: World Student Christian Federation Books, 1973. An excellent discussion of ecological problems in the light of Third World interests for economic equity.

Elder, Frederick. *Crisis in Eden: A Religious Study of Man and Environment*. Nashville: Abingdon, 1970. A pastor uses a biblical perspective to develop a useful distinction between perspectives that include humankind in nature and those that exclude humankind from nature, the latter of which the author rejects on ecological grounds.

Heilbroner, Robert L. *An Inquiry into the Human Prospect*. New York: Norton, 1974. A brilliant ecological analysis by a respected economist and social critic. He comes to conclusions that may be both personally and politically uncomfortable.

Mesarovic, Mihajlo, and Pestel, Eduard. *Mankind at the Turning Point: The Second Report to the Club of Rome*. New York: E. P. Dutton, 1974. Based on the computer model for considering policy alternatives, the book proposes an understanding of growth as organic instead of exponential.

Chapter VI

THE RIGHT TO LIFE AND THE RIGHT TO DEATH

On September 30, 1976, the governor of California signed into law the nation's first statute allowing terminally ill adults to choose to die rather than to have their lives prolonged by medical treatment. This law provides for the preparation of "living wills" by which persons may declare their desire not to be kept alive if and when they face imminent death. Physicians and families who cooperate with this formally registered intention are no longer subject to legal punishment.

Slow death and painful death are certainly not new. A familiar scene is that of family and physician gathered in helpless horror around the deathbed as the drama of suffering is played out before their crying eyes. Would it be surprising if someone standing there should consider administering "timely death" to the one tortured by pain? Such a direct act of killing requires the overcoming of strong natural inclinations and powerfully imbued moral feelings. How often it has been considered is hidden in the consciences of countless caring persons.

To this long-familiar drama is now added a new scene. We are in a hospital room where the presence of persons is overshadowed by tubes and bottles and machines. For a time pain has been held at bay by blessed chemicals, but now the pain returns in force. The new scenario goes on much longer. The machines and chemicals are effective to prolong life, even when they cannot restore life. To someone standing there it now occurs: Why not turn off that machine?

In another room, down the hall or worlds away, there is the same scene, except there is no pain and there are no people in the room. No one? Well, there is still a living body on the bed. There is no sound but a whispering pump. There is no family present. What is the point—only memories and no communication? The nurse comes in rarely, since the machinery is monitored automatically, and lights give warning when attention is needed. Does someone wonder if it might be an act of mercy not to notice when the light comes on?

At the other end of the human life cycle a similar dilemma is often posed. Conception has taken place. A "morning-after" pill could abort the fertilized egg. A little later, it would take a simple medical procedure to accomplish the same result. Still later, a more complicated and less safe procedure would be required to abort the developing organism. This tiny speck of life is in many ways like the unconscious body in the hospital room. It is entirely dependent upon the life-support system that sustains it. If it is separated from this environment, it dies.

The fundamental question raised in both cases is whether there are ever any circumstances of such weight and seriousness that they would justify direct or indirect action resulting in the termination of biologically human life. Surrounding this are a multitude of questions. What is the price of extending life? What justifies the extension of life when its ordinary purposes cannot be fulfilled? Whose life is to be extended—particularly when a decision must be made about whose life is to be saved? Who is to participate in the decision? Should we refuse the "heroic and unusual" methods available either to prolong or to terminate life, because by using them we are playing God, building a new tower of Babel perhaps? Or, are we called by God to subdue nature, including our own bodies, using every available means to provide a more human existence?

These questions take on a fateful seriousness for the woman considering abortion of a fetus known to be defective or endangering her own health. They are intoned like a funeral dirge in the mind of a person watching a loved one die in pain. In these moments of decision, the relation of the quantity of life to the quality of life is stripped bare.

We are focusing here on just two of the many moral questions posed by developments in medical science: abortion and the right to die. These represent real, often horrible moral quandaries faced by thousands of people every day. The purpose of these reflections is obviously not to provide "right answers." There are other, more realistic goals that we can suggest in wrestling with the tangled questions of deliberately ending life. First, we can seek to illuminate these problems by bringing to bear upon them some of the wisdom of the Christian centuries. Secondly, we can reflect upon the various ways of using the alternative principles that emerge. Thirdly, behind this moral purpose is an even more profound religious quest: What is the purpose of human life? *What is the quality of life that gives to its extension in time a meaning?*

In order to think usefully about these issues there is a very practical question, with moral implications, that must be examined: When is human life present or absent? At first glance it would seem to be a simple technical problem for the medical profession to decide. The catch, however, is in the word *human*. For example, there is scientific agreement that there is a continuous development from the moment of conception. From that moment the fetus is separate and distinct from the mother and possesses a genetic makeup different from both the parents. The question is still, When is *human* life present?

Daniel Callahan has classified the many views on this into three possibilities.[1] First, there are those who take a genetic point of view and regard human life as beginning with conception, when the genetic makeup of the organism is fixed. The potentiality for the particular humanity of that organism is then present.

A second group takes the developmental point of view, saying that further development is required before the potentiality is sufficiently present to speak meaningfully of the presence of a human existence. Some would place this point early in pregnancy, others only after considerable development, but all would agree that the precise fixing of the developmental state after which it is useful to call the fetus human is a matter of degree and not a fixed point.

A third group Callahan describes as taking the social-consequences point of view. They understand the nature of *human* not as a matter of biology but as a matter of moral policy to be decided by adult and developed human beings in the light of the social values they wish to maintain.

Obviously, views on abortion will vary considerably according to beliefs about when human life begins. The problem is even more complicated at the other end of the life cycle. When is human life ended? Formerly, it was a simple matter to pronounce clinical death when heartbeat and respiration ceased. Now, however, techniques of resuscitation restore people to life after clinical death, leading to variations in the criteria for deciding when death has occurred.

The significance of these determinations is dramatized by the increasing possibility of transplanting organs. It is important to know immediately when a body is actually dead, since the maintenance of organs in useful condition may otherwise be endangered. On the other hand, it is equally important to protect dying patients against the premature declaration of death.

The determination of the exact time of biological death would, nevertheless, still leave major problems unsolved. Do biological life and human life end simultaneously? Is a person who is in such a deep, irreversible coma that the natural functions continue only by means of artificial support systems humanly alive as well as biologically? Should the use of support systems be continued when there is no longer any hope of restoring meaningful human existence? These questions suggest that a useful understanding of death will be related to a basic understanding of what human life is. That is a moral or religious judgment.

The same three views Callahan describes with reference to the beginning of life apply to life's end. The logic of the genetic position is that abortion is not to be undertaken directly under any circumstances and that everything possible should be done to support life as long as biological life is present. Actually, there are permitted exceptions, such as an abortion that is the unintended by-product of medical treatment intended for the mother's benefit. Another common exception is to withhold "extraordinary or unusual means" to maintain the life of an inevitably dying person.

The developmental position stresses the increasingly personal character of fetal life, so that more and more serious reasons must be involved to justify the termination of fetal life as pregnancy progresses. With regard to the dying person, there is less and less reason to justify extraordinary means to retain life as "meaningful humanness" decreases. This same logic is involved with the social-consequences school, except that there is a wider range of considerations that go into decisions than the presence or absence of humanness in the fetus or the dying person.

There are then great complications in any attempt to determine general principles upon which appropriate decisions can be made. Intervention in the process by which human life comes into and goes out of existence is a very serious moral matter, and yet we cannot fail to respond, certainly not when our own bodies or the bodies of those whom we love or are responsible for are involved. What then are commonly held Christian beliefs that have relevance to this terrifying dilemma? The following four elements in the Christian perspective are cited in almost every discussion of the right to life and the right to death.

1. *The sanctity of human life*. The Genesis story establishes, at the beginning of our religious tradition, the goodness of human life. The creation of the world includes the creation of humankind, and indeed provides for the special place of persons in the order of creation. The psalmist writes, "What is man that thou art mindful of him, and the son of man that thou dost care for him? Yet thou hast made him little less than God, and dost crown him with glory and honor" (Psalm 8:4-5).

That is a very high view of human nature. Indeed, we are made in the image of God. The distortions that result from human sin do not blot out this image, since even in sin we are subject to God's redeeming and forgiving love. No more decisive sign of the value that inheres in human life can be formulated by the religious imagination than that God should give himself for our salvation through Jesus Christ. For this reason, the taking of human life is looked upon as a matter of utmost moral seriousness.

2. *Justice*. The sanctity of human life requires that each of God's creatures receive respect and support from every fellow human being. Justice is the form this obedience takes when it must deal with the multitude of stresses and strains with which human life is beset. That all God's creatures are due precisely the same respect is an ideal hardly attainable in practice. We make judgments daily, if not hourly, that involve discriminations in terms of who can be trusted with what, who is to be rewarded and in what measure, etc. It is extremely difficult to know what equal respect may mean in practice and in specific cases. Equal respect for a number of people may require that even in their best interests we must treat them differentially. The child of one year may be due the same amount of respect as a person of mature years, but the way in which that respect is shown will be vastly different. Justice is the principle by which we translate these complicated considerations into actions intended to result in fairness, mutuality, equity.

3. *Compassion*. There is a basic Christian belief that we are called to loving service to those who suffer and are helpless. Those in need are due not merely the equal concern, which every other human being deserves, but also compassionate concern, which seeks to relieve suffering and to support a quality of life physically and spiritually satisfying to them.

This love is interpreted in a variety of ways. For some, it is the motivation that lies behind the pursuit of justice. For others, it is the principle that adjusts the conflicting demands justice may lay upon us and that judges all our partial achievements. For still others, love is the principle that transcends justice and provides insight into appropriate action in the light of specific circumstances. In all cases, however, the demand of the gospel implies a responsibility to those in extreme need and those who do not have the power to protect their own interests.

4. *Self-determination*. There is a basic commitment to freedom in the Christian tradition. This is grounded in the belief that we are created free to receive or reject God's love. Self-determination is the secular form in which this value comes to us today. In its Christian form, it is not libertarian. Rather, it implies a free acceptance of limitations in order to have an ordered structure within which freedom can be responsibly enjoyed.

These four principles, in either their religious or their secular forms, figure prominently in virtually every debate about abortion and death with dignity. They do not, in and of themselves, determine beliefs on these questions. It is obvious that many proponents of abortion upon demand are emphasizing the right of self-determination of the mother. Opponents of abortion usually emphasize the sanctity of all human life. Others favoring abortion, however, may emphasize the respect for life but define it first in terms of the quality of life available to the mother and to a prospective child rather than primarily in terms of the extension of life in time.

Similarly, those who believe in "pulling the plug" under appropriate circumstances may emphasize compassion for those who suffer and the right of such persons to have their lives ended with dignity if they so wish. They may also see the termination of painful or meaningless life as a mark of respect for life and will want such determinations to be made according to the strict wisdom of justice. Another point of view will emphasize the respect for life as demanding that it should be extended in time without regard to quality, since to make such judgments is to play God and pretend we have more wisdom than is available to us. In this view, God's will for every life is that it should be cherished and maintained, and no situation can justify willful interference with that divine purpose.

One of the important traditions in Western morality has been the idea of natural law, a notion that is frequently important in discussions of abortion and the right to die. In natural law morality, the central focus is on moral principles derived rationally from the structure of reality, including human nature. Thus, actions that run counter to the natural purposes discernible in human structure or biological function are wrong. These structures and functions are indications of divine purposes in creation as well. However, there are wide differences in the rigidity with which the idea of natural law is applied to cases.

The relative rigidity or flexibility with which principles are applied is also a variable in other moral perspectives. Moral principles can be used as rigid rules or as loose guidelines. In the latter case the principles may be almost unrecognizable because they vary so widely with every situation. James Gustafson refers to this approach as "re-inventing the wheel."[2] Each situation is confronted as if there were no previous human experience to enlighten our examination of the issues, as if we have to start from scratch in each new situation to determine the relevant questions and principles that can guide us.

There is, however, an opposite view that has "one shoe for all feet." It is the way of extreme legalism, which first determines the rule that is to apply to any given situation and then applies the rule rigidly and perhaps even heartlessly. These are of course caricatures, and the way of the conscientious person is to find some balance between the general principles or rules and the uniqueness of persons and circumstances involved in any real human dilemma. Some will be closer to one of these poles than to the other. But this remains an important element in moral decision: the relative weight given to traditional wisdom incorporated in rules as against the contextual uniqueness of a given situation.

The following strategies deal only with a very narrow range of problems related to the right to life and the right to death. Among the important questions either left untouched or touched only in passing are: (1) the extensive problems of legal liability; (2) problems surrounding informed consent, the patient's "right to know," and the possible participation of juveniles in decisions about their own treatment; (3) pastoral problems by which the church may mediate between patient, family, health-care professionals, and the interests of society at large. In the face of these many complications, it is important to remember that the purpose of these pages is not to provide an exhaustive exploration of the subject but to model a method by which moral clarification on the issue can be pursued.

It is therefore appropriate to close this discussion with a reminder that what we may think in the relative safety of our present deliberations may or may not be borne out in the intensity of an actual situation. What we decide in advance will not completely and perhaps not even minimally correspond to the realities once we face the actual situations we here view only from afar. This does not mean that we waste our energy in reflecting upon them in advance, since what we do then may in a fundamental way be informed by our conscientious pursuit of the issues now. Rather, the point is to emphasize our freedom in Christ to respond in love in the light of our best understanding of appropriate behavior with each new day. The light of truth will not be exhausted in this or any other moment of reflection, but is open to fresh insight. There is no doubt a grace that is available to us only in actual suffering.

Useful Scriptural References

Genesis 1:26-28
Psalms 8; 90; 116:15-19
Ecclesiastes 3:1-11
Matthew 25:31-46
Luke 10:29-37; 12:16-31

Strategies and Exercises

1. The Degrees of Humanness

Design: Both the abortion and the pulling-the-plug issues raise the question of what it means to be human. Is there a point before which, or beyond which, it is not useful to describe a life as human? The following exercise looks at stages of development and capacities that are frequently mentioned in discussions of humanness, suggests that people rank these items in their definition of humanness, and asks them what sort of life they wish to call human.

Method: Give everybody a copy of the thermometer and the list of characteristics that can define humanness. Go over the instructions together and explain the meaning of any terms that may be unfamiliar to the group. Let people do the exercise privately. Afterward, people can gather in small groups and discuss how their definition of *human* relates to the question of abortion and pulling the plug. If this seems too threatening in your situation, then this issue could be raised by the leader for private reflection.

Sample Sheet:

Put the following characteristics on the thermometer in the order in which you feel they come in the development of the fully human person. Give them more or less space according to how important you think each is in the definition of what it means to be human.

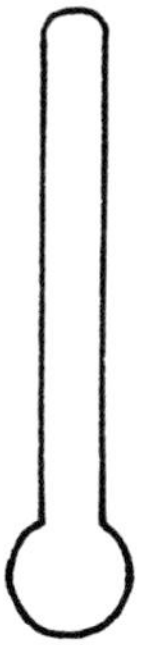

A. Higher brain functions (relating to consciousness)
B. Human form (differentiated body and organs)
C. Ability to think rationally
D. Capacity to enjoy life
E. Genetic existence
F. Ability to love other persons
G. Lower brain functions (nervous system; heart and lungs functioning)
H. Ability to interact with other persons
I. Capacity to respond to God's gracious care
J. Anything else you regard as essential to humanness (specify)

Is there a point below which it is not useful to call a life human? If so, mark it.

2. A Living Will

Design: Increasing attention has been directed toward a document called a living will, which allows people to state their wish, in the case of terminal illness, to be allowed to die without the use of extraordinary or heroic means to prolong their life. In this exercise, group members can explore how they personally feel about signing such a document.

Method: Ask the group to divide into groups of two. Each pair is to have a conversation as if they were two friends discussing whether to execute a living will. Distribute copies of a living will or the following quotation from a typical document of this sort. Afterward, people may wish to discuss the feelings this exercise raised in them.

A Living Will

> If the time comes when I can no longer take part in decisions for my own future, let this statement stand as the testament of my wishes. If there is no reasonable expectation of my recovery from physical or mental disability, I request that I be allowed to die and not be kept alive by artificial means or heroic measures. Death is as much a reality as birth, growth, maturity, and old age—it is the one certainty. I do not fear death as much as I fear the indignity of deterioration, dependence, and hopeless pain. I ask that medication be mercifully administered to me for terminal suffering even if it hastens the moment of death.

3. Who Should Decide?

Design: There is controversy surrounding not only the questions of who should live and who should die, but there is confusion also around the issue of who should be making these decisions. This exercise presents a number of situations in which a decision is called for and asks people to consider whom they would like to make the decision in each case. After doing this, can they state a principle about how they would like to see these decisions made?

Method: Duplicate and distribute the following situations. (If you wish to deal with only abortion or death issues, adapt the situations accordingly.) Explain that you would like people to read each situation and fill in the bar graph below it according to how much weight they think each person or institution should have in making the required decision. If they think that one person should be able to veto the decision reached by anyone else in that situation, they should put a *V* in the part of the box that represents that person's share of the decision process. For example, someone may believe that a doctor and the patient should have equal weight in making the decision, but the patient should be able to veto the doctor's decision if it is not to his or her liking. In this case, the box would be divided in half between the doctor and the patient, and the patient's side would be marked with a *V*. Afterward, questions, such as the following, can be explored:

Did you find you wished different people to make the decision in different situations?

Can you state a general principle for your choices?

How important was the right of self-determination in your choices?

(Note: If a group gets interested in what the content of these decisions might be, a couple of these situations might be fleshed out and role-played or otherwise used as a basis for an exercise on the issues behind such decisions.)

The Situations:

Following is a list of people or institutions who might have a part in any decision on a life or death issue: the patient, family members, doctor, the state (a court of law), other professional advisors (specify). After reading each situation, divide the box into portions that reflect the amount of influence each source should have in that case. Put a *V* in the portion of the box that belongs to anyone who in your opinion should have veto power in that situation.

A seventy-six-year-old man has suffered a massive stroke and is totally paralyzed. He has been wishing to die for some time because he is alone in the world—no family or friends ever visit him. His life could be prolonged for a while, however, if extraordinary means were to be used.

A thirty-six-year-old woman with three young children has terminal cancer. Her life could be extended a few months with a costly, painful treatment. Her husband would like her to have it, but she feels very guilty about the financial burden she would leave behind if she had it and is not sure she wishes to prolong the pain.

A ninety-year-old woman has broken a number of bones in a recent fall, including her hip. She is in great pain, but the doctors will not operate on the hip or give her strong sedatives because these actions might hasten the deterioration of her already frail body. She has been asking her family to get the doctors to put her out of her misery.

A seventy-year-old woman has terminal cancer. She has a loving family who would be happy to care for her through her last days at home. However, she wishes to stay in the hospital and keeps asking the doctors to do everything possible because she does not wish to die.

A twenty-two-year-old man has been brought into the hospital suffering from a drug overdose. The vital signs indicate that he is in an irreversible coma—he might function indefinitely on a respirator but will never regain consciousness. His family has been estranged from him since he took up drugs and will not contribute to the medical costs of sustaining his life.

An eighteen-year-old girl has been brought into the hospital after an automobile accident. She has a severe spinal cord injury, and now it appears that she has also suffered irreversible brain damage. She was put on a respirator immediately upon arrival in the hospital, but now the doctors feel her case to be hopeless. Her parents, however, would like to prolong her life at any cost.

A thirty-five-year-old woman who has three children and was looking forward to resuming a nursing career has just discovered that she is pregnant. She would like to get an abortion, but her husband would like her to have the child.

A thirteen-year-old girl has become pregnant. Her parents think she is too young to have a child and want her to get an abortion. The doctor tends to agree with them. The girl, however, wishes to keep the child and raise it herself.

A forty-two-year-old woman who has wanted a child for years is at last pregnant. Her doctor, however, says tests indicate that the fetus is severely defective, and he would recommend an abortion. She would like to risk having the baby, but her husband tends to think they should follow the doctor's advice.

A woman has just given birth to a child with a spinal gap. The doctors ask the parents to sign a consent form for an operation. They say if they do not operate very soon, the child will die within a few weeks. If they do operate, the child will probably live into its teens but will need many painful operations and extensive home care. It will never have a ''normal'' life. The parents are uncertain they can support this financial and emotional burden.

4. What Would You Say If . . .[3]

Design: This exercise can assist people in clarifying their expectations of different sources of advice in the decision-making process surrounding abortion. What they project as obstacles to abortion may indicate the weight they give to the various sources of advice in the decision-making process.

Method: Give each person six small sheets of paper, each of which carries one of the following headings: *parents; father of the child; minister; doctor; psychologist; social worker*. Then read the following statement and instructions:

> Cindy is a thirteen-year-old high school student who has become pregnant. She comes to you for advice. On the appropriate sheet, list all possible reasons or things that would keep you from *immediately* advising abortion—
> if you were her parents.
> if you were her minister.
> if you were her doctor.
> if you were her psychologist.
> if you were her social worker.
> if you were the father of the child.

After people have had time to make each listing, ask them to analyze their listings to see: (1) which people shared the same obstacles; (2) which people voiced unique obstacles. Then divide into groups of four or five to share these findings and to clarify the possible contributions each source might make in the decision-making process.

5. How Do I Judge the Abortion Issue?

Design: The following strategy presents a number of situations in which a woman might consider abortion. People must decide whether they think an abortion is justified. Afterward, they are asked to formulate the principle or principles that informed their decisions. Did they have one overriding principle, for example, or did they decide each case without reference to any other?

Method: Give each person a copy of the following situations in which abortion is an option. The participants are to put an R next to those situations in which they think the woman is justified in having an abortion and a W next to those where they think she is not. Assure them of anonymity in making their responses.

When everyone is finished, have them reflect privately on such questions as:

Did you have one overriding principle that governed your responses? If so, what was it? If not, how did you make your decisions—did you decide each case individually on its own merits? Or, did you perhaps have a set of principles that governed your decisions? What were they?

The Situations:

In each of the situations below, assume that the pregnancy is in its first trimester (under twelve weeks). Also assume that unless stated otherwise the husband or boyfriend is neutral to or supportive of the woman considering the abortion.

___ A married woman with five children. The last birth was very difficult, and her doctor had advised against having any more children because of the risks to her health.

___ A married woman with six children. Her husband was recently disabled and is now unemployed. They are living on welfare and other state benefits and feel another child would absolutely break them financially.

___ A married woman with three children. She became very depressed after the birth of her last child. She was actually institutionalized for a short while. Both her husband and her doctor feel another pregnancy would institutionalize her again.

___ A married woman with three daughters. She suffered a nervous breakdown two years ago. Both she and her doctor think her mental health is too fragile to have another child, but her husband wants her to have it because he dearly wants a son.

___ A single, eighteen-year-old woman who has just started college. She let herself be talked into intercourse by a smooth-talking senior, whom she has not seen since.

___ A young, single woman who was raped as she came home from work.

___ A twelve-year-old girl who was raped by her stepfather.

___ A prostitute who has become pregnant in spite of her precautions.

___ A very unstable, twenty-five-year-old woman, single, who has had three previous abortions.

___ A thirty-eight-year-old, single career woman who fears a child would ruin her career.

___ A married woman with two children, aged eighteen and twenty. She thought she was past the point of having children and, although financially well off, does not really want another child at this stage in her life.

___ A married woman in her forties who has three grown children. She is not so upset by her unexpected pregnancy as by the tests that reveal that the child is likely to be deformed.

___ A thirty-year-old married woman with no children. She and her husband just recently separated, however, in anticipation of a divorce.

___ A married woman whose husband has repeatedly said that he does not want children.

___ A twenty-six-year-old married woman who would like to pursue her career two more years in order to be more able to return to it after having a family. Her husband, however, is delighted that she is pregnant now.

Now repeat the exercise, assuming this time that the pregnancy is in the last trimester (over twenty-four weeks). Does this change your judgments?

6. Reasons For and Against

Design: In this strategy people are asked to consider the situation of a terminally ill man from four different points of view, pondering the reasons for and against acceding to his wishes to be allowed to die.

Method: Tell people that you wish to explore the case of a terminally ill man from the different viewpoints of four people affected by the situation. Then read the following descriptions.

Charles is fifty-five years old, has terminal cancer, and is in great pain. Even more important to Charles, however, is his fear of destroying the financial future of his wife and son by weeks of hospitalization. He does not wish to die feeling a failure in providing for his family. His wish is to have no future therapy, no operations, no intravenous feedings—only drugs to make him more comfortable.

His wife, Mary, is torn between her desire to have Charles with her a little longer, including a completely unrealistic hope that some medical miracle might save him, and her deep distress at watching him suffer. She has never worked in her life. She knows that her financial future is not bright, but she believes it is immoral for her to consider that.

His son, James, is also torn between wanting to respond to his father's desire to be relieved of the pain and his unwillingness to have his father die. He understands his father's worry about finances, but he cannot see any way to deal with that issue without involving himself in hopeless "conflict of interest." James is certain that he will be unwilling to use the family savings to go to college if it turns out that his mother will need these resources.

The physician, Dr. Jones, knows that there is no use in prolonging Charles's life, but he considers it his duty to prolong life as long as possible in every case. He feels caught in these situations, because he fears criticism from the family if he keeps Charles alive, and he fears their wrath if he does not do everything to keep him alive—no matter what they might say right now. Dr. Jones also fears the criticisms of one of his colleagues who is very vocal about his belief that doctors are being professionally irresponsible when they sentimentally cooperate with a patient's wish to die.

After reading the above descriptions, discuss each of these persons and the reasons for and against doing what Charles is asking *from their respective viewpoints.* Begin by considering the reasons for granting Charles's request from his own perspective, then the reasons against granting his request. As the reasons are offered by the group write them down under the appropriate heading:

Charles		Mary		James		Dr. Jones	
For	Against	For	Against	For	Against	For	Against

When the group has listed a wide range of reasons, ask everyone to make his or her own list of the most important reasons for and against. Which list carries more weight with them? What insights can the Christian tradition offer in this situation? What do they think should be done?

7. Mercy or Murder?

Design: Three courses of action are theoretically possible in relation to a dying patient: heroic or unusual measures may be undertaken to prolong life at any cost; these extraordinary means may be withheld and the patient allowed to die naturally; or, an action may be undertaken that actually hastens the death of the patient. This last course of action is the most controversial and arouses extreme emotion in many people. The following value sheet allows people to reflect privately on this matter.

Method: It is often difficult to maintain a rational discussion on an issue that arouses strong emotions. A sheet with a provocative statement and some follow-up questions which participants may take home and meditate on privately is one way to handle such a situation. The following sheet deals with the issue of active euthanasia.

The Sheet:

Neither physicians nor relatives have been found guilty in court of passive euthanasia (allowing terminally ill patients to die in order to end their suffering). Even in cases of active euthanasia (where a positive act is undertaken to terminate life) convictions are extremely few. These cases are most often disposed of by accepting pleas of temporary insanity, or technical pleas in which the charge is not proven. For example, in *State* v. *Montemarano* (New York, 1973), Dr. Vincent A. Montemarano was tried for murder. He administered a fatal dose of potassium chloride to Eugene Bauer, who was dying of throat cancer. The injection was witnessed by a nurse and recorded on the medical charts. The defense claimed that the drug, which is sometimes used in cancer therapy, was not intended to kill the patient. The jury pronounced the physician not guilty.

1. Do you believe Dr. Montemarano did the right thing?
2. Do you agree with the decision of the court? What are your reasons for agreeing or disagreeing?
3. What are the most likely consequences of the court's leniency in such cases?
4. How would you feel about having Dr. Montemarano as your physician? Would you prefer to have a doctor who you know might consider a course such as this, or one who strictly follows the physician's duty to keep the patient alive under all circumstances?

8. What Should Be Done?

Design: In the following strategy people are asked to suggest ways to handle an unfortunate or morally ambiguous situation. They are then asked to devise the best response to the given situation.

Method: Introduce and read one of the following situations to your group. When you finish, ask everyone to give as many responses as possible that the person in such a dilemma might make. Encourage them to offer alternatives regardless of whether they personally believe such a response would be right, wrong, or too ridiculous to consider seriously. When you have received a wide variety of responses, divide people into groups of three and ask them to come to a consensus in their group, if possible, as to what would be the best course of action to pursue in such a situation. Are there Christian beliefs that influence their decision?

The Situations:

1. You are a medical doctor involved in research and treatment that is increasingly successful in saving genetically defective fetuses. You believe in this work, but you are bothered by two considerations: First, you often save lives when the only expectation is a life of misery and pain; second, you are aware that each success contributes to the pollution of the genetic pool. Such defective persons without your help would not have survived, but now they do survive and sometimes reproduce, introducing their defective genes into the human cycle. What should you do?

2. You are the father of a young girl, a sizable portion of whose brain has been destroyed in an automobile accident. Her heart and respiration are still functioning, but there is no detectable brain activity. In the country where you live a person may be declared dead when brain activity does not record. It is clear that even if she were to survive for a while she would never have any mental capability. A patient in the hospital is in urgent need of a heart transplant and your daughter's cells match closely enough to be a donor. What should you do?

9. The Kidney Machine

Design: Limitations in resources can result in agonizing choices about who should have the right to live. The following situation lets people explore some of these choices. Four people are vying for the use of a kidney machine that has recently become available.

Method: Explain the situation and ask for volunteers to play the four patients. Assign each person one of the roles. After giving them a moment to consider their roles, ask each "patient" to tell the group why he or she should be the one to have access to the kidney machine. When they have each presented their case, divide the rest of the group into panels of three or four persons. These panels represent the health care team which must decide who gets the machine. The panels caucus to make their decisions. After an appropriate amount of time, have the panels report back, telling the person they chose to save and the reasoning they followed in making that choice.

The Situation:

A hospital has four people with kidney trouble, all awaiting the use of a kidney machine. They all know that unless a machine becomes available shortly or they should suddenly be lucky enough to find a donor whose tissue matches theirs, they will eventually die. A machine has just become available and the decision must be made as to who should have it. The people under discussion are:

1. A sixty-year-old man, an influential community leader and appellate court judge, respected for his wisdom.
2. A thirty-five-year-old woman with three children, aged five, seven, and nine. She is divorced and her children's sole means of support.
3. A bright young man of twenty-six, recently married and just out of graduate school. He shows great promise as a public defender.
4. A middle-aged man who is the sole support of his wife and two children. Although he is not drinking now, past drinking clearly contributed to his kidney failure.

Further Suggestions

1. Have people look at the photo essay "Gramp" in *Psychology Today,* February, 1976. What kinds of feelings does the essay arouse in them? Would they consider doing what Gramp did? What do they think of a family that allows a member to carry out such a plan?
2. Develop a full-scale simulation around the case of Dr. Montemarano.

3. Look at various denominational statements on abortion and medical ethics. In particular, study your own denomination's statements. Then, role-play a meeting in which a policy-making body of your church is considering changing one of these statements. What biblical references, Christian beliefs, etc., might support various stances?

4. Describe a crisis situation that involves some issue(s) raised in this chapter. Give people a drawing of a clock and tell them they have only one hour in which to make a decision. Whom would they seek out for guidance? How many minutes would they spend with each source? Divide the minutes on the clock accordingly.

Further Reading

Callahan, Daniel. *Abortion: Law, Choice and Morality*. New York: Macmillan, 1970. An extensive and definitive essay on the legal, moral, and policy issues surrounding abortion.

Nelson, James B. *Human Medicine: Ethical Perspective on New Medical Issues*. Minneapolis: Augsburg Publishing House, 1973. A helpful treatment of a wide range of ethical issues from a broadly Protestant perspective.

Shannon, Thomas, ed. *Readings in Bioethics*. Ramsey, N.J.: Paulist Press, 1976. An excellent selection of articles from a wide range of viewpoints and covering the standard issues in medical ethics—by major Catholic and Protestant writers in the field.

Smith, Harmon L. *Ethics and the New Medicine*. Nashville: Abingdon, 1970. Especially useful in its treatment of abortion and care of the dying in relation to major theological perspectives.

Who Shall Live? Man's Control Over Birth and Death. A report of the working committee to the American Friends Service Committee. New York: Hill and Wang, 1970. A brief but discerning analysis of ethical issues in abortion and the right to death, arguing a position of compassion and liberality on the basis of the Quaker heritage.

Chapter VII

GROUP GOALS AND CONFLICT MANAGEMENT

Death with dignity, the leadership role of women, life-style changes in response to ecological crisis—these are issues that involve varying opinions and may arouse deep emotions. The questions to which we have addressed ourselves in previous chapters are controversial issues in the church. All of them imply some point of view about the role of the church in conflictual matters. However, the role of the church is itself controversial, as the discussion about Christ and culture makes clear. The church can avoid discussion of these difficult questions, but conflict will not thereby be avoided, since the church will still be subject to criticism from those who expect moral leadership on these important questions.

If this is the case, then the setting of appropriate goals for the church and groups within the church becomes extremely important. Moreover, the development of a capacity within the church to handle and use conflict creatively is crucial. We now address ourselves, therefore, directly to these issues, asking whether and how the church can establish a style of response to controversy, a style that enables it not only to survive the conflict but perhaps even to profit from the creative possibilities available in the struggle.

We may note at the outset that conflict in the church is often highly personal. The fact is that these controversial issues can produce emotional stress within the persons who are concerned with them. For example, if we conclude that the ecological crisis threatens the way of life to which we are accustomed, it is not only inevitable but perhaps even useful that we should experience a high degree of personal distress.

Furthermore, these difficulties can create conflict between persons, in families, or in friendship circles. Differences of opinion and judgment, differing decisions about how to maintain or change cherished values—these may be disruptive to relationships. The questions are not trivial, and how such differences are handled is not trivial. It is generally true that the more intensely people are bound to one another, the more potent are the conflicts that arise among them. Conflicts within the church and within church groups may be more or less intense according to the strength of commitment and feeling present between conflicting persons.

Another level on which conflict may arise is in the relationship of the church and its groups to other groups and systems within the society. For example, a particular church may develop a common faith and a mode of action in relation to the matter of abortion. The pursuit of its goals will in all probability bring the group into cooperation with other groups that share these goals and into conflict with groups that oppose them.

Social scientists make an important distinction between *communal* and *noncommunal* conflict.[1] Communal conflict takes place within a basic consensus. Within the church, communal conflict arises when there is a general agreement about the nature and purpose of the church, but there is a struggle over specific meaning or over the application of the consensus. Noncommunal conflict is conflict over the basis of consensus. In the church such conflict may arise when there is no set of common purposes among the parties of the conflict. It is not surprising that conflict becomes more intense when people fear that the basis of consensus is threatened.

We are accustomed to believing that cooperation is the way in which the church can and should achieve common goals. While this is certainly true, there are also positive functions of conflict, which may be lost if our emphasis is solely on cooperation and the avoidance of conflict. First, conflict can aid in forming goals and group identity. Sociologist Lewis Coser asserts that "a certain degree of conflict is an essential element in group formation and the persistence of group life.''[2] The church, like any other group, exists out of a certain sense of what the church is and what it is not. This sense is partly formed by tradition and history, but the nature of the church is forged anew in each new historical situation. The church had its beginnings in a struggle to distinguish itself from Judaism on the one side and Hellenism on the other. From the Council of Chalcedon to the Reformation, the church has been formed in controversy. That struggle continues when the church seeks to be relevant to modern society. In the local parish, general understandings of what *the church* is are translated into specific understandings of what *this church* is in this time and place.

A second important function of conflict is that it can facilitate the solution of concrete problems we face in the church or in our personal and social existence. Competing opinions and judgments can contribute to the development of better solutions than those that would emerge from the deliberations of a single individual or from a group of persons who agree too easily or approach the problem from similar viewpoints. This problem-solving function is sometimes referred to as *realistic conflict,* conflict that deals with an actual and important issue directly.

Not all conflict, however, is realistic. The actual issue of the conflict may be hidden or displaced while the argument revolves around other matters entirely. This is *nonrealistic conflict.*[3] Often, people are simply angry at one another. They may have old, unresolved hurts, or they may be reacting to the frustration of a difficult situation. Even here conflict can serve a positive function. Thus, the third function of conflict to which we may call attention is the possibility for it to release tensions. This ''blowing off steam,'' taking place early and moderately, may prevent tensions from building up to the point at which disastrous forms of conflict are inevitable.

Although these three positive functions of conflict are possibilities, it is also clear that conflict can have a destructive effect. People do get hurt, groups are devastated, goals and purposes can be lost in chaos. The choices we make about how to respond and handle conflict are value choices of great importance. The various styles of response to conflict can be described in terms of two variables: (1) the relative importance given to people and relationships and (2) the relative importance given to goals and purposes. These variables can be related to each other in five different ways, representing different styles of handling conflict.[4]

1. *Relationships are more important than goals.* In this style the individual is primarily concerned with how the conflict may affect relationships with others in the group and outside of the group. Since these relationships may be damaged by open and intense conflict—perhaps beyond repair—it is necessary to cooperate with others in the pursuit of their goals rather than to pursue one's own goals vigorously.

2. *Goals are more important than relationships.* In a conflict situation, usually someone is right and someone is wrong. To ensure that the proper and appropriate goals are achieved, one should vigorously pursue one's own best judgment. The use of both persuasion and power is natural in this process.

3. *Both goals and relationships are important and an adjustment must be made between them.* Goals should be pursued for the good of all. It is thus necessary to compromise with the views of others. Everyone cannot possibly be fully satisfied, but persuasion and flexibility will allow everyone to express their views and feelings, and to be satisfied at least part of the time.

4. *Goals and relations are both important and are mutually supportive.* It is not necessary to sacrifice commitment either to one's goals or to relationships, since it is often possible to pursue them both. In fact, working through differences can result in more complete achievement of the goals of everyone involved and thus more satisfying relationships in the long run. To accomplish this, conflict must be brought out into the open, to be dealt with directly and in mutual trust.

5. *Differences must be tolerated.* Conflict between persons and

groups pursuing different goals is a fact of life. The outcome cannot be much influenced by any of the various ways people suggest for dealing with conflict. There are really only two alternatives in a conflict situation: either tolerate it or withdraw from it.

An individual may tend to choose one of these styles more than another. However, we all choose all of them at one time or another. More important than which style we choose first may be the question of which style we fall back on when the pressure builds up. What do we do when our preferred style is not working? How long do we maintain that style before trying another? Do we have one style in personal conflict and another in group or intergroup conflict? These are important questions which may determine the way in which conflicts develop for us in the churches.

Toward a Christian Response to Conflict

What values are there in the Judeo-Christian tradition that may be useful to us if we wish to understand and develop a creative style of response to conflict in the church? Obviously the range of ideas that can be useful is as broad as the tradition itself. Here we choose three basic themes as preliminary suggestions.

1. *The Christian doctrine of the person.* The Christian view of the person involves both a recognition of the created goodness of humanity and the sinful perversion of that goodness. This is the ambiguity of existence which forms the battleground for forces of good and evil. Conflict represents this ambiguity: We both understand and do not understand where our true good lies. We struggle for high and holy goals, which are perverted by our own insecurity and anxiety. We ride roughshod over the needs of our neighbors, disrespecting the goals for which they struggle.

Our view of conflict must take account of this ambiguity, the sinfulness of our highest purposes and best intentions. Our goals are relativized in the light of the divine intention for our lives. The human harmony to which we are called is fractured by our stubborn assertions of power and autonomy. On the other hand, the dimly perceived purposes for which we strive are a part of the divine calling to seek a more human and just existence for ourselves and for others. Conflict becomes both a judgment on our sinful self-assertion and, at the same time, a promise that our efforts are not in vain.

2. *History as the scene of God's struggle with sin and death.* The history of Israel is the history of struggle—of the nation surrounded by enemies on every side, of the nation faced with false prophets and faithless people who threatened its covenantal relationship to God. The covenant itself represents a continual struggle. The prophets charge king and people with unfaithfulness to the covenant. There follow repentance and reconciliation and a new covenant. The new covenant is then violated and the cycle begins again!

In the New Testament this history of the divine struggle reaches a new level in the Incarnation. The God who gives himself to his people on the cross is contending with the forces of sin and death. The depth of this agony is represented by the cry of Jesus when he experienced himself as abandoned by the very God who called him to that fate.[5] Here, obviously, is no sentimental view of conflict, which romanticizes and idealizes. Neither is it a view that sees conflict as being without redeeming possibilities. God chose conflict as the mode of redemption. He places himself in the midst of the struggle. The Crucifixion symbolizes the fact that hope is available in the depth of despair. If we have hope only when things are going well, our hope is available only when we do not need it.

3. *Reconciliation.* The end of the drama of salvation is not on the Cross, however, but in the meaning that is given to the Cross by the Resurrection. Sin and death are not triumphant, but conflict and suffering are the necessary preconditions of a Resurrection faith. We must understand the Cross in the light of the Resurrection. Otherwise, it depicts the story of a struggle that ought to have been avoided at all costs, since it ends in death and defeat. Actually, the story marks the end of bondage to "the law of sin and death" (Rom. 8:2). That is the meaning of the Christian drama of salvation.

Reconciliation is an imperative of the Christian faith: We are called to be reconciled to God and our neighbor. "If you are offering your gift at the altar, and there remember that your brother has something against you, leave your gift there before the altar and go; first be reconciled to your brother, and then come and offer your gift" (Matt. 5:23-24). However, if reconciliation is a command, it is first of all a statement of fact. We *are* reconciled in Christ. This may guard against the interpretation of the command as a call to servile surrender to the forces of evil. The meaning of redemptive love is not that evil is allowed to run its course unopposed, but that the way of reconciliation is through struggle and suffering. Conflict is not an option to be avoided. Neither is it a goal to be pursued. It is the way through which grace often leads us to repentance, convicting us of our sin but promising redemption beyond the present pain and hopelessness.

The content and meaning of the Christian faith is the subject of sermons and classes in the church, but these formal occasions are not the only places where the faith is formulated and communicated. The purposes of the church are also formulated and refined in boards and committees, congregational meetings, and pastoral calls. At the point where decisions are being made and action planned, the nature of the church is emerging. The many controversial subjects that have been dealt with in this book may be approached in situations planned around the specific subject. On the other hand, these devices may be used as an aid to education and decision in the organizational structure of the church. For example, some of the strategies on Christ and culture can be used in board and committee discussions.

The strategies of previous chapters have been organized around particular issues. Those that follow in this chapter are organized primarily around various formats for dealing with goal definition and conflict. The content should be varied in order to deal with specific subjects that are becoming points of conflict. The strategies can be adapted to match the nature of the controversy currently facing a church group.

It may be useful to recall the fundamental assumption on which the use of this method is based: The people in our churches are fundamentally intelligent and well-intentioned people who are searching for a deeper Christian faith. They must be trusted to achieve, within an atmosphere of trust and freedom, an increasingly mature faith and responsible course of action. If leaders know in advance what conclusions they want the group to come to, the use of this method will only lead to frustration. If, alternatively, people are assisted in isolating the commonalities of Christian faith that they share and the ambiguities and uncertainties that remain, the possibility for more truth and light to emerge among them is very great indeed. They may become the people of God searching for a way through the wilderness in the belief that there is a creative destiny in their journey.

Useful Scriptural References

Genesis 32:1-33:4
Isaiah 42
Amos 7:10-17
Matthew 10:34-42
John 2:13-20
Acts 15
II Corinthians 2:1-11
Luke 4:16-30; 6:27-38; 17:1-4

Strategies and Exercises

1. The Crystal Ball

Design: This strategy is for use in groups taking a long-term view of themselves. It can be used at an all-church meeting, such as an annual congregational meeting, or for a church council, an education committee, etc. People consider a series of statements about what their organization or institution might be like in five, ten, or twenty-five years.

Method: Have a brainstorming session in which people offer statements that might be true of the group, organization, or institution in a given number of years. Statements should not be censored at this stage. All possibilities, however unlikely, should be written on a large piece of paper or blackboard. Future group activity, character, or composition may be noted.

When no more suggestions are forthcoming, ask people to choose privately the three statements they personally would most *like to come true* and the three statements they think will probably *be true*. Collect these hopes and predictions anonymously and make a group profile of each. Discuss. How unified is the group when viewing the future? Do people think their hopes will come true? What does this say about group optimism? Are there any goals or strategies that could be agreed upon to achieve the hopes of the group?

2. What Might We Do?

Design: This strategy is designed to help a group in its consideration of possible goals. Like the preceding one, it can be used in many settings in the church. People are asked to choose the goals they would most like to see pursued and to debate the relative merits of the three or four most popular goals.

Method: Supply a list of possible goals for your group. Have everyone choose the one goal they would most like to see fulfilled and write it on a piece of paper. If the group is small, put the statements into a box and ask each person to draw one statement out and give all the reasons for pursuing that goal he or she can in two or three minutes.

If the group is large, collect the responses and find the three or four goals that most people supported. Divide into three or four subgroups and assign each subgroup one of these goals. Have the groups caucus to prepare a convincing case as to why the goal they have been assigned should be made top priority. Give each group three or four minutes to present its case. (You may allow a one-or two-minute rebuttal period for each group after all the cases have been presented.) If at the end you feel a need to have some public affirmation of where people really stand, ask them to move to the group whose goal they would actually be most willing to support. Do not allow argument to ensue at this stage, however.

3. Goal Analysis

Design: This exercise can be done as a follow-up to one of the preceding exercises when two or three conflicting goals each seem to present an attractive alternative to pursue. People are asked to sort out the advantages and disadvantages of each goal and to rate how important each of these are to them personally.

Method: List the two or three goals that are real possibilities for the group. Depending on the size of the group, have people, either individually or in small groups, list all the advantages they can think of for pursuing each goal in one column and all the disadvantages in another column. Do this with each alternative presented. When finished, master lists can be made, listing all the advantages and all the disadvantages unearthed by the entire group.

Then ask everyone individually to rank how important each advantage and each disadvantage seems to them. They should give a 2 to a strong advantage or a −2 to a strong disadvantage, a 1 or a −1 to a mild advantage or disadvantage, and a 0 to an advantage or disadvantage that is not important to them. The ensuing discussion may include the following issues:

Do people find the advantages and disadvantages cancel one another out on any goal?

Are there any things about which the group in general feels strongly?

Could any disadvantages be overcome?

Any goal that emerges as a likely priority of the group can have its disadvantages examined more closely. A brainstorming session may follow in which the group tries to isolate courses of action that might remove these disadvantages as barriers.

4. "World Communion Sunday"

Design: The story below is concerned with the relation between internal group conflict and external goals. It poses a dilemma about which small groups are asked to reach agreement. It is ideally followed up by the next exercise, Conflict: A Tool or a Curse? The use of the story format stirs feelings as well as intellect. In the effort to come to consensus, people must express their positions, listen to others' positions, and then negotiate, distinguishing between what is essential to them and what can be compromised.

Method: Tell the group that you are going to read them a story. They are to listen carefully since you will ask them to do something afterward. When you have read the story through once, ask them to rank the four characters in it (Linda, Henry, Janet, and George) according to whom they like best. Number 1 should be the one they like most, number 4 the one they like least. This does not mean they really have to like their first choice, but that in comparison to the others, they like this person best. Now read the story again, being careful not to repeat or emphasize anything unduly. Do not answer any questions about it, since uncertainty over facts may become an important part of the ensuing dialogue.

When you have read the story the second time, and participants have ranked the characters, have them divide into groups of three. (This strategy does not work well with groups of any other size.) Ask them to share their rankings within the groups and to give their reasons for liking one character better than another. When they have done that, they are to attempt to reach a consensus as to who is indeed the "best" character and who the next best, etc. The point is not to outargue one another, but to try to hear all the reasons given, to see which they did not think of or what information they did not hear, and to attempt to build a consensus together. Encourage the groups to find the points on which compromise can be made without ignoring important ideas or feelings. Discourage argument and emphasize listening to others. At the end it is usually interesting for the triads to report their results since the groups often reach more than one consensus.

The Story:

Linda, Henry, Janet, and George are members of a committee organizing a presentation to the church for World Communion Sunday. Recently the committee has been having some difficulty functioning effectively. Henry has been objecting increasingly to Linda's direction of the committee. He has said that she is ignoring suggestions and riding roughshod over them all in order to get her agenda into the presentation. Linda denies this; she says that she has been trying only to get an effective presentation organized by their deadline. If they quibble about every little detail, there will be no presentation when the time comes. Henry's constant objections are obstructing the process.

Janet says that while she personally has appreciated Linda's leadership, she does feel that the tensions between Henry and Linda should be worked through. After all, it is unreasonable to expect the congregation to become more sensitive to the plight of others if they cannot even be sensitive to one another within this small committee. Learning to be caring of others is really more important than producing the perfect presentation.

George reacts quickly to Janet's suggestion. He is emphatic that airing the conflict can only lead to disaster. He says it will both make matters worse between Henry and Linda and lead to a poor presentation. Henry and Linda should bury any personal conflict they might have, and any conflicts on substantive issues should be decided by a vote of the committee as soon as they realize a conflict has arisen.

5. Conflict: A Tool or a Curse?

Design: This exercise presents people with a series of statements to consider about the role of conflict in group process. It is particularly useful as a follow-up to the above, "World Communion Sunday."

Method: Duplicate and distribute the following statements about conflict. Ask people to think about the statements privately and to record whether they mainly agree or disagree with each. If the group has just done the exercise with the story "World Communion Sunday," ask everyone (after responding to the statements) to look at their rankings of the people in the story and consider which character would have responded most nearly as they did. Was this the character they ranked most highly? If not, can they think of any reasons for liking another character better than the one they seem to agree with most nearly?

The Statements:

Below are some statements about the role of conflict in groups. Read each statement carefully and put *A* by it if you agree with it in general and a *D* by it if you disagree with it in general.

___ Personal differences must be worked through if a group is to function effectively.

___ Conflict is always harmful to group functioning and goal attainment.

___ If a conflict can be worked through, frequently a group functions more effectively than if it had been ignored.

___ Conflict on issues of importance to a group can be healthy and beneficial.

___ Personality conflicts must be avoided if a group is to function effectively.

___ It is more important that members of a group learn to work together harmoniously than that they produce significant results.

___ It is more important to obtain significant results in a group than to avoid conflict.

6. Four Pictures[6]

Design: This exercise allows people to express nonverbally how they understand the group to be functioning, or how they wish to function in the group. It is useful because people will sometimes draw things that they would not otherwise express. (Some people may not be able to admit that they do not wish to be part of a group, but they may be able to draw and talk about a picture that shows this.)

Method: Make available to everyone one large or four smaller pieces of paper and felt pens or crayons for drawing. Ask the participants to draw four pictures, each of which answers one of the four questions you ask. Use either the organizational or the personal questions depending on the needs of your group. It is best to have the four questions written out somewhere so that people can refer to them while drawing. Emphasize that the pictures do not need to be works of art. They are to represent people's feelings rather than meet critical artistic standards.

Give some notion of the time allowed for drawing so that people do not labor over one picture and neglect the other three. (Twenty minutes should be sufficient.) When almost all have finished, have people get into pairs and share their pictures.

Note: Since people are not accustomed to such "childish devices," it may be necessary to build an appropriate atmosphere before undertaking such a nonverbal strategy.

The Questions:

Organizational	*Personal*
Where is the group now?	Where am I in *(the group)?*
Where does it want to be?	Where do I want to be?
What are the obstacles in its path?	What are the obstacles in my way?
What can help it along?	What is helping me?

7. Expectations and Responsibilities

Design: Frequently organizations experience conflict and ineffectiveness because people are unclear about what is expected of them or have unfulfilled expectations of others. This exercise is designed to improve communication between groups or factions that are having difficulty meshing expectations and responsibilities.[7] A few simple questions are asked each party and a discussion ensues.

Method: Identify the various parties—persons or groups—who seem to be unclear about what is expected of them or who seem disappointed by the performance of other parts of the organization. Have these parties meet together. For example, a board might meet with a staff, a Christian education committee with the Sunday school teachers, a youth group with its adult leaders, a church council with the deacons, etc. Give each group four large sheets of paper and pens.

Each group should put one of the following four questions at the top of each piece of paper:

1. What are *our* (X's) responsibilities?
2. What do we expect of ________ (Y)?
3. What does ________ (Y) expect of us?
4. What does ________ (Y) think we expect of them?

If a board and a staff were meeting together, the above questions would be filled in like this:

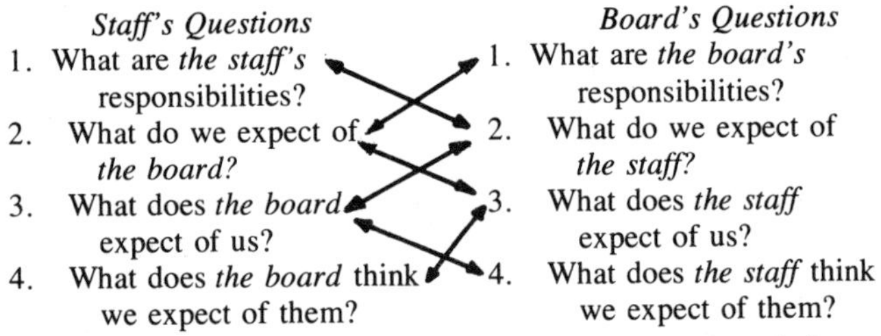

Staff's Questions	*Board's Questions*
1. What are *the staff's* responsibilities?	1. What are *the board's* responsibilities?
2. What do we expect of *the board?*	2. What do we expect of *the staff?*
3. What does *the board* expect of us?	3. What does *the staff* expect of us?
4. What does *the board* think we expect of them?	4. What does *the staff* think we expect of them?

Since the wording and numbering of these questions is important, it may be easier for the leader to write out the questions for the respective groups before the meeting begins.

Each group should then list their responsibilities and expectations under the appropriate question. The questions should be answered in the order presented. Sometimes groups have trouble answering these questions because they disagree among themselves as to what their responsibilities are or what they expect of the other party. In this case, it is useful to have them list those things on which they are generally agreed under the questions and to put the items under dispute on a separate sheet of paper. A group may discover that their problems with another group may have more to do with their own conflicting expectations than with the outside group itself. Isolating and resolving these inner group conflicts may improve their relations with others.

After answering these questions, the groups should get together and compare their responses. In particular, they should compare the questions connected by the arrows. Cross comparisons of questions 1 and 2 will reveal direct conflicts in expectations of the two groups. Comparisons of questions 2 and 3, and of 3 and 4, will reveal various levels of misunderstanding. In this way, communication gaps, conflicts, and misunderstandings may be identified. Does the board expect things of the staff that the staff does not feel are its responsibilities, or vice versa? Or, does the staff think the board expects things of it that the board in fact does not expect? These few questions can reveal a large number of issues that simple discussion may clarify, or which can go on a future agenda if the issues seem too massive to settle in one session.

8. Opinion Poll

Design: This strategy can help members of a large group develop a clearer picture of the group as a whole. It can also help to expose unspoken opposition that may be hindering group functioning. People are asked to respond *anonymously* to a number of issues of concern to the group or institution. Then a group profile is made of the responses.

Method: Make a list of statements on issues of concern with which people can agree or disagree. After each statement put the numbers 1 2 3 4. Provide a key, such as, 1=strongly agree; 2=mildly agree; 3=mildly disagree; 4=strongly disagree. Duplicate this paper. A sample paper might look like this:

Our church should spend more money on evangelism. 1 2 3 4
Our church needs fewer Bible-study groups. 1 2 3 4
Our church needs more involvement with the local community. 1 2 3 4
Our church needs to be more concerned with educating its own members on social issues. 1 2 3 4

People are then asked to circle the number that most clearly reflects their stand on each issue. When they are finished, they deposit their papers in a ballot box. These responses are tabulated and a profile is made of the entire group. People may then discuss the profile. Are there any surprises? How do they feel about the group now? Do they wish to say anything about their own responses? (Do not force people to speak about themselves because they may feel tricked and become angry.)

9. Dealing with Discord

Design: This strategy can help church people sort out their attitudes toward conflict in terms of religious ideas. Participants are invited to ponder a variety of approaches to conflict in the church.[8] Then they are asked to apply these approaches to a given conflictual situation.

Method: *Stage I.* Duplicate and distribute the five statements below. Explain that most of us probably use all these approaches to conflict at one time or another. They might consider, however, the degree to which they act or want to act out of each one. If they rank them from their most favorite to their least favorite, it may reveal how they prefer one method but fall back on other methods when the first does not seem to be working.

The Statements:

A. The Bible teaches that we ought to turn the other cheek and not resist evil; therefore, in the church, we should seek to avoid conflict and learn to surrender our own will and determination.

B. Jesus was in constant conflict with his opponents because he unswervingly followed God's will; therefore, we should expect conflict and should struggle to fulfill God's will in the life of the church.

C. The church should be a caring community after the biblical example, but care will involve conflict; therefore, we should seek in love to struggle through our differences, deepening our fellowship and refining our goals.

D. The church is an imperfect community of "saved sinners," and we should expect there to be conflict; therefore, compromise between our differences is the best interpretation of the gospel in the life of the church.

E. The biblical understanding of human nature recognizes the inevitability of sin and evil, even in the life of the church; therefore, there is nothing we can do about conflict except learn to accept it in Christian humility.

Method: *Stage II.* Read the following description of a conflictual situation to the group:

The neighborhood in which your church is located has changed ethnically and economically. The membership has mostly moved away.

Another church has offered to buy the building for almost enough money to enable your church to move out with its membership. The offer to buy is good for only twenty-eight days. The church must decide by then, but the membership is hopelessly split on what to do.

Now have everyone draw a twenty-eight-day calendar. Ask them to choose which approach toward conflict they would use first and put the letter (A, B, C, D, or E) in each of the days they would pursue that style of conflict participation. Then have them decide which approach they would adopt next, and place the letter in each of the days they would use it. Have them continue to do this until they have filled all twenty-eight days on the calendar. Then ask them each to choose another person in the group with whom to compare calendars and share their reasoning. Are there any of the five approaches that they have not used? Does this conversation make them want to change any part of their decision?

Further Suggestions

1. Have the leadership core of your church take "The Conflict Management Survey" (see below in Further Reading). Organize a weekend around the learnings available in this very useful instrument.
2. If people are having trouble listening to or hearing one another on a conflictual issue, adapting the format of The Mirror of Faith in chapter 3 can be useful. People pair off to discuss the controversial issue. One person begins by offering a brief statement of his or her position. The other person must reflect—restate—this position before earning the right to make his or her own statement.
3. If group goals are not coming to fruition and group activity sometimes seems to contradict stated goals, it may be useful to do a values grid. An issue is stated and the group analyzes which of Louis Raths's seven processes of valuing they have gone through on that issue. (An example of a values grid sheet can be found in *Values Clarification* by Simon, Howe, and Kirschenbaum.)

4. If group discontent revolves around how time or resources are being spent, do an organizational time or resource pie. Use the format suggested in The Budget Pie in chapter 5. If time is the issue, make a list of those things that consume the bulk of the group's time (e.g., administration, program planning). Have people divide up the pie according to how much time they see the group spending in each of these areas. Are there any surprises? Can anything be done to change the nature of the pie?
5. Have a person take the role of a proponent of a view under consideration in your group and sit in the "hot seat." The rest of the group poses difficult questions concerning this view to the hot-seat occupant, who tries to field them as best he or she can.

Further Reading

Hall, Jay. *The Conflict Management Survey*. Conroe, Texas: Teleometrics International, n.d. An evaluation instrument of conflict styles, but contains a brief and incisive discussion of conflict theory in the pages describing the scoring system.

Jamieson, David J. *Conflict*. St. Louis, Mo.: Church Leadership Resources, 1970. An excellent series of papers analyzing conflict sociologically, in the New Testament, theologically and institutionally in the church.

Leas, Speed, and Kittlaus, Paul. *Church Fights: Managing Conflict in the Local Church*. Philadelphia: Westminster Press, 1973. Emphasis upon struggles in the local church which are analyzed with insightful comments and suggestions.

LeFevre, Perry. *Conflict in the Voluntary Association*. Chicago: Exploration Press, 1975. A case study and follow-up analysis of conflict in a suburban church.

"Conflict I," *The Register*. LIX, 4, May 1969.

"Conflict II," *The Register*. LX, 2, December 1969. Chicago Theological Seminary. A series of articles analyzing conflict in the church and alternative styles of response and describing the natural history of disruptive fights in local congregations. Especially valuable is the article by Charles Dailey in "Conflict II" entitled "The Management of Conflict."

NOTES

Chapter I

1. Louis Raths, Merrill Harmin, Sidney Simon, *Values in Teaching* (Columbus, Ohio: Charles E. Merrill, 1966), pp. 28-29. The approach of values clarification is based on the pragmatism of John Dewey. In the adaptations we are making we have attempted to be freer of this instrumentalism. This does not mean that Christian faith is incompatible with instrumentalism. Rather, our adaptations are intended to make it a matter of choice what the method of clarifying values is to be. Pragmatism, although a very popular and almost universal perspective in our society, is only one among several available options.

Chapter II

1. Two very useful volumes have become available too late to influence the preparation of the present manuscript: Maury Smith, O.F.M., *A Practical Guide to Value Clarification* and Howard Kirschenbaum, *Advanced Value Clarification*. Both are published by University Associates, LaJolla, CA, 1977.

Chapter III

1. H. Richard Niebuhr, *Christ and Culture* (New York: Harper, 1956), p. 1.

2. *Ibid.*, p. 2.

3. This game is based upon the therapeutic method of Carl Rogers but is widely used in this form in encounter groups and in values clarification strategies.

4. Sidney Simon, Leland Howe, and Howard Kirschenbaum, *Values Clarification: A Handbook of Practical Strategies* (New York: Hart, 1972), pp. 366-37.

5. *Ibid.*, p. 228.

6. Donald E. Miller, Graydon F. Snyder, Robert W. Neff, *Using Biblical Simulations* (Valley Forge: Judson Press, 1973), pp. 153 ff. This is the first of two volumes of biblical simulations.

Chapter IV

1. The two kinds of research relevant here are sexological investigations and studies of gender differentiation. Useful simplifications of the first kind are *The Sex Researchers* by Edward Brecher and *Understanding Human Sexual Inadequacy* by Fred Belliveau and Lin Richter. A simplification of the latter type of research is found in *Sexual Signatures* by John Money and Patricia Tucker.

2. Adapted from Eleanor S. Morrison and Mila Underhill Price, *Values in Sexuality* (New York: Hart, 1974), pp. 70-71.

3. We are indebted to Julia Less Wagstaff for technical assistance in the preparation of this simulation.

4. We have here used the translation of the Thecla story from *The Apocryphal New Testament*, trans. Montague Rhodes James (Oxford: Clarendon Press, 1924). A more modern and definitive version of the Acts of Paul can be found in *New Testament Apocrypha*, 2 vols., ed. Hennecke-Schneemelcher, trans. R. McL. Wilson (Philadelphia: Westminster Press, 1965).

Chapter V

1. Mihajlo Mesarovic and Eduard Pestel, *Mankind at the Turning Point: The Second Report to the Club of Rome* (New York: E. P. Dutton, 1974), p. 123.

2. Donella H. Meadows *et al. The Limits to Growth* (New York: Universe Books, 1972), pp. 48, 51.
3. Mesarovic and Pestel, *Mankind at the Turning Point,* p. 166.
4. Robert L. Heilbroner, *An Inquiry into the Human Prospect* (New York: Norton, 1974), p. 127.
5. Mesarovic and Pestel, *Mankind at the Turning Point,* p. 147.
6. Heilbroner, *An Inquiry into the Human Prospect,* p. 140.
7. Adapted from Morrison and Price, *Values in Sexuality,* pp. 107-8.
8. These are the three points of Sermon L on "The Use of Money," *Works of John Wesley* (New York: Emory and Waugh, 1831).

Chapter VI

1. Daniel Callahan, *Abortion: Law, Choice and Morality* (New York: Macmillan, 1970), chapter 11.
2. James Gustafson in unpublished remarks, September 25, 1975, at a conference on "Medical Ethical Issues in Long Term Care," Oak Forest Hospital, Oak Forest, Illinois.
3. We are indebted for this exercise to the Reverend Joseph E. McCormick, O.S.A.

Chapter VII

1. Lewis A. Coser, *The Functions of Social Conflict* (Glencoe, Ill.: The Free Press, 1967), p. 75.
2. *Ibid.,* p. 31.
3. *Ibid.,* p. 49.
4. This typology is an adaptation of that developed by Jay Hall in "The Conflict Management Survey" (Conroe, Texas: Teleometrics International, n.d.).
5. This discussion of the Crucifixion and the Resurrection is influenced by Jürgen Moltmann, *The Crucified God,* trans. R. A. Wilson and John Bowden (New York: Harper, 1974), especially chapter 5.
6. This exercise is adapted from one developed by Drs. Philip and Phoebe Anderson.
7. The theory behind this exercise is that of R. D. Laing and found in R. D. Laing, H. Phillipson, and A. R. Lee, *Interpersonal Perception* (New York: Springer, 1966).
8. This exercise represents a translation of the social categories of Jay Hall's typology into religious language.